Medical English
Clear & Simple

A Practice-Based Approach to English for ESL Healthcare Professionals

Medical English
Clear & Simple

A Practice-Based Approach to English for ESL Healthcare Professionals

Melodie Hull, RPN, MSc, MEd (TESOL), BA, PID
Nursing Faculty
College of the Rockies
Cranbrook, British Columbia, Canada
Nursing Tutor, Distance Education, Transitions to Nursing and Health Program
Thompson Rivers University
Kamloops, British Columbia, Canada

International Adviser to the Department of Languages
International University of Business, Agriculture, and Technology
Dhaka, Bangladesh

Nurse-Educator and Consultant
Clayton International Consulting
Cranbrook, BC, Canada

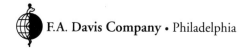
F.A. Davis Company • Philadelphia

F.A. Davis Company
1915 Arch Street
Philadelphia, PA 19103
http://www.fadavis.com

Printed in the United States of America

Last digit indicates print number: 10 9 8 7 6 5 4 3 2 1

Acquisitions Editor: Jonathan Joyce
Director of Content Development: Darlene D. Pedersen
Senior Project Editor: Padraic J. Maroney
Design and Illustrations Manager: Carolyn O'Brien

As new scientific information becomes available through basic and clinical research, recommended treatments and drug therapies undergo changes. The author(s) and publisher have done everything possible to make this book accurate, up to date, and in accord with accepted standards at the time of publication. The author(s), editors, and publisher are not responsible for errors or omissions or for consequences from application of the book, and make no warranty, expressed or implied, in regard to the contents of the book. Any practice described in this book should be applied by the reader in accordance with professional standards of care used in regard to the unique circumstances that may apply in each situation. The reader is advised always to check product information (package inserts) for changes and new information regarding dose and contraindications before administering any drug. Caution is especially urged when using new or infrequently ordered drugs.

Library of Congress Cataloging-in-Publication Data

Hull, Melodie.
    Medical English clear and simple: a practice based approach to English for ESL healthcare professionals/Melodie Hull.
        p.; cm.
    Includes bibliographical references and index.
    ISBN 978-0-8036-2165-7 (alk. paper)
    1. Readers—Medicine. 2. English language—Conversation and phrase books (for medical personnel)
    3. English language—Textbooks for foreign speakers. 4. Medical personnel, Foreign—United States. I. Title.
        [DNLM: 1. Terminology as Topic—Problems and Exercises. 2. Communication—Problems and Exercises.
    3. Language—Problems and Exercises. W 18.2 H913m 2010]
        PE1127. M4H85 2010
        428.6'402461—dc22

                                                                        2009042818

This book is dedicated to two very important and influential
people in my life:

My very good friend, Patty Sangri, of the Universidad
Tecnologica de Cancun, who gave me my first job in English for
Specific Purposes and who opened
this whole new world to me.

My wonderful husband, Steven, whose unwavering love
and faith in me, as well as his incredible patience and support,
has made this book possible.

THANK YOU

I met Melodie Hull, the author of this book, in 2006 when we all attended the International Symposium on English for Medical Purposes in Beijing, China. As one of the keynote speakers, she roused my attention when I read her research abstract. It offered a brief overview of literature on how the actual goals of the curriculum of English for Medical Purposes are defined. In the symposium, her speech was a great success and provided all the researchers, especially Chinese researchers, in the medical English field opportunity for critical thought regarding current curriculum design. In addition, her wit, her wealth of knowledge and experience, and her enthusiasm for the medical English field impressed all the attendees. In the following years, we have kept in touch with each other. I have gradually come to know many of her works, all of which are greatly applicable and in great demand. On behalf of all Chinese medical English researchers, I genuinely appreciate what Melodie has done and will do in this field.

Medical English Clear & Simple is designed to help learners of medical English at an advanced level. The intended readers are medical and medical English students, medical professionals, and those involved in the medical field who have a strong desire to improve their medical English.

This book guides readers through eight main sections, enabling them to explore and develop skills within certain systems or medical fields. Each unit enables readers to engage more actively with medical matter or content and encourages them to develop their own skills in medical English reading, listening, speaking, and writing. Throughout the book, topics are extended, interwoven, and deconstructed, with the readers' understanding strengthened by tasks and follow-up questions. For the learners to take full advantage of the material, the book has included what the author believes is most needed by them. Exercises and learning activities offer language-learning conditions that enrich their communicative competence and skills within the context of their careers. Written by an experienced researcher in the field, *Medical English Clear & Simple* is an essential resource for students and researchers of medical English.

I, Xie Yu, sincerely wish that by reading and using this book, you will have a pleasant and instructive experience in improving your medical English.

Xie Yu, MA
English for Medical Purposes Lecture
Capital Medical University
Beijing, PRC

Congratulations on the publication of this important book.

Melodie Hull is a friend, colleague, and previous employee. While teaching nursing full time at a local university college, she worked as a staff nurse part time in one of my mental health care facilities. As I got to know her, I discovered her interest in teaching English for nursing and medical purposes. Her approach to the subject was (and is) quite unique. Her vision of the need for functional, career-specific English for health professionals is commendable and one which I share. This book does just that! I, like Melodie, appreciate the need for nurses or doctors to be involved in the creation and design of this type of material and coursework and have always supported her in her endeavors to fill this need. We agree that English for Medical Purposes materials should be based in the context of the health professions at all times. Melodie is committed to best practices in health care and realizes that language skills and competencies play an enormous role in the delivery of safe, ethical, and professional care. Indeed, she believes this so strongly that beyond nursing, she has added a graduate degree in TESOL to her credentials to ensure her material is well-grounded in theory and practice.

Medical English Clear & Simple is a comprehensive introduction to the language of the health professions. In my opinion, it is well suited to the needs of international medical graduates who wish to complete a residency in Canada, the USA, or to work in an English-speaking milieu eventually. It is also well suited for internationally educated nurses and nursing students whose first language is not English. The text offers essential terminology for working with colleagues and patients, but it does more than that: the communication focus is paramount for career success in an English-speaking country. This book accomplishes that.

Ronald I. Wong BS, MD
Family Physician, registered in Vancouver BC, Canada, and Kingston, Jamaica
Graduate University of British Columbia Medical School
Internship at King's County Hospital, Brooklyn, New York
Family Practice Residency, Good Samaritan Hospital, Cincinnati, Ohio,
and Ravenna General Hospital, Ravenna, Ohio, USA

This is no ordinary text. Melodie Hull's years of experience in international nursing, education, and theater arts provide an innovative approach to English-based medical terminology. The author's expertise in this area is evident in the selection of content and sequencing of tasks, but it is the love of learners and the desire to see them succeed that shines in the gentle, down-to-earth guidance included in the learning activities. By incorporating activities that address the various senses, the author taps into different learning styles and preferences, rather than relying solely on pronunciation and memorization. Her appreciation for the learner's need to feel confident comes through in the design of activities that engage the adult in using new terms in a variety of contexts. Upon completion of this text, a learner can go to the workplace knowing he or she will effectively use medical terminology in verbal and nonverbal communications. This is the text that I wish I had written myself.

Sharon L. Andersen, RN, BSN, MSN, MEd, EdD
Clinical Nurse Specialist in Adult Mental Health
Proprietor, Crone's Nest Educational Consultants
Retired Nursing Instructor, Kwantlen Polytechnic University
and University of British Columbia, Canada

Having used a previous book by Melodie Hull, I was honored to have been asked to write this foreword for the new textbook that she has written. This new work is a comprehensive book designed for non-native English-speaking students in health-care programs. *Medical English Clear & Simple* fulfills a need since it is health care oriented, but ESL/EFL accessible. As there are more and more non-native speakers of English medical professionals in the USA, the need for such a book has become critical. *Medical English Clear & Simple* assists students toward success in health-care programs by providing opportunities for reading, writing, speaking, and listening within their health-care career. It provides ample opportunities to apply what has been learned and helps students build their health-care related vocabulary.

Medical English Clear & Simple is a useful resource as a communication teaching tool for instructors in the health-care field and as a refresher or a professional development course for international health-care professionals.

Melodie Hull has achieved her purpose of providing a valuable resource for health-care students or professionals who are of non-English speaking backgrounds. *Medical English Clear & Simple* is the answer to the needs of health-care or ESL/EFL instructors who are looking for a comprehensive book that will help their students improve their health-related language skills.

Barbara Jonckheere
Lecturer/Academic Senate Representative
American Language Institute
University College and Extension Services
California State University, Long Beach

In *Medical English Clear & Simple*, Melodie Hull has presented a practical step-by-step guide for learning career-specific English with a communication focus. The guide is a valuable resource, especially for students in health studies programs and health professionals who are of non-English speaking backgrounds.

In reviewing the draft copy of the Annotated Table of Contents and the Introduction, as well as a discussion about the book with the author, I have come to appreciate the communicative focus of the text, integration of cultural concepts of health and wellness, and opportunity for critical thinking through exercises provided in the book.

The content is organized in eight units using a medical systems format that is familiar to internationally educated health professionals. Having my basic nursing education (BScN) from India and 40 years of experience in nursing education as a teacher and an administrator in Canada has given me the understanding and appreciation of the value of meaningful and effective verbal and written communication skills for health professionals. The author's approach to a workbook format in the book provides opportunity for learning to communicate English within the context of the health-care system.

I recommend this book to students in health studies programs who are of non-English speaking backgrounds and foreign-educated health professionals.

Chinnama Baines, RN, BScN (CMC, Madras, India), MScN (UBC, Canada), PhD (GU, MO, USA)
Nursing Education Consultant
(Retired Dean of School of Nursing, UCC (Thompson Rivers University),
Kamloops, BC, Canada

Reneé T. Burwell, ASN, BSN, MSEd, EdD
Coordinator of Health Science Programs
Charlotte Technical Center
Port Charlotte, Florida

Susan C. Engle, RN, MSN
Medical-Surgical Nursing Instructor
Napa Valley College
Napa, California

Nancy J. Gay, RN, BSN
Instructor, Nurse Aide Training Program
Pickens Technical College
Aurora, Colorado

Deborah S. Gilbert, MBA, EdS, RHIM
Associate Professor of Office Administration
   (Medical Assisting and Medical Transcription)
Dalton State College
Dalton, Georgia

Jacqueline Guhde, MSN, RN, CNS
Assistant Professor of Clinical Nursing
The University of Akron College of Nursing
Akron, Ohio

Deborah B. Hadley, RN, MSN, CNOR
Nursing Instructor
Alcorn State University
Natchez, Mississippi

Sharyn Haran, Med
Instructor, Business and Office Occupations
   (Business and Allied Health; Medical Office
   Clerk Program)
South Seattle Community College
Seattle, Washington

Sharon Harris-Pelliccia, Registered Physician
Assistant, Board Certified, BS
Department Chair, Medical Studies
Mildred Elley
Latham, New York

Joanne Hartzell, Certified Professional
Coder, BS
Director Practical Nursing
Lanier Technical College-Forsyth
Cumming, Georgia

Aprille Haynie, MSN, RN
Evaluation Committee Chairperson, Advanced
   Medical-Surgical Nursing and Nursing
   Leadership Course Coordinator
Huron School of Nursing
East Cleveland, Ohio

Marlene Rogers Hancock, RN, MSN
Instructor
Lane Community College
Eugene, Oregon

Anita L. Huse, RN, MSN, EdD
Nurse Educator and Owner
Huse Healthcare Educational Consultants
Londonderry, New Hampshire

Jule B. Monnens, RN, MSN
Program Director, Nursing
Community College of Denver
Denver, Colorado

Sharon Moore, RN, BSN, Graduate
Certificate in Nursing Education, Certified
Medical-Surgical Registered Nurse
Practical Nursing Program Coordinator
Forsyth Technical Community College
Winston-Salem, North Carolina

Tara L. Narcross, PhD
Coordinator, Language Institute and Basic
   English Department
Columbus State Community College
Columbus, Ohio

Cindy Neely, MSN, RN
Nursing Campus Clinical Laboratory Coordi-
   nator and Professor of Nursing
Oklahoma City Community College
Oklahoma City, Oklahoma

Diane O'Hara, BSN, MS, EdD
Healthcare Services Specialist
Erie 2–Chataqua-Cattaragus BOCES School of
   Practical Nursing
Derby, New York

ACKNOWLEDGMENTS

It is with pleasure that I take a moment here to acknowledge people who have been significant influences on my work. First, I want to honor Dr. Sharon Andersen, my friend, colleague, and mentor who taught me so much about writing nursing degrees, curricula, and courses. I can't thank her enough. She is truly my hero. A very special thanks to Jonathan Joyce, Acquisitions Editor at F.A. Davis who first approached me about my work with English for nurses and medical professionals. His openness to a new paradigm for teaching career-specific language and his understanding of the need for this book have been instrumental in the development of the final product. He saw my vision and ran with it. I am forever grateful. Also at F.A. Davis, I want to say thank you to Padraic Maroney, Senior Project Manager, whose valuable guidance and great sense of humor made completion of the manuscript a pleasure. And thank you to Barbara Tchabovsky, Development Editor, for all her work, including those grammar and accuracy checks for both English and Medicine. Thank you also for her patience and ability to make sense of my writing and ideas. Incredible work!

Melodie Hull

Melodie Hull, Author

CONTENTS

INTRODUCTION

Welcome to *Medical English Clear & Simple,* a career-specific language resource.

This book has been written in response to a growing need for career-specific language skills training in health care. While many English language books for nurses or other health professions tend to focus on medical terminology, *Medical English Clear & Simple* does not. The author believes the narrow focus offered by a vocabulary-building focus based strictly on medical terminology lacks a communication focus. As a result, it is generally ineffective in meeting the communicative and functional needs of English Second Language or English Foreign Language (ESL/EFL) health professionals. *Medical English Clear & Simple* encourages a broader, communicative and functional use of English that includes opportunities to think critically and in a reflective, analytical manner required in nursing and the health professions.

PURPOSE AND AUDIENCE

Medical English Clear & Simple has been designed for those students in health studies programs or health professionals who are of non-English speaking backgrounds (NESB). It is an excellent companion text or resource for student success in health studies. Individuals wishing to find work in the USA or Canada will find the book an invaluable resource and study companion for professional licensure exams.

Medical English Clear & Simple deals specifically with the teaching and learning of career-specific English for health professionals. The book is directed at the level of English for Specific Purposes and assumes the learner will have an intermediate level of English language competency and skills. The text also presupposes a definite, distinct language and culture for health professionals consisting of general English, professional and academic English, as well as colloquial English related to patient care.

Readers do need a minimum intermediate command of the English language. Prior technical knowledge in one of the health disciplines is a necessity, or the reader should be concurrently enrolled in a health sciences or health studies program.

This textbook lends itself to use by health and/or language instructors. Both will find the inclusion of an Answer Key with accompanying rationale very helpful should they not have these dual qualifications. It is recommended that instructors should have a knowledge and skill base in English for Specific Purpose or advanced, general ESL/EFL. **A background in nursing, medicine, or any allied health profession would be an absolute asset and is recommended by the author.**

APPROACH

This book is different. It was conceived to answer some key questions about the language needs of health professionals of non-English speaking backgrounds. These were:

* How can students of non-English speaking backgrounds be assisted toward success in co-occurring health studies/health sciences programs through language?

* What language skills are of priority importance to health professionals wishing to live and work in English-speaking North America?

* How are safe practices and quality care influenced positively or negatively by English language competencies and skills in the health-care setting?

* What value do health professionals from countries other than the United States of America and Canada place on the interpersonal relationship between the patient and the care provider?

- To what degree is optimal health-care delivery dependent on the ability of the care provider to speak both professional and colloquial, common English?

- What cultural factors influence professional practice in health-care delivery?

- How can these differences in professional health-care practices, if they exist, be addressed through language learning?

- How can NESB health professionals be assisted to learn to use English within the context of Canadian and American health-care systems and culture?

Communication and the ability to work as a health professional safely and effectively in the English language are key philosophical concepts of the text. Developing the capacity to interact with professional colleagues, treatment teams, clients (patients), families, and the community are considered essential language skills required by the learner and are addressed throughout the exercises and learning activities within this book.

The pedagogical approach of the text is to teach medical English in a lexical and communicative manner, combined. To be understood and to be able to understand is paramount to the provision of safe, competent care. Safety to practice is a core concept threaded throughout the text. The book is unique in this.[1] *Medical English Clear & Simple* comprehensively teaches career-specific language as a subspecialty of English for Specific Purposes, building not only a language repertoire, but also the ability to use language in meaningful ways.

AUTHENTICITY OF MATERIAL

Melodie Hull's background as a health professional and in health education allows her the privilege of firsthand linguistic experience within this context. She is also a qualified teacher and materials designer in Teaching English to Speakers of Other Languages (TESOL) at the graduate level. This absolutely makes *Medical English Clear & Simple* unique. Readers will find the material and exercises truly relevant to their work and studies.

ORGANIZATION OF THE TEXT

Medical English Clear & Simple proceeds in a progressive, step-wise fashion. Units contain three distinct sections, one flowing into the other. At each step, the reader is invited to discover, explore, and use language within the context of American and Canadian health care. Generally, the units are arranged as follows:

- Anatomy and Physiology

- Chronic or Acute Diseases or Conditions

- Treatments, Interventions, and Assistance

There are two exceptions to this organizational format. Chapter 1 introduces the context and culture of health care and its professions. Chapter 8 focuses on pharmacology and medication administration.

COMPONENTS AND FEATURES

Medical English Clear & Simple focuses on the knowledge, skills, and competencies required for practice, including principles of safe practice, while building English language skills.

---

[1]*Safety to Practice* is a concept used by nursing educators to guide and assess nursing students. It speaks to their responsibility to act as gatekeepers for the profession. *Safe practice* is what nurses actually do.

Themes of the text:

1) safety to practice

2) culture of health professions

3) culture and context of health-care delivery in Canada and the USA

4) focus on the adult (with the addition of an interview and case study of an ill child)

5) interprofessional communication

6) professional, interpersonal communication with clients (patients), families, and the public

Medical English Clear & Simple also includes:

- reading, writing, listening, and speaking exercises

- professional, academic, technical, and colloquial lexis, including anatomy and physiology, naming equipment, reading lab reports, and understanding diagnostics

- dialogues, interviews, and opportunities for pair and group work

- case studies

- the language of treatment and caring interventions, including pharmacology and medication administration

- the skills of charting, information reports, procedures, clinical pathways, and flow charts

- exposure to diverse clinical settings including hospitals, clinics, and a pharmacy

- readings and exercises that build cultural competency

- grammar highlights and reviews

- vocabulary alerts

- pronunciation hints using phonetics and audio links to *Taber's Cyclopedic Medical Dictionary*, 20th Edition, F.A. Davis Company

- suggested audio-video clips on the Internet to enhance listening and speaking skills

- concept reviews and discussions

- reading and writing in various genres

- reading for gist

- interpreting and writing journal abstracts

- critical thinking exercises at the end of each chapter provide an opportunity to apply essential content

- reflective questions and essay writing comparing and contrasting the reader's professional practice and culture with that of the USA and Canada

- an answer key that includes rationale for safe, competent practice within the culture and context of Western health care (i.e., Canada and the USA)

STUDENT GUIDE

Medical English Clear & Simple has been written with you in mind. The workbook format has dedicated spaces for your answers and responses. Each and every unit is designed to:

- provide opportunities for reading, writing, speaking, and listening all within the context of your career in health care

- support your ongoing learning by providing practical applications for new vocabulary and language skills

Example:

WRITING EXERCISE

    A) Use your new vocabulary. Write a sentence or two by combining these words in a meaningful way.

men	muscles	injury	lifting	pain
relief	ice	heavy	back	

_____

_____

    B) Use a key word from the previous exercise to complete a new sentence.
       1) Tisha's arm hurts today. She may have strained a _____ playing baseball yesterday.

- provide practical applications for language and medical knowledge, combined

- assist you to build a comprehensive and continuous language repertoire in the context of the health professions and delivery of health care

- include photos and illustrations that promote clarity and understanding of new material

- present opportunities for reflective and personal writing exercises to help you explore your own thinking and approach to your professional practice in the mode of the English language

Example:

WRITING EXERCISE—REFLECTIVE QUESTIONS

The text talks about the changing lifestyles of women in North America over the past 50 years and suggests that this has caused a greater incidence of coronary artery disease. What are your thoughts about this? How does it compare with your country of origin? Write your reflections here.

_____

_____

_____

- assist with professional writing through skill-building techniques of learning structure and form and choosing appropriate terminology

- develop multiple-choice test-taking skills

Example:

Multiple Choice

5) Professional caring means having high standards of care, knowledge, and skills to help people meet their health-care needs.
   In this context, *professional caring* can best be described as
   a) requiring advanced education, training, and preparation.
   b) a function that can be done by anyone with compassion and a will to help.
   c) simply a synonym for caring.

6) Veronica has high standards of cleanliness for herself, her home, and her job. In this context, *high standards* can best be described as
   a) she is messy.
   b) she doesn't wash or clean very often, only once a month.
   c) her goals.

7) If you forget to change a patient's dressing, does it affect your conscience? In this context, *conscience* can best be described as
   a) a moral sense of being right or wrong.
   b) make you think you are overworked.
   c) laziness.

- give opportunities to develop or enhance your critical thinking skills
- provide Pronunciation Hints with phonetic spellings based on *Taber's Cyclopedic Medical Dictionary,* 20th Edition, F.A. Davis Company

Example:

BOX 1-4 PRONUNCIATION HINTS

To understand the pronunciation guides for each of the following words, please refer to *Taber's Cyclopedic Medical Dictionary* (F.A. Davis Company).

domains – dō-**măn's**

unique – ū-**nē-k**

leprosy – **lĕp'**rō-sē

Alzheimer's – **ălts'**hī-mĕrz

conscience – kon'**shŭntz**

epilepsy - **ĕp'**ĭ-lĕp"sē

- encourage you to link to *Medical English Clear & Simple* on Davis Plus online for supplemental language exercises

- assist you with pronunciation by linking you to *Taber's Cyclopedic Medical Dictionary*'s audio features on the Davis Plus website.

- include a quick and easy Glossary of Terms on the *Medical English Clear & Simple* Davis Plus link.

- include an Answer Key that offers the rationale or reasoning for many of the questions and exercises to ensure your full understanding

Example:

Unit 8 Answer Key:

Understanding Intramuscular Injections

1) at the dorsal gluteal site (also known as the gluteus medius or gluteus maximus). Note: This site is no longer a preferred site for an intramuscular injection. However, many older patients and immigrants are familiar with it and will request that it be used. Clinical judgment by the health professional (usually the nurse in this situation) will determine if the patient can or cannot have the medication here and why. The patient's choice must always be considered.

INSTRUCTOR'S GUIDE

Thank you for choosing *Medical English Clear & Simple*. You have found a wonderful resource for teaching! Readings, dialogues, and case studies predominate in the text, introducing the use of language to assess, confer, consult, interpret, interview, explore perception and perspective, and provide rationale. The focus is to teach communication in career-specific contexts. Exercises also include questioning, narratives, testimonies, and reflective discussions all within the bounds of health and health care. A complete list of these can be found in the Table of Contents.

This book is best suited for co-occurring language and health studies courses. Its content closely reflects content in introductory and/or first-year nursing, medicine, and other health professions programs. As a companion to these, *Medical English Clear & Simple* can absolutely enhance student success. It is also well suited for any upgrading or refresher programs for internationally educated nurses, as well as international medical graduates and so on who wish to either (1) immigrate or work in health in the USA or Canada, (2) participate in a clinical practicum here, or (c) speak to or correspond with American and Canadian health professionals. Finally, you will also find this book helpful as an excellent resource for those health professionals interested in learning English as a new language for personal and/or professional development purposes.

Medical English Clear & Simple is designed in a cumulative, comprehensive fashion. Vocabulary and linguistic skills introduced in one unit are further developed in succeeding ones. With this in mind, the author recommends proceeding through the material in the order in which it has been designed.

Welcome! Let's begin our study of *Medical English Clear and Simple.*

Unit 1 provides multiple opportunities for the reader to become acquainted with the American and Canadian approaches to health. It introduces language used in the context of health and health care, providing a foundation for use of the language in situations specific to health-care careers. It also aids in the development of an awareness of Western health care and the Western view of professionalism and professional expectations in health care. The use of appropriate terms and expressions in clinical situations is also included. While this context is reflected throughout this and subsequent units, Unit 1 provides the foundation.

Unit 1's focus and main subdivisions are Concepts of Health and Wellness, Professional Caring, The Drugstore, and Calling the Doctor's Office. Subsequent chapters focus on specific body systems and the correct and appropriate use of language in caring for clients in specific situations.

SECTION ONE   Concepts of Health and Wellness

This section introduces health and wellness through American and Canadian cultural perspectives. It includes two reading selections, each followed by reading exercises and by speaking, listening, and writing exercises designed to improve your communication skills.

Reading Selection 1-1

Read the following in its entirety. Many words may be new to you. The exercises that follow will help you learn their meaning.

PERSPECTIVES ON HEALTH CARE IN THE NEW MILLENNIUM

In the United States of America and in Canada, perspectives on health care have changed over the last 30 years. Today, the public sees itself as a consumer of health-care services and products. This means that when individuals seek advice or treatment, they often come well-informed about their health issues and needs. Today's patient expects to be treated as an intelligent, competent person by the doctor, nurse, and other health-care professionals. No longer is the patient a passive receiver of health care. The new patient comes with information, education, and an inquiring mind.

Professionally, today's view of health care is concerned with health promotion and disease prevention. It is no longer disease-focused or cure-focused. Health care is concerned with quality of life. In this new perspective, it extends beyond health challenges and basic medical care to lifestyle adaptations to ensure optimal health. Healthy living programs in schools, businesses, and community agencies are an example of health promotion initiatives. Health-care professionals and governments at all levels collaborate with communities and patients/health-care consumers not only to promote health but also to provide the best health care possible.

 READING EXERCISES

The following reading exercises challenge your ability to understand the general meaning of the selection, to learn new vocabulary and be able to expand on it, and to use new words in sentences.

Understanding the General Meaning

Read the text again. Think about it. Do you understand it? What is the general meaning of the text? What is its focus?

_____

_____

_____

Building Vocabulary

Take a moment now to review what you have just read. Circle any words that are new to you. Write them down here. In a moment, you may see them again in exercises that will help you understand their meaning. If not, at the end of this section, feel free to use your dictionary.

_____

_____

_____

Determining Meaning from Context. To build vocabulary, study the following words or terms taken from this text. Discover all you can about them by looking at them in context. Choose the correct meaning. Finally, take a look at how these words or terms expand in English.

1. Lifestyle *(adjective; noun, singular)*

In context:
a) He lives a busy lifestyle. He works long days and parties all night.
b) A healthy lifestyle includes a balance between work, rest, play, and diet.
c) Lifestyle adaptations are often necessary to ensure health and wellness.

Meaning: *Lifestyle* can best be described as
a) way of life
b) good or bad
c) alive or dead
d) what style or fashion of food or clothes you like

Word expansion:
a) Nurse Wong's *lifestyle* is very different from her colleagues. She likes to work nights and sleep all day. (noun)
b) I would prefer a leisurely *lifestyle;* however, I have to work. (noun)
c) I would prefer *to style my life* after Mother Teresa—work hard, be dedicated, and really, really help people. (conditional (would prefer) + verb, infinitive (style) + noun (life) combine as a verb phrase)
d) The nurse suggested *lifestyle adaptations* to the client to help control his newly diagnosed diabetes. (adjective)

2. Consumer *(noun)*

In context:
a) She buys her food at the grocery store. She is a regular consumer there.
b) Sometimes I think I am a consumer of information. I can't get enough.

Meaning: The term *consumer* can best be described as
a) when your nose is plugged
b) a customer, client, or patient
c) a person who purchases, uses, or eats a product
d) both (b) and (c)

Word expansion:
a) He was so hungry; he *consumed* all the food in the house. (verb, past tense)
b) She cannot think. She *is consumed* by pain. (verb, present tense continuous)
c) They have a *consummate* relationship. It's perfect. (adjective)
d) I am guilty of *consuming* too much junk food. (gerund, present participle used as a noun)
e) He is a careful *consumer,* always checking the quality and prices of what he purchases. (noun)

3. Issue *(noun, verb)*

In context:
a) Today's health issues include contraception and antibiotic-resistant organisms.
b) Students love to debate political issues.

Meaning: The word *issues* can best be described as meaning
a) the main topics, results, or points of interest in a subject
b) things you sneeze into
c) giving
d) none of the above

Word expansion:
a) I hope they *will issue* my working visa for Canada. (verb, future tense)
b) The computer *is issuing* your results right now. Please wait. (verb, present tense continuous)
c) They *issued* my driver's license in 1992. (verb, past tense)
d) *Issuance* of a passport requires your birth certificate and other identification. (noun, singular)
e) The nurse had many *issues* she wanted to discuss with her supervisor. (noun, plural)

4. Needs *(noun, verb)*

In context:
a) A person's primary needs include food, clothing, and shelter.
b) What are your patient's needs right now? Treatment or rest?
c) He needs to find a way to pay off his debts.

Meaning: *Needs* can best be described as meaning
a) something you want
b) something you require
c) lack of food and water
d) desire

Word expansion
a) Jack is emotionally *needy.* He follows his girlfriend around like a puppy dog. (adjective)
b) I *need* a vacation. No, not really. I just want one. (verb, present tense)
c) Do you donate money to the *needy?* (noun)
d) There are many *needy* people in the world. (adjective)

5. Passive receiver *(noun, verb)*

In context:
a) Why doesn't she complain about her treatment instead of just passively receiving it?
b) She is so compliant. She accepts everything. She really is a passive receiver of her life.

Meaning: The term *passive receiver* can best be described as
a) outspoken
b) submissive and acted upon
c) disinterested and apathetic
d) unconscious

Word expansion:
a) In some countries, nurses are the *passive receivers* of physicians' orders. In the United States and in Canada, nurses have a responsibility to question orders if they think they are wrong. (noun)
b) How can you sit there and *passively receive* the insults of that person? (adverb [passively] + verb present tense [receive])
c) *Passive reception* requires the ability to be submissive and just allow things to happen to you. (term, adjective + noun, combined)

6. Health promotion *(noun [identifying a concept]; adjective)*

In context:
a) Nurses are always involved in health promotion in the community.
b) The government sponsors health promotion by advertising healthy lifestyle choices on TV.

Meaning: The term/concept *health promotion* can best be understood as meaning
a) an activity that only doctors do
b) teaching and providing information about healthy living
c) a TV advertisement campaign
d) when you are healthy

Word expansion:
a) I *am promoting health* each time I teach a patient about healthy eating. (verb, present tense, continuous + object of verb)
b) How do you *promote health* with your patients? (verb, present tense + noun)
c) The community has begun to sponsor many *health promotion* meetings and activities. (adjective + noun form term)
d) Community officials and health-care professionals joined in planning activities for *health promotion.* (noun)

7. Prevention *(noun, adjective)*

In context:
a) Prevention of starvation is a priority for the World Health Organization.
b) Disaster prevention is the concern of environmentalists and politicians.

Meaning: *Prevention* can best be described as
a) gathering knowledge about a subject
b) inoculation
c) taking positive action to avoid a terrible illness or situation from occurring
d) taking political action by blockading or marching

Word expansion:
a) The city of Vancouver, British Columbia, hopes *to prevent* a bridge disaster if an earthquake should occur. They have ordered structural repairs to all bridges. (verb, infinitive)
b) Can measles be *prevented?* (verb, past tense)
c) *Preventing* the spread of HIV/AIDS is a global issue. (gerund, present participle used as a noun)

8. Disease *(noun)*

In context:
a) The disease of polio has been eradicated in North America.
b) Do you suffer from a disease?

Meaning: The word *disease* can best be described as
a) pathological change in organs or tissues revealed by particular signs and symptoms
b) an illness that last only 3 days
c) something only children and old people get
d) a condition that is always curable

Word expansion:
a) We wanted to save the ovaries, but they were too *diseased*. We removed them. (adjective)
b) Some *diseases* are infectious; others are not. (noun, plural)

9. Cure *(noun)*

In context:
a) Canadians Drs. Banting and Best didn't find the cure for diabetes; they found a treatment that saved many people's lives.
b) There is no cure for the common cold.

Meaning: The noun *cure* can best be described as
a) treating the symptoms of a disease
b) a particular method of treatment designed to restore health
c) remission
d) none of the above

Word expansion:
a) If a doctor could restore health to 100%, she could say she *cured* the patient. (verb, past tense)
b) Bob had prostate cancer but says he is now *cured*. (adjective)
c) Scientists are interested in *curing* AIDS as well as preventing it. (gerund, present participle used as noun)
d) Some herbs have *curative* factors. (adjective)
e) Some diseases, such as Huntington's disease, are *incurable*. (adjective)

10. Collaborate *(verb)*

In context:
a) It is important for the nurse and doctor to collaborate on a plan of care for the patient.
b) If we collaborate, we can get this job done quickly.

Meaning: The word *collaborate* can best be described as
a) being efficient
b) being responsible
c) taking turns
d) working together and planning together

Word expansion:
a) The multidisciplinary health-care team worked in *collaboration* to help the patient through rehabilitation. (noun, object of preposition "in")
b) The hospital *is collaborating* with Social Services to ensure the rights of the child are protected. (verb, present tense, continuous)
c) Luckily, the insurance company *collaborated* with us and paid the medical bills for Joe. (verb, past tense)
d) The health-care team used a *collaborative* approach to the patient's care and he improved quickly. (adjective)

Using New Words in Sentences. Use a key word from the previous exercise to create a new sentence.

1) _____ (Bob, addictive)
2) _____ (nurses, not)
3) _____ (promotion)
4) _____ (overweight, excessive)
5) _____ (unhealthy, youth)
6) _____ (political, health care)

SPEAKING EXERCISE

Read the following completed sentences aloud. Ask a peer or teacher to help you with pronunciation. Proceed to the Pronunciation Hint section following. This will also help.

Bob says he is not unhealthy, but he is most certainly very overweight. He is obese. Members of multidisciplinary research teams are trying to collaborate and find a cure for addiction and obesity.

PRONUNCIATION HINTS
To understand the pronunciation guides for each of the following words, please refer to *Taber's Cyclopedic Medical Dictionary* (F. A. Davis Company).

unhealthy – ŭn-**hĕlth**-ē

overweight – ō-vur-**wăt'**

addiction – ă-**dĭk'**shŭn

multidisciplinary – mŭl"tī-**dĭs'**ĭ-plĭ-năr-ē

obese – ō-**bēs'**

LISTENING EXERCISE

If you would like to hear more native English speakers from Canada and the United States, search the Internet for radio stations located there. Many radio stations have programs dedicated to the subject of health and wellness. Try to find one. Listen carefully by Internet or radio to hear many of the words you have just learned.

WRITING EXERCISE

Use your new vocabulary. Write a sentence or two by combining these words and names in a meaningful way.

Dr. Banting	collaborated	disease
Dr. Best	cure	famous
treatment		

_____

_____

_____

Reading Selection 1-2

Read the following aloud or silently to yourself.

HEALTH IS A STATE OF OPTIMAL WELL-BEING

It is a " . . . a state of complete physical, mental, and social well-being and not merely the absence of disease or infirmity. . . . to reach a level of optimal physical, mental and social well-being, an individual or group is able to realize aspirations, to satisfy needs, and to change or cope with the environment. Health, therefore, is seen as a resource for living, a positive concept emphasizing social and personal resources, as well as physical capacities."

—World Health Organization[1]

READING EXERCISES

This time you are asked questions to test your general understanding of the reading selection, asked about the meaning of specific words, and provided with an opportunity to practice answering multiple-choice questions—the type of question most frequently used on nursing exams—as a way of building vocabulary.

Understanding the General Meaning

In your own words, answer the following questions based on your reading.

1) What is the gist of this reading? The main point?

_____

_____

2) Is this academic language easy or difficult for you to read? Please explain.

_____

_____

Building Vocabulary

Take a moment now to review what you have just read. Consider the vocabulary list below. Do you understand these words? Think about them. In a moment, you will see them again in exercises that will help you understand their meaning. If need be, at the end of this section feel free to use your dictionary for clarification.

optimal	state
infirmity	needs
realize	capacities

A variety of exercises—mix and match, explaining the meaning of words, and multiple choice—can be used to expand your vocabulary

Mix and Match.   Consider what you have just read. Complete the exercise in Box 1-1 by matching a term or phrase from the text to the English language explanation. To do this, you must consider the meaning of words in the context of Western health care. You might be interested to know that not only are these terms and phrases very commonly used by health professionals, but they also appear on national licensing exams.

---

[1] Definition available at the World Health Organization website, http://www.who.int/aboutwho/en/definition.html

BOX 1-1 Mix and Match

Draw a line from the term or phrase in the left column to the explanation in the right column.

TERM OR PHRASE	EXPLANATION
optimal well-being	dreams and goals
physical well-being	the ability to feel comfortable among other people; social ease and skills
mental well-being	physical fitness; a healthy, active body
social resources	emotional stability; free from mental or emotional disturbance
to satisfy needs	physical/emotional surroundings
aspirations	the ability to accomplish what must be done to survive and grow
environment	personal sense of wellness

Sentence Completion.   Complete the following sentences using your own words.

1) Frederica has very poor vision, yet she says her health is very good. That is her subjective opinion. **Subjective** means _____

2) The test results for Mrs. Ortega have arrived from the laboratory. When you read them you discover she does not have diabetes and she is in optimal health in general. In this case, optimal health is defined objectively. **Objectively** means _____

3) The medical concept of **physical fitness** means _____

Exam Writing in North America Cultural Context

Students planning to write a licensing exam such as the Nursing Certification Licensing Examination (NCLEX) in the United States or the Canadian Registered Nurse Exam (CRNE)/Canadian Nursing Examination (CNE) in Canada will enjoy the opportunity to practice multiple-choice questions. These national exams include 75% to 100% multiple-choice questions.

Multiple Choice.   Complete the following multiple-choice questions that deal with the subject of health. This mock test provides an opportunity to see a variety of usages for the new vocabulary. Choose the best answer.

1) *Health* can best be described as
  a) physical well-being.
  b) spiritual well-being.
  c) not being disabled or ill.
  d) a positive state of mind and body.
  e) all of the above

2) The patient with diabetes says he is in *good health*. This means
   a) he feels well and his diabetes is under control.
   b) he is foolish.
   c) he is disabled and doesn't know it.
   d) he needs to get a doctor's opinion.

3) The elderly patient is very, very thin. She has not eaten a proper meal in 1 week. She is in poor health. *Poor health* is best described as
   a) too lazy to buy groceries.
   b) improper nutrition and health care.
   c) being in the hospital.
   d) she's okay. It is alright to be very thin.

4) Mrs. Anderson is in failing health. She is 94, has cancer, and now has pneumonia. *Failing health* can best be described as
   a) no family visits her.
   b) lack of nutrition and exercise.
   c) in deteriorating condition and may die.
   d) needs to see a doctor.

5) My mom is in relatively good health. She has arthritis and eczema, but otherwise she is well. *Relatively good health* means
   a) able to function and have a quality of life that suits her.
   b) deteriorating condition and may die.
   c) she is my relative and is in good health.
   d) none of the above

6) I am a nurse. It is important for me to give good health care to my patients. Giving *good health care* can be described as
   a) providing the best professional treatment, skills, compassion, and caring activities possible.
   b) providing basic physical care only.
   c) following doctors orders only.
   d) none of the above

SPEAKING EXERCISE

Return to the reading that defines health. Read it aloud now, even if you are reading alone. If you are able to record your voice, please do so. Then listen back. Check your pronunciation with the box below or ask a native English speaker to help you.

PRONUNCIATION HINTS
To understand the pronunciation guides for each of the following words, please refer to *Taber's Cyclopedic Medical Dictionary* (F. A. Davis Company).

health – **hĕlth**   ŏ

optimal – **ŏp'tĭm-ăl**

aspirations – **ăs-pĭ-rā'shŭnz**

LISTENING EXERCISE

At this point in *Medical English Clear and Simple,* you have some homework. You are encouraged to speak to a native English-speaking health professional if you know one or to watch an English language television show or film set in an American health-care setting. Listen. The purpose of this exercise is simply to begin to familiarize yourself with how English is spoken in the context of health care.

WRITING EXERCISE—A REFLECTIVE QUESTION

As you can see from the reading selections and exercises, health is considered holistically from a Western perspective. Biological, psychological, sociological, environmental, and spiritual factors are all considered in its definition. How is health defined in your country of origin? Write a short paragraph here.

_____

_____

_____

SECTION TWO # Professional Caring

Now that we have taken a look at culturally bound concepts of health and wellness in Canada and the United States, this section introduces the concepts of professional caring and the roles of professional caregivers. The meaning of holism and holistic care are explored. Exercises provide opportunities to compare and contrast how the Western model of health-care delivery applies to that of other countries. Please remember that although some of the readings that follow are based in nursing, they are relevant to all health-care professionals.

Reading Selection 1-3

Read the following. If an opportunity arises, discuss it with friends. Offer your own thoughts and opinions. Make comparisons with your own country or others to enrich the discussion.

PROFESSIONAL CARING

Professional caring is based on a foundation of providing support for people in need as well as promoting their personal growth and development. This can mean progressing from a position of physical and/or emotional health challenges to a position of wellness. Earlier in this chapter, we reviewed the definition of health and discovered that it includes the biological, psychological, sociological, and spiritual aspects of a person's lived experience. Health also includes the element of environment: factors that can help or hinder an individual's ability to meet everyday challenges and enjoy quality of life.

According to the International Council of Nurses (ICN), nurses have four responsibilities: preventing illness, restoring health, alleviating suffering, and promoting health (ICN 1975). These are the domains of professional caring, and they apply to all health professions. In the United States and Canada, we often refer to Jean Watson's theory of Transpersonal Caring.[1] She, like others, sees that nursing and medicine have moved from the medical model of care to a model that includes valuing the transpersonal relationship between the caregiver and care-receiver—that professional caring is a standard of practice. It includes compassion, competence, confidence, conscience, and commitment.

[1]University of Colorado School of Nursing, Transpersonal Caring and the Caring Moment Defined, http://www2.uchsc.edu/son/caring/content/transpersonal.asp

Additionally, a number of theories of health-care practices support multicultural care. Evident in our health-care philosophy, this is the belief that health professionals require a level of cultural competency to provide the best care: a solid understanding of sociocultural practices from around the world. This knowledge helps them provide an additional level of empathy and promotes trust, respect, and optimal health outcomes.

READING EXERCISES

The following reading exercises challenge your ability to understand the meaning of the selection and to learn and use new vocabulary.

Understanding the General Meaning

1) Read the text again. Think about it. Do you understand it? What is the general meaning of the text? What is its focus?

_____

_____

2) Although the reading talks about nursing, it claims to be applicable to other health professions. For example, the four responsibilities of nurses are described. Are these the same professional characteristics of other health professions? If so, name those professions.

_____

_____

Building Vocabulary

Take a moment now to review what you have just read. Circle any words that are new to you. Write them down here. In a moment, you may see them again in exercises that will help you understand their meaning. If not, at the end of this section, feel free to use your dictionary.

_____

_____

Multiple Choice. Here are some words to review. Do you understand them? Try to discover their meaning from their context-based use in the reading selection and in the stem of the question. Again, these are multiple-choice questions, the most common type of question you'll find on nursing exams.

1) I am a competent nurse.
   In this context, *competent* can best be described as
   a) learning about a subject.
   b) skilled, knowledgeable, and capable.
   c) unsure of how to treat new problems.

2) Canada is a multicultural mosaic while the United States is more of a melting pot.
   In this context, *melting pot* can best be described as
   a) each culture being valued as separate to mainstream culture.
   b) an expectation that all new immigrants assimilate into mainstream culture.
   c) only Caucasians are valued.

3) My father faces the health challenge of diabetes.
   In this context, *health challenge* can best be described as
   a) He is sick and should be in the hospital.
   b) He is afraid of this illness and cannot cope. He needs a full-time nurse.
   c) He has a chronic illness that he must treat and be aware of as he goes about his life.

4) My father's lived experience of diabetes has been positive. He is quite comfortable with it.
   In this context, *lived experience* can best be described as
   a) His unique, personal experience with this health challenge. It has been one of acceptance and adaptability.
   b) He hates his diabetes.
   c) His personal experience of living with diabetes has been bad and he considers himself a sick person.

5) Professional caring means having high standards of care, knowledge, and skills to help people meet their health-care needs.
   In this context, *professional caring* can best be described as
   a) requiring advanced education, training, and preparation.
   b) a function that can be done by anyone with compassion and a will to help.
   c) simply a synonym for caring.

6) Veronica has high standards of cleanliness for herself, her home, and her job.
   In this context, *high standards* can best be described as
   a) she is messy.
   b) she doesn't wash or clean very often, only once a month.
   c) cleanliness is an important goal for her.

7) If you forget to change a patient's dressing, does it affect your conscience?
   In this context, *conscience* can best be described as
   a) a moral sense of being right or wrong.
   b) making you think you are overworked.
   c) laziness.

Using New Words in Sentences. Use the following words or phrases in complete sentences.

1) demonstrate a high level of competency

_____

2) challenge, epilepsy

_____

3) standards, care, professional

_____

_____

SPEAKING EXERCISE

Read the following sentences aloud. Ask a peer or teacher to help you with pronunciation. Proceed to the Pronunciation Hints section following. This will also help.

These are the domains of professional caring and apply to all health professions.

Ravinder has a unique, personal experience with this health challenge of leprosy. It has been one of acceptance and adaptability.

Mr. Heinrich has severe Alzheimer's disease. He is not competent to manage his own finances.

PRONUNCIATION HINTS

To understand the pronunciation guides for each of the following words, please refer to *Taber's Cyclopedic Medical Dictionary* (F. A. Davis Company).

domains – dō-**măn's**

unique – ū-**nē**-k

leprosy – **lĕp'**rō-sē

Alzheimer's – **ălts'**hī-mĕrz

conscience – **kon'**shŭntz

epilepsy – **ĕp'**i-lĕp"sē

LISTENING EXERCISE

Ask a peer or colleague to read the few sentences in the Speaking exercise back to you. Listen carefully. In a multicultural context, you will be exposed to people with many different accents. Are you able to understand what the person says if you are not allowed to look at the written word at the same time?

WRITING EXERCISE—REFLECTIVE WRITING

Think about all that you have read and learned so far. Write your personal thoughts and feelings about both the content and context.

_____

_____

_____

Reading Selection 1-4

Read the following text about holistic care. Notice any words that are new to you. They will be important to you in the upcoming exercises.

HOLISTIC CARE

Each individual's response to illness and health can be different. Today, health professionals acknowledge this and use holistic health assessments when working with patients. The positive **outcomes** of **prescribed** treatments are often very dependent on that patient's lifestyle, culture, and access to good health care prior to, during, and after **initial** contact.

Holism is a philosophy in which an individual cannot be separated from all the parts of his or her life. This includes family, culture, environment, community and occupational relationships. All aspects **interrelate** to affect the quality of life of an individual. These come together to become part of an individual's lived experience.

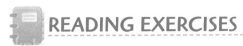

READING EXERCISES

As with previous reading selections, the exercises that follow will help you understand the meaning of the passage and learn new vocabulary.

Understanding the General Meaning

Read the text again. Think about it. What is holistic health?

_____

_____

_____

Building Vocabulary

Take a moment now to review what you have just read. Write the words that you see highlighted into the spaces below. Then define them in your own words. In a moment, you may see them again in exercises that will help you understand their meaning. If not, at the end of this section, feel free to use your dictionary.

_____

_____

_____

_____

   To build vocabulary you need to be able not only to identify new words and their meaning, but also to be able to explain the words to others and use them properly. These exercises will help you do that.

Mix and Match.   Recognizing words that have a similar meaning is one way to build vocabulary. Complete the exercise in Box 1-2 to help you do this.

BOX 1-2 Mix and Match

Connect the word or term in the left column with the definition in the right. Look for definitions or words of similar meaning. Draw a line between the matching terms.

COLUMN 1	COLUMN 2
community relationships	a sum of personal beliefs
lived experience	all aspects; sum of all parts
philosophy	social connections
outcomes	family doctor
isolation	necessary or very important
general practitioner	results
essential	alone/separated from others
dependent	reliant upon
initial	first; taking the lead
holistic	unique, personal experiences that lead to unique actions, beliefs, and lifestyles

Explaining the Meaning of Words.   Read the following to expand new vocabulary. Find the meaning of each statement based on what you've just learned as well as the simple context of the statement.

1) Health professionals such as doctors and nurses value the relationships they build with their clients or patients. What does this mean?

_____

2) The core of the helping relationship is the rapport the health professional builds with the client. It is built on trust, respect, warmth, and empathy. What does *rapport* mean?

_____

3) The philosophical underpinning of all health care is the value we all place on life. What does *underpinning* mean?

_____

4) Philosophically and morally health professionals are concerned with helping people who cannot fully help themselves. What does *morally* mean?

_____

SPEAKING EXERCISE

Return to the reading Holistic Care. Read it aloud now, even if you are reading alone. If you are able to record your voice, please do so now. Read slowly to clearly enunciate your words. Check your pronunciation with the box below or ask a native English speaker to help you.

BOX 1- 4 PRONUNCIATION HINTS

To understand the pronunciation guides for each of the following words, please refer to *Taber's Cyclopedic Medical Dictionary* (F. A. Davis Company).

acknowledge – ak-**now**-lj

outcomes – **owt**-kō'm-z

dependent – dē-**pĕn**-dĕnt

initial – ĭn-**ĭsh**'ăl

philosophy – fĭ-**lŏs**'ō-fē

aspects – **ăs**'pĕkt's

interrelate – ĭn"tĕr-rē-**lāt**

LISTENING EXERCISE

Now is the time to listen to your self-recording or listen to a co-learner's recording. Check your pronunciation with the box (above) or ask a native English speaker to help you.

WRITING EXERCISE—REFLECTIVE WRITING

Compare and contrast the value placed by the doctor on the relationship between the patient and doctor in your country of origin with that of the United States and Canada.

_____

_____

Compare and contrast the value placed by the nurse on the relationship between the patient and doctor in your country of origin with that of the United States and Canada.

_____

_____

Draw a conclusion. From all that you have learned about the philosophy and practice of holistic care, write a statement about whether or not this is new and/or useful for you to know. Explain.

_____

_____

_____

Reading Selection 1-5

Read the following paragraph. It identifies members of the health-care team.

HEALTH-CARE PROFESSIONALS: MEMBERS OF THE HEALTH-CARE TEAM

Health professionals do not work alone. They work on multidisciplinary care teams that are client-focused. As a whole, the team manages the client's care. In so doing, they are able to provide a fully integrated plan that includes the client in all decision-making. Coordination of care is valued and all members of the team work together toward optimal health outcomes for the client. These health-care teams include registered nurses, doctors, physiotherapists, dieticians, social workers, occupational therapists, and various other specialists; many of these professionals are known by abbreviations, such as RN for registered nurse. No one voice on the team is of less value than the other. Each member has equal input and is respected for his or her professional expertise. While doctors may make final clinical decisions for some aspects of care, they do so in consultation and collaboration with the team and the client. They do not work completely independently.

READING EXERCISES

The following exercises will help you to understand and interpret the reading and build new vocabulary.

Understanding the General Meaning

Answer the following questions related to the general meaning and gist of the paragraph you have just read. Answer True or False. Remember you are working in the context of Canadian and American health care.

1) Doctors have full authority over all aspects of patient care.
   a) True
   b) False

2) Physiotherapists are never invited to participate in health-care teams.
   a) True
   b) False

3) Collaboration within the health-care team does not include the patient.
   a) True
   b) False

4) Patients have no choice in the type of care they receive.
   a) True
   b) False

5) Nurses and dieticians may each have something valuable to add to the care planning done for patients.
   a) True
   b) False

Interpreting the Reading

Based on this reading, answer the question: What is the core message communicated in this paragraph?

_____

_____

Building Vocabulary

It is important to know how to expand and use the new words you are learning. You can do this by using them in sentences. It is also essential to recognize commonly used abbreviations.

Sentence Completion. Using the words or their derivatives from the present exercise, fill in the blanks in the following sentences.

1) Ling Wu is new in town and needs a family doctor. She must look under the heading _____ in the yellow pages of her phonebook.

2) Rochelyn was in a car accident a few weeks ago. She pulled a muscle in her upper arm. Now she attends _____ three times per week to help improve muscle strength in her arms.

3) Winston is having difficulties adjusting to the separation from his wife and kids since the divorce last month. He is feeling suicidal. At the medical clinic today, he is referred to the _____ for assessment and care.

4) Azeim studied the respiratory system, gas exchanges, biology, physiology, and technology in a 4-year degree program to become a _____.

5) The Ngoba family really appreciated the kind and competent care their elderly family member received from the _____ on the medical unit at the hospital. Today their mom is being discharged. The Ngobas have brought the _____ a small bouquet of flowers in thanks.

6) GinGin has just completed a 1-year practical nursing program. Now she must write the national exams to obtain her _____ to practice.

Mix and Match. Test yourself to see if you can determine the correct abbreviation for professional titles by completing the exercise in Box 1-3.

BOX 1-3 Mix and Match: Abbreviations for Members of the Health-Care Team

Match the abbreviation with the professional title of members of the health-care team with their description. See how many you can recognize. Test yourself.

PROFESSIONAL TITLE (ABBREVIATED)	DESCRIPTION OF PROFESSIONAL
OT	registered nurse: a person who practices professional nursing; may or may not be specialized
RN	social worker: concerned with patient's living arrangements, finances, and personal support networks
MD	medical doctor
SW	registered psychiatric nurse: a person who practices professional nursing; specialized in mental health and addiction care[1]
RT	occupational therapist: promotes health and wellness through occupation and purposeful activity
RPN	physiotherapist: concerned with patient's movement and function
LPN	licensed practical nurse: subordinate to RNs and RPNs yet fully qualified within own scope of practice and licensing to provide certain patient care
PT	general practitioner: a physician with a general focus, most often seen as a family doctor
GP	respiratory therapist concerned with patient airways and their function OR a recreation therapist concerned with patient activity and quality of life

[1]The designation RPN is often found in British commonwealth countries such as Canada. In the United States, the psychiatric nurse is an RN with master's degree preparation in this specialty.

Speaking Exercise

Reading aloud helps us overcome the shyness and discomfort that may come when trying to pronounce new words in English. The method of breaking a paragraph up into sentences is an excellent strategy to practice speaking. Try this procedure. Use the Pronunciation Hints listed below the exercise as a guide.

1) Practice reading one sentence at a time to improve your ability to read short paragraphs more fluently.

First, read the following sentence three times before proceeding to the next sentence.

I am a member of the health-care team.

Now read the following sentence three times before proceeding to the next sentence.

I am a health professional.

Now read the following sentence three times before proceeding to the next sentence.

I, too, work in a hospital.

Now read the following sentence three times before proceeding to the next sentence.

I am frequently asked to see patients who have had injuries to their head and face from a motor vehicle accident.

Now read the following sentence three times before proceeding to the next sentence.

Who am I?

Now read the following sentence three times before proceeding.

I am a dental surgeon.

2) Now read all of the sentences together. Repeat reading the paragraph aloud as many times as you like to feel comfortable and competent with it.

I am a member of the health-care team. I am a health professional, I, too, work in a hospital. I am frequently asked to see patients who have had injuries to the head and face from a motor vehicle accident. Who am I? I am a dental surgeon.

PRONUNCIATION HINTS

To understand the pronunciation guides for each of the following words, please refer to *Taber's Cyclopedic Medical Dictionary* (F. A. Davis Company).

professional – prō-**fĕsh'**ŭn-ăl

patients – **pā'**shĕnts

surgeon – **sŭr'**jŭn

dental – **dĕn't**-ăl

vehicle – **vē'ĭ**-kl

LISTENING EXERCISE

Use the Internet as a resource for learning. On your web browser, search for short audio-visual clips (video clips). Listen as many times as you like, but be sure to listen to an example of a native English speaker so that you may study pronunciation and oral presentation. You might like to try this site: *Health Care Professionals—Pt 1* at http://www.youtube.com. This video clip is narrated by a native English speaker and he introduces a couple of health professionals for whom English is not their first language. Listen carefully to those speakers as they talk about their careers. How do their varying accents affect your ability to understand what they are saying? If you have an accent when you speak English, how will this affect your own ability to be understood in the workplace?

WRITING EXERCISE

Take a moment to think about the speaking exercise you have just completed. The process is called *chaining*. What do you think about this method? Are you familiar with it? Do you find it helpful? Write your comments here, using full sentences.

Reading Selection 1-6

Read the following aloud or silently to yourself. Note that the verbs are highlighted. While reading, try to see if you can determine why this has been done. You will also find that this reading is written in an interview style with the health-care professional as the interviewer. All health professionals need to gain historical data from their clients and should become skilled on how to interview a client. This exercise is designed to simulate that process.

PROFESSIONAL CARING: HISTORY TAKING AND THE ILLNESS EXPERIENCE

To complete this reading exercise, pretend that you are now 20 years of age. Then, imagine that you are being interviewed by a health professional. She or he wants to know about your childhood experience of having the measles. You do remember it. You were 8 years old at the time. This is an exercise in the use of the past tense.

1) At the age of 8, what **did** you think you **had?**
   a) I thought I had a rash.
   b) I had a rash.
   c) My mom said measles.

2) What **did** you think **made** you sick?
   a) I ate bad food.
   b) I thought I ate something I was allergic to.
   c) I went to bed quickly.

3) How **did** you decide that you **were** sick? What **were** your signs and symptoms of illness?
   a) Mom told me.
   b) I had a rash and a high fever.
   c) High fever. Rash.

4) What **did** this illness do to your body?
   a) It made me have spots.
   b) It made me sleepy.
   c) I had a lot of red spots, my eyes hurt in the light, and I was itchy.

5) How severe **was** this illness? For example, **did** you have to go to the hospital or **take** a few days off from school?
   a) Severe. I had to stay home from school for 2 weeks.
   b) Not bad. I didn't miss school.
   c) Severe. I stayed home.

6) What **were** the main problems that this illness **caused** for you? Think holistically.
   a) No school.
   b) Not being hungry.
   c) I was itchy and unhappy and couldn't go to school.

7) At 8 years old, what kind of treatment **did** you think you should have?
   a) Ice cream.
   b) My mom gave me aspirin and ice water and lotion for my itchiness.
   c) I thought I should have ice cream, candies, watch TV, play, and lay in bed whenever I wanted to.

8) What kind of treatment **did** you actually get?
   a) My mom gave me some aspirins, ice water to drink, and some lotion for my itchiness. I had to stay in bed and couldn't watch TV for a few days.
   b) Bed rest.
   c) I didn't get to watch TV.

9) **Did** the treatment help?
   a) No.
   b) Yes.
   c) Yeah, I guess so.

10) Who **did** you ask for help? **Did** they treat you?
   a) I asked my mom. Yes, she did.
   b) I asked the school teacher.
   c) My dad.

11) What **was** the treatment? **Did** it make you feel better?
   a) I took some pills and stayed home to rest. Yes, it made me feel better.
   b) Pills and yes.
   c) I didn't get any treatment.

12) **Did** you receive a prescription for your illness? What **was** it?
   a) I don't know. I was only 8.
   b) Aspirin.
   c) I got bed rest.

13) Where **did** you **get** your medication?
   a) Drugstore.
   b) The doctor ordered it.
   c) I got it from my mom.

14) How **did** you **take** your medication?
   a) I didn't take any.
   b) The doctor ordered it.
   c) My mom crushed the pills and put them in honey for me to swallow.

15) Who **was** your caregiver at home?
   a) Nobody.
   b) My mom and my family.
   c) I didn't have a nurse.

READING EXERCISES

As with the other reading selections, the following exercises will help you zero in on the general meaning of the interview you have just read and build vocabulary.

Understanding the General Meaning

It is extremely important in health care that professionals read, write, and listen to questions and answers accurately. Serious treatment mistakes can be made when this does not occur. Answer the following questions based on the reading selection.

1) What is the general subject of the interview you have just read? _____

2) What is the purpose of an interview like the one you just read? _____

3) What is the time focus or time frame of this interview? _____

4) Whose perspective is being elicited? Who is providing the subjective report of the illness experience? _____

5) Imagine an interview like this with a 28-year-old pregnant woman. What would then be the immediate purpose of this interview? _____
_____

Building Vocabulary

The history-taking interview requires use of the past tense. It is critical that the health professional uses the correct tense for the correct time in history. To do otherwise might lead other members of the health-care team to understand the patient has these recorded symptoms right now. This will affect the type of care the patient will receive.

To build vocabulary successfully you must be aware of the different tenses of verbs. Here we present a review of the present and past tenses of some common verbs and then ask you to use them in sentences.

Review of Some Verb Tenses. Review the following tables of the present and past tenses of some common verbs. Reflect back on the interview reading to see how past tenses were used.

Table 1-1 Present and Past Tenses of the Verb "to be"	
PRESENT	PAST
I am	We were
You are	You were
He (she, it) is	He (she, it) was
We are	We were
They are	They were

Table 1-2 Present and Past Tenses of the Verb "to have"	
PRESENT	PAST
I have	I had
You have	You had
He (she, it) has	He (she, it) had
We have	We had
They have	They had

Table 1-3 Present and Past Tenses of the Verb "to do"	
PRESENT	PAST
I do	I did
You do	You did
He (she, it) does	He (she, it) did
We do	We did
They do	They did

Table 1-4 Present and Past Tenses of the Verb "to cause"	
PRESENT	PAST
I cause	I caused
You cause	you caused
He/she/it causes	He/she/it caused
We cause	We caused
They cause	They caused

Table 1-5 Present and Past Tenses of the Verb "to make"	
PRESENT	PAST
I make	I made
You make	You made
He/she/it makes	He/she/it made
We make	We made
They make	They made

Sentence Completion. Complete the following sentences using the correct form of the verb.

1) In 1979, Miriam _____ her fourth child. Then she _____ her tubes tied so she would not have any more babies.

2) Rhianna _____ 12 years old when she _____ her tonsils removed. This procedure is called a tonsillectomy.

3) When she _____ the chicken pox, she _____ a very itchy rash. She _____ to scratch all of the time but her mother _____ her to do it. She _____ want her daughter to have scars afterwards.

4) Jane's mother _____ her chicken soup when she _____ the mumps as
   a kid. It _____ too difficult for her to swallow solid food at the time.
5) The nurse _____ me get out of bed after surgery, but I _____ want to.
   I was afraid of the pain.

SPEAKING EXERCISE

Find a partner. Using the same health history interview, interview your partner about an illness
he or she had in the past. The Pronunciation Hints box below will help.

PRONUNCIATION HINTS

To understand the pronunciation guides for each of the following words, please refer to *Taber's Cyclopedic
Medical Dictionary* (F. A. Davis Company).

treatment – **trēt′mĕnt**

swallow – **swăl′ō**

tonsillectomy – **tŏn-sĭl-ĕk′tō-mē**

mumps – **mŭmps**

LISTENING EXERCISE

Listen to a friend talking about an illness he or she had when he or she was a child. He or she
may or may not be speaking in English. Listen for cues such as tone of voice to decide whether
or not this was a serious event for the person. Active listening includes the ability to perceive
meaning through attending to nonverbal behavior as well as the spoken word.

WRITING EXERCISE—REFLECTIVE WRITING

We use language to achieve different purposes. The social purpose of different types of texts is referred to as its *genre*. Telling what has happened (recounting) is a common genre. So are explaining and describing. They are useful grammatical forms when the health professionals need to talk
about the patient's situation or condition with the health-care team. You have now been introduced to the genre of the health interview for history-taking.

Jot down a few notes. Identify what has been most meaningful for you working with the interview genre.

_____

_____

_____

The Drugstore

We are still building a contextual framework for health care and the health professions. In this section there are many opportunities to learn about drugstores, pharmacists, and prescriptions. This material has value to you as an individual as well as to your patients. You will be introduced to procedures, recounting (telling), and explaining. Reading comprehension exercises focus on specificity and are grounded in safety-in-practice concepts for health professionals.

Reading Selection 1-7

Read the following in its entirety. Many words may be new to you.

DRUGSTORES AND PHARMACISTS

In the United States and Canada, prescriptions are **filled** by a pharmacist at a drugstore. In other countries the drugstore may be referred to as the chemist's or the pharmacy. Sometimes Americans and Canadians say "pharmacy," too. The drugstore sells more than simply medication. It also has merchandise for health and home care, cosmetics, greeting cards, snack foods, and various other novelties and sundries. The business focus of a drugstore is to sell health and wellness products and merchandise.

Pharmacists are highly educated professionals with university **degrees** that include clinical *practica*. The total amount of time to become a pharmacist is 6 to 8 years. A pharmacist dispenses medication ordered by a doctor; however, he or she also sells over-the-counter medication (OTC). Pharmacists are client-focused. They spend a good deal of time in communication with client, teaching and informing them about medications and their safe **usage**.

There are no drugstores in hospitals. A pharmacy is located within the hospital and the hospital pharmacists **dispense** the medications for all patients based on the written or verbal orders of a doctor. Health professionals working within the hospital often call these pharmacists for advice or clarification on medication orders.

READING EXERCISES

As you read through this text, you formed an opinion about its purpose and learned some specific terms. Let's try them now in some exercises.

Understanding the General Meaning

1) What is the goal of this text?

_____

_____

2) Take a moment to think about what you have just read. What genre do you think it portrays? Explain.

_____

_____

Building Vocabulary

As you read the text, you noticed that some words were highlighted. Write them here and define them by yourself or with the help of a teacher or peers. These words will appear again later.

When they do, check your answers. Were you right? Were you able to comprehend their meaning simply from reading the text?

_____

_____

_____

_____

Determining Meaning from the Context.   To build vocabulary, study the following words or terms taken from this text. Discover all you can about them by looking at them in context. Then, choose the correct meaning. Finally, take a look at how these words or terms expand in English.

1. Filled *(verb, past tense)*

In context:
a) I got my prescription filled at the pharmacy.
b) My tire was low, so I filled it with more air.

Meaning: The word *filled* can best be described as meaning
a) to re-supply or return to original level
b) put pressure in or on something
c) ate too much
d) the job of a pharmacist

Word expansion
a) I *was filling* the patient's prescription when the phone rang and interrupted me. (verb, past tense continuous)
b) What do you want me *to fill?* Both prescriptions? (verb, infinitive)

2. Referred to *(verb)*

In context:
a) I was referred to the pediatrician after my baby was born.
b) Miss Harris is the teacher, but she prefers to be referred to as Janine.

Meaning: The term *referred to* can best be described as
a) suggesting a new way or new opinion be gotten or used
b) looking something up in a textbook
c) asking about resources
d) none of the above

Word expansion:
a) Can I please have a *referral* to physiotherapy for treatment, Doctor? (noun)
b) I am going *to refer* you to the eye specialist, Miss Abramowski. (verb, infinitive)
c) In *reference* to your comments earlier, I would like to say that I was not involved in that activity. (idiom)

3. Degrees *(noun, plural)*

In context
a) Doctors have science and medicine degrees from a university.
b) You earn a diploma in high school and a degree in a college or university.

Meaning: In this case, *degrees* can be described as
a) temperatures
b) measurements on a scale

c) documents of achievement

d) signs of graduation

Word expansion:

a) Is he a *degreed* psychologist or simply a counselor? (slang use of noun as an adjective)

b) When did you obtain your *degree?* (noun)

c) Keep this medication at room temperature or above 32 *degrees* Fahrenheit. (noun)

4. Dispenses *(verb)*

In context:

a) The psychologist dispenses good advice.

b) The pharmacist dispenses medication and advice.

Meaning: The verb *dispenses* can best be defined as

a) gives out, passes out, or provides

b) sells

c) counts and measures

d) something only a pharmacist can do

Word expansion:

a) A *dispensing* optician is a person licensed only to prepare your eyeglass from a prescription. (adjective)

b) When *dispensing* medication, you should not be distracted. It's a safety issue. (verb, present tense continuous)

c) She *dispensed* the medication at the hospital pharmacy, but she told me I can get a refill for my prescription at my local drugstore. (verb, past tense)

5. However *(conjunctive adverb)*

In context:

a) I wanted to go to university; however, I didn't have the money.

b) I wish I could take a holiday now; however, I have to work to save money for it first.

Meaning: In this context the word *however* can best be described as

a) unfortunately

b) not possible

c) in spite of

Word expansion:

However is a conjunctive adverb and does not expand.

6. Over-the-counter *(noun phrase, adjective)*

In context:

a) Some drugs require a prescription, but others can simply be bought over-the-counter.

b) I can go to the local drugstore and buy certain medications without ever speaking to my doctor or pharmacist. These are over-the-counter medications.

Meaning: The term *over-the-counter* can best be described as meaning

a) drugs that do not require a prescription and can be bought freely in a store

b) drugs you must ask the pharmacist to pass you over his or her counter top

c) drugs that you need a prescription for

Word expansion:

a) Do you know the difference between *OTC* and controlled drugs? (abbreviation)

Sentence Completion.   Complete the following sentences to the best of your ability, expanding your use of the new vocabulary.

1) A very large company that manufactures medications is referred to as a _____ company.

2) Many people do not take their medications as _____. They miss a dose or stop taking them too soon.

3) My neighbor always buys her allergy medication _____. It doesn't require a prescription.

SPEAKING EXERCISE

Return to the Building Vocabulary exercise. Find a partner. Take turns reading each of the six main words and the "in context" sentences out loud to each other. The Pronunciation Hints box below will help.

PRONUNCIATION HINTS

To understand the pronunciation guides for each of the following words, please refer to *Taber's Cyclopedic Medical Dictionary* (F. A. Davis Company).

degrees – dĕ-**grē′**z

dispenses – dĭs-**pĕns**-ĕz

pharmacist – **făr′**mă-sĭst

pharmacy – **făr′**mă-sē

prescription – prē-**skrĭp′**shŭn

LISTENING EXERCISE

Continue to work with your partner, only this time turn your back to him or her. Listen without looking and without reading. What do you learn about yourself and your ability to understand what is being said in English?

WRITING EXERCISE

Your reading has been written in the *factual genre* and is an *information report*. Its goal is to present information about something. In this case, that something is drugstores and pharmacists. As part of their daily duties, health professionals write many information reports. Take a look at the reading again, checking its format. Compare the format of the reading to information in Box 1-4. Can you see the structure and form?

BOX 1-4 Information Reports

Structure
    A general statement is given to identify the topic.
    A description of behaviors, purposes, and location is given.
Textual features
    Information is organized into paragraphs.
    Key words are repeated throughout the paragraphs (e.g., pharmacists).
Grammatical features
    Present tense verbs are used to identify and classify the topic (e.g., is, are).
    Adjectives help build descriptions of behaviors, roles, purposes, and locations.
    Circumstances of place are included to describe the location as well as the behaviors in those locations.

Using the format and suggestions given in the box, write an information report here. (You may write just one paragraph, if you like.) Use the topic: The Emergency Department.

_____

_____

_____

_____

_____

_____

Reading Selection 1-8

Read the following dialogue aloud or silently to yourself.

FILLING A PRESCRIPTION

Customer: Hi! I've got a prescription here I'd like filled.

Pharmacist: OK, what's your name, please?

Customer: Jane Hansworth.

Pharmacist: How do you spell that?

Customer: Hansworth, H - a - n - s - w - o - r - t - h; Jane, J - a - n - e .

Pharmacist: And your home address? Phone number?

Customer: 125 Blueberry Lane, Surrey, B.C. 853-729.

Pharmacist: OK. Are you [allergic] to any medications?

Customer: Yes, penicillin.

Pharmacist: Thank you. I'll write that down on your file. Your prescription will be ready in about 5 minutes.

******

Pharmacist: Jane Hansworth? Your prescription is ready.

Customer: Here I am.

Pharmacist: OK. This is cyclobenzaprine. Have you ever taken this medication before?

Customer: No.

Pharmacist: Fine. Well, let me tell you a little bit about it. First, your doctor wants you to take one tablet; that's 10 mg of cyclobenzaprine when your back pain is really bad, but do not take more than three pills a day. Try to space them out every 4 to 6 hours or so.

Customer: OK. I hope they work. My back is killing me. I was in a car accident last week.

Pharmacist: Well, Jane, cyclobenzaprine is an excellent muscle relaxant. But because it does such a good job, you should be aware that you may feel very sleepy on it. Don't drive and don't drink any alcohol when you have taken a pill. That could make the effects even worse. You may have some trouble concentrating when you use cyclobenzaprine, so avoid working with machinery or things that use a lot of concentration, like your sewing machine or anything that might cause an accident if you're not completely alert.

Customer: Thanks, I'll remember that. But my plans are just to go home and lie on the couch and watch TV for a couple of days until my back feels better. So long!

 READING EXERCISES

Health professionals must be specific in their questions and in remembering the details of the client's answers.

Understanding the General Meaning

Multiple Choice. Your answers to the following questions will reveal your general understanding of the reading selection.

Choose the correct answer in these multiple-choice questions.

1) Who needs their prescription filled?
   a) The pharmacist.
   b) A doctor.
   c) Jane Hansworth.
   d) The chemist.

2) Who ordered a prescription medication?
   a) Jane Hansworth.
   b) A doctor.
   c) The pharmacist.
   d) The physiotherapist.

3) What kind of drug is cyclobenzaprine?
   a) A sedative.
   b) Something for fever.
   c) A muscle relaxant.
   d) An antibiotic.

4) Why is Jane taking cyclobenzaprine?
   a) She's very tired.
   b) She has back pain.
   c) She likes it.
   d) She was in a car accident.

5) How often should Jane take this medication?
   a) Only when she wants to.
   b) Only at bedtime.
   c) Once per day.
   d) At 4 to 6 hour intervals, if needed.

Interpreting the Reading

Why have these two people come together? In other words, what is the purpose of their communication?

Building Vocabulary

Determining Meaning from Context.   Try to discover the meaning of the next few words through context. Then follow the directions as they appear in these multiple-choice questions.

1. Pharmacist *(noun)*

In context:
a) The pharmacist is on duty in the drugstore.
b) The pharmacist dispenses drugs.

Meaning: A *pharmacist* is best described as
a) a job for a man
b) a department in the hospital
c) not a person, but a place
d) a university-educated specialist in pharmacology

Word expansion:
a) *Pharmacology* is the study of properties of medicines. (noun)
b) The *pharmacological* properties of D5W are dextrose and 5 parts water. (adjective)
c) The hospital *pharmacy* is open 24 hours a day. (noun)
d) Large *pharmaceutical* companies do research. (adjective)

2. Prescription *(noun)*

In context:
a) The doctor wrote a prescription for Tylenol #3 with codeine.
b) Only a pharmacist can fill a prescription.

Meaning: A *prescription* can best be described as
a) all types of medications
b) an order for a medication that only a doctor or qualified medical, dental, or nursing pro-
    fessional can order
c) as a kind of nutrient
d) the person who dispenses medication

Word expansion:
a) Doctors and some nurse practitioners have *prescriptive* powers. They can write *prescriptions*.
    (adjective; noun, plural)
b) The doctor has written a *prescription* for a muscle relaxant. (noun)
c) The doctor *prescribed* a sedative for his patient. (verb, past tense)

3. Allergic *(adjective)*

In context:

a) Joe is allergic to bee stings. One sting could kill him within 3 minutes!
b) I can take tetracycline for an antibiotic, but I am allergic to penicillin. Don't give it to me!

Meaning: The word *allergic* can best be described as
a) not preferable
b) difficult to take
c) an abnormal reaction to a substance
d) a state of fear

Word expansion:

a) Melodie has an *allergy* to lobster. It makes her throat swell shut and she has difficulty breathing. (noun)

b) Elisa had an *allergic* reaction to strawberries. She broke out in hives: little red, itchy bumps on her skin. (adjective)

c) The springtime brings many airborne *allergens*. Flowers and trees make some people sneeze and sniffle. (noun)

Mix and Match.   The exercise in Box 1-5 will help you recognize words of similar meaning—synonyms.

BOX 1-5 Mix and Match: Synonyms

Match the term on the left with the word of similar meaning—a synonym—in the right column.

WORD	WORDS OF SIMILAR MEANING OR SYNONYMS
drugstore	client
prescription	chesterfield or sofa
customer	pharmacy
cyclobenzaprine	giving me a lot of trouble or pain
druggist	pharmacist
tablet	focus
space them out	take at intervals of time
couch	doctor's order
"killing me"	muscle relaxant
sleepy	drowsy
concentrate	pill

SPEAKING EXERCISES

Read the following completed sentences aloud. Ask a peer or teacher to help you with pronunciation. Proceed to the Pronunciation Hints section following. This will also help.

Pharmacology is the study of properties of medicines.

Large pharmaceutical companies do research.

I can take tetracycline for an antibiotic, but I am allergic to penicillin. Don't give it to me.

PRONUNCIATION HINTS

To understand the pronunciation guides for each of the following words, please refer to *Taber's Cyclopedic Medical Dictionary* (F. A. Davis Company).

pharmacology – făr"mă-**kŏl**'ō-jē

pharmaceutical – făr-mă-**sū**'tĭ-kăl

tetracycline – tĕt"ră-**sī**'klēn

antibiotic – ăn"tĭ-bī-**ŏt**'ĭk

allergic – ă-**lĕr**'jĭk

LISTENING EXERCISE

Make an audio recording of the dialogue. Then listen back to it without following along with the written script. Identify where and when you hesitated or stumbled on words. Go back and review them. Practice saying them aloud.

WRITING EXERCISE—EXPLANATORY WRITING

Study Box 1-6 and then proceed through the questions to learn more about how to write in this genre.

1) In the dialogue, Jane has a social purpose: she wants the pharmacist to do and to understand something. She uses the genres of explaining and recounting. So now, in your own words, briefly tell us what happened in this dialogue. (Approximately 50 words)

_____

_____

_____

_____

2) The pharmacist in this dialogue uses the genres of explanation and procedure. In a few words or less, identify these.

_____

_____

_____

3) In your own words, provide an explanation for why you personally might go to a drugstore.

_____

4) In your own words, tell the procedure for taking a tablet. Be specific and identify all the steps in the procedure.

5) Jane is using language to achieve a particular purpose. What is that purpose?

6) Jane explains something to the pharmacist.
   a) What does she explain?

   b) Why does she explain it?

Reading Selection 1-9

We are now going to expand our language usage to that of reading and writing prescriptions. Read the following aloud or silently to yourself.

WRITING A MEDICATION ORDER

The proper form for writing a medication order or a prescription is shown in Box 1-7.

These are actually steps in the process of writing the order. We could look at it this way:

Step 1: Identify the drug by name.
Step 2: Identify the prescribed amount of the drug to be taken or used.
Step 3: Identify the route by which it is to be given. For example, it might be given by mouth (orally), spray, drops, injection, or ointment.
Step 4: Identify the frequency of administration. For example, how many times per day or per hour will this drug be taken?

Here is an example:
   You want to give the antibiotic ampicillin 250 milligrams by mouth four times per day.

BOX 1-7 Content of a Prescription

Drug → amount → route → frequency or time

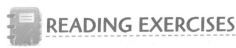

READING EXERCISES

The following exercises will help you in understanding and being able to write prescriptions.

Understanding the General Meaning

In your own words, what have you just read? If you have understood the reading correctly, you will be able to write the steps of the medication order procedure here. Do so now.

BUILDING VOCABULARY

Completing Prescription Orders Using the Steps in the Process.   Complete the following prescription orders by placing them in the correct order. Review the steps given above before beginning. You will need to add some of your own words to make the prescription order clear to the reader.

1) bedtime each night   sedative medication   mouth   10 milligrams

2) lunch   insulin   before   injection   every day   10 units

3) mornings   anti-arrhythmia   50 milligrams   mouth

4) ointment   twice daily   over affected area   5 milligrams   Itchaway

5) Seeclear   drops   right eye   2 three times per day

SPEAKING EXERCISE

Refer to the previous exercise. Try to read each and every prescription order without stopping and without hesitating. This is generally quite difficult for students of non-English speaking backgrounds. Rest assured—it gets better and easier the more you practice. The Pronunciation Hints box below will help.

PRONUNCIATION HINTS

To understand the pronunciation guides for each of the following words, please refer to *Taber's Cyclopedic Medical Dictionary* (F. A. Davis Company).

sedative – **sĕd'**ă-tĭv

injection – ĭn-**jĕk'**shŭn

milligrams – **mĭl'**ĭ-grăm'z

arrhythmia – ă-**rĭth'mē**-ă

ointment – **oynt'**mĕnt

LISTENING EXERCISE

Listen to a partner say these medication orders (prescription orders) to you. Pretend you are listening to the doctor give orders by telephone. Can you understand what the person is saying? What did you learn from this exercise?

WRITING EXERCISE—REFLECTIVE WRITING

In bulleted format, identify the most salient or most important elements of this section. What really stands out as interesting in the context of your profession or in the content of this section?

_____

_____

_____

SECTION FOUR Calling the Doctor's Office

In this final section of Unit 1 we explore how language is used in the context of a patient phoning the doctor's office to make an appointment. In the context of an injury, vocabulary focuses on naming signs and symptoms, inquiry, and assessment. Health professionals working in clinics will appreciate the need for this type of initial screening by a medical office assistant (MOA) or nurse prior to having the patient come in for an appointment with a doctor. An introduction to equipment and treatment modalities is briefly introduced to build language repertoire.

Reading Selection 1–10

Read the following dialogue aloud or silently to yourself. Work with a partner if possible.

PHONE CALL TO A DOCTOR'S OFFICE

Scene: The phone rings at the doctor's office. The medical office assistant (MOA) answers.

MOA: Doctor Smith's office.

Patient: Yeah, hello. Can I talk to the doctor, please? I think I've got an infected foot.

MOA: Well, Dr. Smith is tied up with a patient right now. Maybe I can help you. What seems to be the problem?

Patient: Well . . . I stepped on a nail. And now the spot is all green and oozing pus or something.

MOA: When did you do this?

Patient: Oh, about 3 days ago. I cleaned it right away but . . . gee . . . it's looking pretty bad now. And, it's sore. Sometimes it even throbs.

MOA: Yes, I see. Maybe you should come in to see the doctor. Let me check for an opening today.

Patient: Thanks.

MOA: OK. Dr. Smith can see you at 2:30 this afternoon. Will that work for you?

Patient: 2:30 . . . Let me think a minute. I'll need to get a ride. . . . Yes . . . OK, I'll be there at 2:30. I can make it.

MOA: All right. May I have your name please?

Patient: Yes. It's Melinda Jugaru. M-e-l-i-n-d-a J-u-g-a-r-u.

MOA: Thank you. We'll see you then at 2:30 this afternoon, Melinda. Do you know our address?

Patient: You're on the corner of 108th Avenue and 152nd Street, aren't you?

MOA: Yes, that's right. You can't miss us.

Patient: Thank you. Bye.

MOA: Good-bye.

READING EXERCISES

It is important to not only understand the general meaning of a reading selection (or conversation) but also to understand—and remember—the specifics, which can be very important when assessing and treating a patient. (Remember: in a previous reading selection, the patient told the interviewer she was allergic to penicillin; that is an example of a specific detail that is very important, influencing treatment decisions.)

Understanding the General Meaning

Very generally, explain what this dialogue is about. What is the main theme or topic?

_____

Understanding Specifics

Based on the dialogue, complete the following short answer questions. You do not need to make full sentences. You must be very specific.

1) Melinda has an injury. What is it? _____
2) What is the patient's problem today? _____
3) Who is the patient calling? _____
4) What does the patient want? _____
5) What does the patient get? _____
6) When will Melinda see the doctor? _____
7) What does the patient think is wrong with her? _____
8) How long has the patient had this injury? _____
9) What are the signs and symptoms here? _____
10) Based on your own professional knowledge, what treatment will Melinda likely receive from the doctor? _____
11) Where is the location of the injury? _____
12) Did you notice the MOA did not say "Hello" or "Good Morning"? Do you think this is proper etiquette or proper behavior for a health professional? Explain.

_____

_____

Building Vocabulary

All of the exercises given below—determining meaning from general context, mix and match exercises, and multiple-choice exercises—will help you expand your vocabulary.

Determining the Meaning from the Context.   Review the following words taken from the dialogue. Identify the meaning based on the examples from that reading and from the "in context" sentences herein.

1. Infected *(verb, past tense)*

In context:
a) The wound is infected. It has a green, foul-smelling discharge.
b) Keep that wound clean. You don't want it to get infected.

Meaning: The verb *infected* can best be described as meaning
a) dirty
b) contaminated with disease-producing matter
c) diseased

Word expansion:
a) An *infection* can be spread by poor hand-washing practices. (noun)
b) Every year, influenza *infects* thousands of people. (verb, present tense)
c) Nurses, laboratory technicians, and doctors must be cautious around *infectious* materials if they don't want to spread them to other people. (adjective)

2. Sore *(adjective)*

In context:
a) I stubbed my little toe on the chair. Now it is really sore!
b) My tongue is sore. I bit it. Ouch!

Meaning: The word *sore* can best be described as
a) redness and swelling
b) swollen
c) causing low level pain

Word expansion:
a) I can feel some *soreness* in my muscles today. It's probably because I ran a marathon yesterday. (noun)
b) Can you please look at this *sore* on my arm? Is it infected? (noun)

3. Throbs *(verb, singular)*

In context:
a) I am in love. Every time I see my boyfriend, my heart throbs!
b) When Mary gets a migraine, she says her head throbs.

Meaning: The verb *throbs* means
a) bangs
b) stops
c) pulses or pulsates

Word expansion:
a) The *throbbing* in my big toe is a result of the blood rushing to it. I stubbed it on the chair. (noun, gerund)

4. Nail *(noun)*

In context:
a) A carpenter uses a nail and a hammer.
b) A nail is made of iron.

Meaning: The word *nail* can best be described as
a) to hit
b) a pointed piece of manufactured metal used to connect materials
c) the hardened area at your fingertips

Word expansion:

a) In the emergency room, it is possible to see a patient who has been *nailed* by a pneumatic hammer at his construction site. This is very serious. (verb, past tense)

b) When *nailing* two pieces of wood together, you will need a hammer. (verb, present continuous)

5. Pus *(noun)*

In context:

a) There is pus coming out of that wound.

b) If you squeeze a boil, pus will pop out.

Meaning: The word **pus** can best be defined as

a) a fluid-like substance that contains dead cells, tissue, and leukocytes

b) to press against or move forward

c) contaminant fluid discharge that signifies infection

Word expansion:

a) She had a *pustular* lesion on her arm. (adjective)

Multiple Choice.   Complete the following multiple-choice questions. The answers will help confirm that you have understood the terms. You will also find new ways to use the words or to describe them.

1) In this story, a *nail* refers to
   a) part of your finger tip.
   b) slow movement.
   c) a sharp metal object used for connecting pieces of wood.

2) The proper way to explain *oozing* is to say
   a) discharging.
   b) leaking.
   c) spotting.

3) The better term for *pus* is
   a) drainage.
   b) gangrene.
   c) purulent discharge.

4) The term *gee* is often heard at the beginning of a sentence, or alone.
   Gee is
   a) an exclamation or expression of surprise or wonder.
   b) an abbreviation for Jesus.
   c) a word that doesn't mean anything.

5) "An opening today" simply means
   a) there is an available time to see you today.
   b) the door is open.
   c) the clinic is open.

6) Another way to say your throat is *sore* is to say that it
   a) is infected.
   b) is red and swollen.
   c) hurts.

7) Sometimes you need to "get a ride" home from work.
   This means
   a) you must ask someone to provide transportation for you.
   b) you must take the subway.
   c) you must hitchhike.

8) People who suffer bad headaches often say their head *throbs*.
   This means
   a) they can't concentrate.
   b) they can feel and hear a pulsing sensation in their heads.
   c) there is drumming in their heads.

9) When I walk, I *step*.
   This means
   a) I touch the ground.
   b) I run.
   c) the action of a leg in walking or running where the foot is going up or down.

10) Another way of saying you need *help* is to say you need
    a) a tutor.
    b) a prescription.
    c) assistance.

11) When assessing an injury, you must find the *spot* on the body where it occurred.
    In this context, the word *spot* means
    a) location or site.
    b) discoloration.
    c) area.

Mix and Match.   The exercise in Box 1-8 will help you become familiar with some expressions commonly used in day-to-day health-care settings.

BOX 1-8 Mix and Match: Commonly Used Expressions

Find the meaning for the following words. Draw a line from column 1 to column 2.

COLUMN 1	COLUMN 2
tied up	get a ride there
right away	busy
pretty bad	will that work for you?
is that possible?	not good
an opening	an available time
find someone to drive me there	immediately

Sentence Completion Exercise. Take a look at the following graphics. They are pictures of equipment a person might use when he or she has a musculoskeletal injury or condition that affects the musculoskeletal system. Can you name them in English?

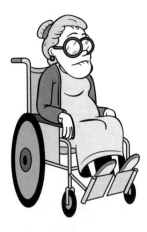

1) This patient is using a _____.
   a) bike
   b) stretcher
   c) scooter
   d) wheelchair

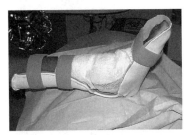

2) This patient should not put weight on his ankle. He is wearing a _____.
   a) cast
   b) cane
   c) protection
   d) splint

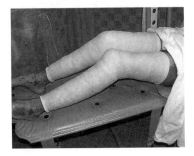

3) This patient broke his legs. He needs to wear a _____.
   a) pair of pants
   b) shorts
   c) cast.
   d) cane

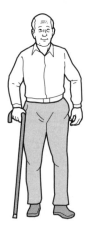

4) This patient walks with a limp. He needs a _____ for balance.
   a) cast
   b) splint
   c) walker
   d) cane

Introduction to American and Canadian Health Care and Cultural Concepts of Health and Wellness

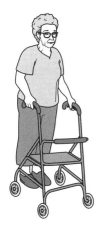

5) Sometimes when you get older you need help walking. This equipment is called a _____.
   a) cane
   b) support
   c) walker
   d) aid

SPEAKING EXERCISE

Read the completed sentences above aloud. Ask a peer or teacher to help you with pronunciation. Proceed to the Pronunciation Hints section following. This will also help.

PRONUNCIATION HINTS

To understand the pronunciation guides for each of the following words, please refer to *Taber's Cyclopedic Medical Dictionary* (F. A. Davis Company).

musculoskeletal – mŭs′kū-lō-**skĕl**′ĕ-tăl

splint – **splĭnt**

stretcher – **strĕch**′er

LISTENING EXERCISE

Continue to work on your listening skills. Ask a partner to read a role in the dialogue. Sit with your back to him or her and try to not read along.

WRITING EXERCISE—REFLECTIVE WRITING

Answer the following questions. Take a few moments to write these down. Complete this exercise and share with a co-student, a teacher, or a health-care colleague. Enter into a discussion. Practice your new English.

1) List some common antibiotics. _____

2) How are antibiotics administered? _____

3) Does Melinda's foot wound need to be covered? _____

_____

4) This patient may require a very special stat treatment. What might that be? _____

5) Why might she need this special treatment? _____

_____

ANSWER KEY

Concepts of Health and Wellness

 READING SELECTION 1—PERSPECTIVES ON HEALTH CARE IN THE NEW MILLENNIUM

Understanding the General Meaning

There have been changes in the way people think about health and health care. We are now more concerned with promoting health and wellness to prevent illness and disease rather than focusing on treatment and cure only.

Building Vocabulary

Multiple Choice

1) a, 2) d, 3) a, 4) b, 5) b, 6) b, 7) c, 8) a, 9) b, 10) d

Using New Words in Sentences. The following are examples of sentences you may have constructed.

1) Bob has an addictive lifestyle.

2) Modern nurses collaborate with doctors; they are not submissive to them.

3) Health promotion is a focus of care.

4) The patient is overweight from excessive eating.

5) Some youth are unhealthy due to inactive lifestyles.

6) Political decisions often affect the delivery of health care and health services.

Writing Exercise

Dr. Banting and Dr. Best collaborated to find a cure for the disease of diabetes. They are famous for finding a treatment.

 READING SELECTION 2—HEALTH IS A STATE OF OPTIMAL WELL-BEING

Understanding the General Meaning

Examples of answers. Please check to see that you have understood what you have read, in general.

1) Main point: Health is about how well you, personally, think you are. This includes how you think and feel about your body, your mind, your spirit, and the environment you live in.

2) Academic language note: The language in this reading is quite academic and very commonly used by health professionals in formal writings.

Building Vocabulary

Mix and Match

BOX 1-1	Mix and Match: Answers
TERM OR PHRASE	**EXPLANATION**
optimal well-being	personal sense of wellness
physical well-being	physical fitness; a healthy, active body
mental well-being	emotional stability; free from mental or emotional disturbance
social resources	the ability to feel comfortable among other people; social ease and skills
to satisfy needs	the ability to accomplish what must be done to survive and grow
aspirations	dreams and goals
environment	physical/emotional surroundings

Sentence Completion

1) Subjective means that this is someone's very personal opinion and may not be a scientific fact. It is Frederica's personal opinion.

2) Objectively means that personal opinion is not considered. In this case it means there is scientific evidence or proof that determines a conclusion.

3) Medically, physical fitness means the ability of the body to function at its most optimal level.

Multiple Choice

1) d, 2) a, 3) b, 4) c, 5) a, 6) a

Professional Caring

 READING SELECTION 3—PROFESSIONAL CARING

Understanding the General Meaning

1) Caring is the core component of all health care and has a very broad definition.

2) Some other health professions that include the four responsibilities described for nurses—namely, preventing illness, restoring health, alleviating suffering, and promoting health—include physiotherapists, respiratory therapists, medical doctors, and many others. These four responsibilities are common philosophical foundations of most, if not all, of the health professions.

Building Vocabulary

Multiple Choice

1) b, 2) b, 3) c, 4) a, 5) a, 6) c, 7) a

Using New Words in Sentences.   The following are examples of sentences you may have constructed.

1) Doctors are expected to demonstrate a high level of competency in patient care.

2) Some people face the daily challenge of living with epilepsy.

3) Legally and morally, all health professionals have standards of care they must follow.

 # READING SELECTION 4—HOLISTIC CARE

Understanding the General Meaning

Holistic health is a way of thinking about health that includes all aspects of it: biological health, psychological health, sociological health, spiritual health, and environmental health.

Building Vocabulary

Mix and Match

BOX 1-2 Mix and Match: Answers

COLUMN 1	COLUMN 2
community relationships	social connections
lived experience	unique, personal experiences that lead to unique actions, beliefs, and lifestyles
philosophy	a sum of personal beliefs
outcomes	results
isolation	alone/separated from others
general practitioner	family doctor
essential	necessary or very important
dependent	reliant upon
initial	first; taking the lead
holistic	all aspects; sum of all parts

Explaining the Meaning of Words

1) These health professionals believe that building and maintaining an interpersonal relationship with a patient is very important to providing good care.

2) In this context, rapport means a relationship of mutual understanding, trust, and willingness to work together for someone's health.

3) In this context, underpinning means the foundation or basis.

4) Morally refers to what is personally ethical or accepted as right or wrong. Morals can be subjective or objective. They can be personal or professional. Morals can be part of individual, family, group, community, or cultural beliefs.

READING SELECTION 5—HEALTH-CARE PROFESSIONALS: MEMBERS OF THE HEALTH-CARE TEAM

Understanding the General Meaning

1) b - false, 2) b - false, 3) b - false, 4) b - false, 5) a - true

Interpreting the Reading

The core message of this reading is that health care is provided by a team made up of many types of professionals who all have the same goal of helping the patient achieve wellness.

Building Vocabulary

Sentence Completion

1) physicians

2) physiotherapy

3) registered psychiatric nurse

4) respiratory therapist

5) registered nurses or licensed practical nurses/nurses or care team

6) license

Mix and Match

BOX 1-3	Mix and Match: Abbreviations for Members of the Health-Care Team: Answers
OT	occupational therapist: promotes health and wellness through occupation and purposeful activity
RN	registered nurse: a person who practices professional nursing; may or may not be specialized.
MD	medical doctor
SW	social worker: concerned with patient's living arrangements, finances, and personal support networks
RT	respiratory therapist concerned with patient airway and their function OR a recreation therapist concerned with patient activity and quality of life
RPN	registered psychiatric nurse: a person who practices professional nursing; specialized in mental health and addictions care
LPN	licensed practical nurse: subordinate to RNs and RPNs yet fully qualified within own scope of practice and licensing to provide certain patient care
PT	physiotherapist: concerned with patient's movement and function
GP	general practitioner: a physician with a general focus, most often seen as the family doctor

Answering the Interview Questions

To complete the interview, you must have kept in the role of yourself to provide subjective data. If you answered from your mother's point of view, you have not used your own opinion. When health professionals interview a client/patient, it is essential *not* to put our own words and values into the mouths of the clients.

1) **a**

   Rationale: This question uses the verb *think*. You must reply using that verb in its proper form.

2) **b**

   Rationale: This question uses the verb *think*. You must reply using that verb in its proper form.

3) **b**

   Rationale: This question leads you to the answer by asking YOU how you came to the conclusion you were sick.

4) **c**

   Rationale: You are being asked to describe what happened to your body.

5) **a**

   Rationale: Measles are highly contagious. The Public Health Department does not allow anyone with the measles to go to school.

6) **c**

   Rationale: Once again, you are being asked for your subjective opinion about your experience in the past.

7) **c**

   Rationale: At 8 years of age, you would not have thought about medications. It is likely you would have felt physically unwell and emotionally sorry for yourself. To cheer yourself up, you might have wanted special foods and privileges. Once again, to answer this question successfully you need to think of yourself at this young age.

8) **a**

   Rationale: At 8 years old you were able to understand what the treatment from mother was.

9) **a**

   Rationale: This is the only treatment for measles. The question begins with the word "did" and requires a yes or no answer.

10) **a**

    Rationale: This is a two-part question and requires a two-part answer.

11) **a**

    Rationale: The question asks "what was the treatment," not name the treatment. The answer, then, must say what you did. Again, this is a two-part question that requires a two-part answer.

12) **a**

    Rationale: At 8 years old it is very, very unlikely you knew whether or not you had a prescription. Subjectively, you probably didn't know.

13) **c**

    Rationale: Subjectively, at 8 years old, you would have gotten this medication from your mom. You are not being asked where she got it from. Medical English requires absolute specificity in listening to, understanding, and responding to questions. This is just a practice example of how this is so.

14) **c**
Rationale: This is often common with children's medication if there is no liquid form available.

15) **b**
Rationale: Your mother or family member in the home would most likely have been the one who took care of you during your experience with the measles.

Understanding the General Meaning

1) The subject of the interview is your own (the reader's) personal, subjective recount of your experience with the measles when you were a child. Recounting means recalling and telling a story or experience.

2) The purpose of the interview is to inquire about your (the reader's) past experience with an illness. This information will be important to a patient's clinical record and forms part of the health history component of any hospital admission or intake interview.

3) The time frame for this interview is the past: the childhood of the person being interviewed (the interviewee).

4) The interviewee is answering question from her perspective and is providing subjective data.

5) The purpose is to identify or listen for the word "measles." Rationale: Any health professional who hears this word come from a pregnant patient would immediately explore the situation further to find out which kind of measles she has had, if there were any lasting effects from the illness, and/or if the person has ever been immunized against any type of measles since then. It is absolutely a safe practice measure required of all health professionals. We cannot be sure that the general public can differentiate between one type of measles and the other. We must listen carefully and follow through.

Building Vocabulary

Sentence Completion

1) had, had

2) was, had

3) got, had, wanted, forbade, didn't

4) gave or fed, had, was

5) made, didn't

The Drugstore

 READING SELECTION 7–DRUGSTORES AND PHARMACISTS

Understanding the General Meaning

1) The social purpose or goal of this reading is to inform the reader about drugstores and pharmacists. It also identifies the relationships between the two.

2) This reading portrays the factual genre. It is an information report.

Building Vocabulary

Multiple Choice

1) a, 2) a, 3) c, 4) a, 5) a, 6) a

Sentence Completion

1) pharmaceutical

2) prescribed

3) over-the-counter

 WRITING EXERCISE

An example of writing in an information report about the Emergency Department is given below:

> Sometimes when you are sick or injured, you go to the Emergency Department at the hospital. This is a place where ambulances police and families bring patients who need immediate treatment. If you just have a cold or sore stomach, you don't go to the Emergency Department. It's a very busy place.
>
> The medical team working in "emergency" consists of doctors, nurses, laboratory technicians, and care aides. They are caring and very efficient. They all help assess the patient and then the doctor makes the final diagnosis. Most often, the team treats the patient and then the patient is discharged to his or her home. Sometimes, the patient is transferred to another unit of the hospital to stay.
>
> Here in Box 1-4 Answers is the same report with the key features important for a factual genre information report (as shown in Box 1-4 in the text) identified.

BOX 1-4 Features of an Information Report Applied

1) Structure
  a) General statement to identify the topic
    Example: *Sometimes when you are sick or injured, you go to the Emergency Department at the hospital.*
  b) Description of purpose
    Example: *This is a place where ambulances and police and families bring patients who need immediate treatment.*

2) Textual features
  a) Information is organized into paragraphs
  b) Key words are repeated throughout the paragraphs
    Example: *emergency department, patient, hospital, team*

3) Grammatical features
  a) Present tense verbs are used to identify and classify the topic
    Example: *go, bring, are, treat*
  b) Adjectives help build descriptions
    Example: *immediate, final*
  c) Circumstances of place describe the location and behaviors in those locations
    Example: *where, this is a place, when you, if you just have . . . don't go, working in . . .*√

READING SELECTION 8—FILLING A PRESCRIPTION

Understanding the General Meaning

1) c, 2) b, 3) c, 4) b, 5) d

Interpreting the Reading

Simply, the dialogue is about someone who wants something from another person. They communicate for that purpose.

Building Vocabulary

Multiple Choice

1) d, 2) b, 3) c

Mix and Match

BOX 1–5 Mix and Match: Synonyms: Answers	
WORD	WORDS OF SIMILAR MEANING OR SYNONYMS
drugstore	pharmacy
prescription	doctor's order
customer	client
cyclobenzaprine	muscle relaxant
druggist	pharmacist
tablet	pill
space them out	take at intervals of time
couch	chesterfield or sofa
"killing me"	giving me a lot of trouble or pain
sleepy	drowsy
concentrate	focus

 WRITING EXERCISES

1) Jane's primary social purpose for going to the pharmacist is to get her prescription filled. She wants him to do this for her.

2) Explanation: the pharmacist explains the purpose of the drug and what type of medication it is.
Procedure: the pharmacist teaches the client the proper procedure for taking the medication safely.

3) Personal response. It might be something like: "I had a prescription for an antibiotic from my doctor to be filled, and I also wanted to buy over-the-counter aspirin."

4) I should take the pill when my back pain is really bad, but not less than 4 hours apart, and I should not take more than a total of three pills each day. I should not drink alcohol while taking the pill and I should not do anything like driving or working with machinery since the pill may make me sleepy.

5) Her purpose is to get her prescription filled so she can have some pain relief.

6) a) She explains her need for pain relief.
   b) She explains it to reinforce her need for the medication. This is not necessary because she already has a prescription from the doctor. However, many customers wish to discuss their circumstances with the pharmacist. In that way, the pharmacist can provide any additional teaching or medication-related advice that is appropriate.

 ## READING SELECTION 9—WRITING A MEDICATION ORDER

Understanding the General Meaning

I have just read about the process of writing a medication order in an abbreviated form.

Building Vocabulary

1) Sedative medication 10 milligrams by mouth each night at bedtime.

2) Insulin 10 units by injection every day before lunch.

3) Anti-arrhythmia 50 milligrams by mouth, mornings. This can also be written as anti-arrhythmia 50 milligrams by mouth each morning.

4) Itchaway ointment 5 milligrams twice daily over affected area (of skin).

5) Seeclear 2 drops three times per day to the right eye.

Calling the Doctor's Office

 ## READING SELECTION 10—PHONE CALL TO A DOCTOR'S OFFICE

Understanding the General Meaning

The lady wants to have her injury assessed and treated.

Understanding Specifics

1) She stepped on a nail.
   Rationale: Stepping on the nail is the injury. Her medical condition is that this wound is infected. So, the correct answer is that she stepped on a nail.

2) She has a wound that is not healing.
   Rationale: She describes an injury and her current signs and symptoms. She describes the status of the wound. It is not healing and she is aware of this although she does not say so, specifically.

3) She is calling the doctor.
   Rationale: Think carefully here. Who does Melinda ask to speak to? Who does she want to get advice from first and foremost? The doctor, not the medical office assistant.

4) She wants to talk to the doctor.
   Rationale: As previously noted, she is calling the doctor and asks for him/her. This is the first thing she wants in the dialogue.

5) She gets to speak to the MOA and she gets an appointment with the doctor. She did NOT get to speak with the doctor on the phone.

6) She will see the doctor at 2:30 this afternoon.

7) She thinks her foot is infected.
Rationale: You are being asked what Melinda thinks is her problem. This requires a "subjective report" from the patient, Melinda. It is always possible her foot is not infected. After all, she has not yet been seen by a doctor. It may be that she has a piece of glass, dirt, or debris in her foot as well as developing an infection.

8) She's had the injury for approximately 3 days.

9) The wound is green, oozing, throbs, and is sore. Note: Melinda is describing the signs and symptoms of an infected wound.

10) The doctor will cleanse and cover the wound, write her a prescription for an antibiotic, and possibly give her a tetanus shot because she stepped on a rusty nail.

11) It is on the sole of her foot.

12) Yes, it is true. The MOA didn't greet the caller. Although this may not sound polite at first, it is acceptable to answer a telephone in a health facility by first identifying it by name. It would be quite acceptable to say "hello" or "good morning" following that.

Building Vocabulary

Determining Meaning from Context

1) b, 2) c, 3) c, 4) b, 5) c

Multiple Choice

1) c, 2) a, 3) c, 4) a, 5) a, 6) c, 7) a, 8) b, 9) c, 10) c, 11) a

Mix and Match

BOX 1-8 Mix and Match: Commonly Used Expressions: Answers

COLUMN 1	COLUMN 2
tied up	busy
right away	immediately
pretty bad	not good
is that possible?	will that work for you?
an opening	an available time
find someone to drive me there	get a ride there

Sentence Completion

1) d, 2) d, 3) c, 4) d, 5) c

 ## WRITING EXERCISES

Some suggested answers follow.

1) Some common antibiotics are penicillins, tetracycline, sulfa drugs, and Keflex.

2) Antibiotics may be administered by mouth (p.o.), by intravenous (IV) or intramuscular (IM) injection, and sometimes in a cream or ointment applied to the skin.

3) Yes, she needs to cover it now that it is infected. However, current practices in wound care show that keeping a wound open/uncovered is actually beneficial to healing. In this case, Melinda must get back to her home. To do so, she must cover her wound. Once at home, she may be able to uncover it and leave it open. Proper medical terminology would be to say she needs to cover the wound with a clean dressing. It does not have to be sterile.

4) She is likely to receive a tetanus shot to prevent tetanus. However, this will depend on whether she has had one previously and when this occurred.

5) She stepped on a dirty, rusty, contaminated piece of metal. The soil provides a good reservoir for tetanus and the nail provides a mode of transmission.

UNIT 2

Throughout the three sections of Unit 2 there are multiple opportunities to acquire vocabulary, learn grammar, and practice communication skills in the context of discussion about the musculoskeletal system. The unit progresses from a review of basic anatomy and physiology to identifying, naming, and describing body movements, posture, gait, ambulation, and position. Next, there is an introduction to the language of diagnostics and assessments related to bones and bone fractures. Finally, you will be introduced to dialogue and interview styles that require use of the targeted language. Remember, Unit 2 builds upon Unit 1. Expect to see that continuation throughout the book.

SECTION ONE Anatomy and Physiology

This section introduces the language of body systems. It starts with a brief introduction to terms used to describe the anatomy and physiology of the human body on the level of the cell, body cavities, body systems, and the whole organism. It then explores the human skeleton and muscles. Opportunities to build language skills include labeling, explaining, telling, and describing.

Reading Selection 2-1

Read the following in its entirety. Many words may be new to you. The exercises that follow will help teach their meaning.

ORGANIZATION OF THE BODY

The body is organized into cells, tissues, organs, and systems. A cell is an aggregate (a collection) of protoplasm: organic material and fluid. It contains a nucleus or nuclear material. A cell is the smallest unit of life for all plants and animals. Groups, or aggregates, of similar cells acting together to perform specific functions make up tissues. Primary tissues in the body are the epithelial, connective, skeletal, muscular, and nervous tissues. Organs are parts of the body that have specific functions. They are made up of specific types of tissues. Some organs like the lungs and kidneys are in pairs, but for the most part, organs are single entities. They are organized into body systems. Some examples of organ systems are the cardiovascular system, the musculoskeletal system, and the digestive system.

 ## READING EXERCISES

The following exercises will help you understand the general meaning of what you have just read as well as build vocabulary.

Understanding the General Meaning

Read the text again. Think about it. Do you understand it? What is the general meaning of the text? What is its focus?

_____

_____

Building Vocabulary

Take a moment now to review what you have just read. Have you noticed a lot of scientific or technical language? Write those words down here and then proceed through the exercises to discover their meaning. If you do not find all of the words that challenge you in the exercises, please refer to your dictionary before beginning the next section.

_____

_____

_____

Determining Meaning from Context. Discover all you can about these words by looking at them in context. Choose the correct meaning. Finally, take a look at how these words or terms expand in English—for example, how a noun like **function** can be expanded to an adjective—**functional,** to another noun—**functionary,** to a verb—**function,** and still yet to another adjective—**dysfunctional** (by adding the prefix _dys_ [not]).

1. Cavities _(noun, plural)_

In context:
a) I have to go to the dentist. I have a couple of cavities in my teeth.
b) The intestines are located in the abdominal cavity.

Meaning: The word _cavity_ can best be described as meaning
a) painful
b) old
c) rotten
d) a hollow space

Word expansion:
a) The abdominal _cavity_ is also known as the cavum abdominis (noun).
b) The process of forming a cavity is known as _cavitation._ (noun)
c) The structure started _to cave_ in. (verb, infinitive)

2. Functions _(noun, plural)_

In context:
a) How many functions does your computer keyboard have?
b) My function as a nurse is to care for people and help them achieve a positive state of well-being.

Meaning: _Function_ can best be described as meaning
a) job or responsibility; duty or performance
b) utilization
c) mechanical technique
d) useful

Word expansion:
a) Replacing the patient's right hip has returned her ability _to function_ independently. (verb, infinitive)

b) I'm sorry. I'm not *functioning* very well today. I have not had enough sleep this week. (verb, present continuous)

c) Dr. Anderson is the *functionary* here. He is the Chief Executive Officer of the hospital: an official. (noun)

d) This equipment is *dysfunctional.* Please have it repaired. (adjective)

3. Primary *(adjective)*

In context:

a) The primary focus of care for a fractured bone is to set it.

b) Primary care requires the nurse to take direct responsibility for all care for each assigned patient only.

Meaning: The word *primary* can best be described as

a) first in time or order

b) last in time or order

c) not very important

Word expansion:

a) The treatment team is *primarily* concerned with the patient's emotional health rather than physical health. (adverb)

b) *Primary* care occurs when the patient makes his or her first contact with the health-care system. (adjective)

c) A *primary* hemorrhage occurs at the time of the injury. (adjective)

d) People are said to be in their *prime* at their period of greatest health and strength. (noun)

4. Epithelial *(adjective)*

In context:

a) The epithelium is made up of epithelial cells.

b) Epithelial cells are irregular in shape and have a single nucleus.

Meaning: The word *epithelial* can best be described as

a) a Latin term for skin

b) a description of the makeup of epithelium

c) carcinoma

d) none of the above

Word expansion:

a) *Epithelial* tissue forms the outer surface of the body and lines the body cavities, tubes, and passageways that lead to the exterior of the body. (adjective)

b) A malignant tumor consisting of epithelial cells is known as an *epithelioma.* (noun)

c) The skin is composed of a layer of epithelial cells called *epithelium.* (noun)

5. Connective *(adjective)*

In context:

a) Things that connect or bind together and provide support are connective.

b) Connective tissues are the most abundant of all tissue types in the body.

Meaning:

The description of *connective* can best be explained as meaning

a) joining or associating

b) being similar and matching

c) passing an electrical impulse or wave

d) all of the above

Word expansion:

a) *Connective* tissue consists of just a relatively few cells, but it contains a great deal of intra-cellular substance. (adjective)

Mix and Match.   To test your knowledge of English, see if you can draw meaning from the examples provided in this exercise. Use the following three mix-and-match exercises in Boxes 2-1, 2-2, and 2-3 to help you. Work with a partner, if you like.

BOX 2-1 Mix and Match: Types of Tissues

Draw a line from the type of cell to its function.

TYPE OF CELL	FUNCTION
epithelial	stretches, contracts, and allows movement
connective	receives and carries impulses to and from the brain
muscle	external/inner surface of body skin and membranes
nerve	anchors, connects, and supports other tissues, tendons, ligaments; highly vascular

BOX 2-2 Mix and Match: Body Cavities

Draw a line from the body cavity to the organs it contains.

CAVITY	ORGANS
abdominal cavity	bowels, reproductive organs
thoracic cavity	brain
cranial cavity	heart, lungs
oral cavity	tongue
pelvic cavity	intestines, liver, stomach, kidneys

BOX 2-3 Mix and Match: Common Names for Body Cavities

Draw a line from the anatomical term for a body cavity to its common term.

ANATOMICAL TERM	COMMON NAME
abdominal cavity	pelvis
thoracic cavity	belly
cranial cavity	chest
oral cavity	head
pelvic cavity	mouth

PRONUNCIATION HINTS

thoracic – thō-**răs'ĭ**k

cranial – **krā'**nē-ăl

abdominal – ăb-**dŏm'ĭ**-năl

cavity – **kăv'ĭ**-tē

epithelia – ĕp"ĭ-**thē'**lē-ă

The Musculoskeletal System

SPEAKING EXERCISE

Return to the three mix-and-match exercises. Practice reading your answers aloud in complete sentences. First, use the verb *contain*. Then, do the same exercise, but substitute the verb *consists of*. Follow this example. The Pronunciation Hints box will help.

The abdominal cavity contains the stomach and intestines.

LISTENING EXERCISE

Ask a peer, teacher, or native English speaker to read any part of this section aloud to you. Do NOT read along with them. Listen only. What do you notice about the way they speak? What lesson do you learn from listening to another?

WRITING EXERCISE—A REFLECTIVE QUESTION

Think back in your life to the time you studied anatomy and physiology (A&P). Using some of the vocabulary you have just studied, write a short paragraph about that. For example, you might want to say which topics in the A&P course you did or did not like.

Reading Selection 2-2

Read the following in its entirety. The exercises that follow will help teach the meaning of many terms used.

THE MUSCULOSKELETAL SYSTEM

The skeleton comprises the first part of the musculoskeletal system—the bones. There are 206 bones in the human body and they comprise the skeleton. The skeletal system is responsible for supporting the weight of the body, for posture, and for gait. Muscles comprise the second part of the system. They are responsible for most body movements. There are three main types of muscle—skeletal, smooth, and cardiac. Skeletal muscles are sometimes called striated muscles because of their striped appearance when seen under the microscope. They attach to bones of the skeleton and are under voluntary control. This allows us to engage in physical activities such as walking, running, smiling, winking, and grasping. Skeletal muscles also allow us to manipulate things like holding a pencil or buttoning a shirt. Smooth muscles comprise the walls of organs such as the liver, spleen, and kidneys. They are responsible for the transport of nutrients and other materials through the body. Smooth muscles are not under voluntary control. We cannot make them work. Cardiac muscle is also involuntary. This particular type of muscle allows the heart to pump and accommodate (respond) to changes in the entire body that require it to pump faster or more slowly.

READING EXERCISES

As with the previous reading selection, you can use the exercises below to improve your understanding and vocabulary.

Understanding the General Meaning

Read the text again. Think about it. Do you understand it? What is the general meaning of the text? What is its focus?

_____

_____

_____

Building Vocabulary

Take a moment now to review what you have just read. Write down any words you have not understood or would like to clarify. Then work through the following exercises to discover their meaning.

_____

_____

_____

_____

Determining Meaning from Context. To build vocabulary, study the following words taken from the reading. Discover all you can about them by looking at them in context. Choose the correct meaning. Finally, take a look at how these words expand in English.

1. Muscle *(noun, verb)*

In context:

a) I carried a heavy suitcase yesterday and now the muscle in my arm hurts.

b) If you run in a marathon, every muscle in your body will be forced to work.

Meaning: The word *muscle* can best be described as

a) body tissue capable of contracting to produce motion

b) the heart

c) effort and force

d) deltoid

Word expansion:

a) That man *was muscling* his way through the crowd. He was very rude. He pushed every-body. (verb, past continuous)

b) Look at that young woman. She is an athlete. Her body is very *muscular.* (adjective)

c) *Muscular* dystrophy is a disease marked by progressive wasting of muscles (adjective of dys-trophy, but the two words used together function as a noun, naming a specific disease)

d) The *musculature* of the body refers to the health and status of all body muscles. (noun)

> **VOCABULARY ALERT** If a word begins with the prefix *myo,* it refers to something *muscular.*

2. Voluntary *(adjective)*

In context:

a) Smiling is a voluntary method of communicating friendship.

b) The ability to raise your hand is under voluntary muscle control. Just think about it and do it.

Meaning: The word *voluntary* can best be described as meaning

a) lack of personal control over muscles
b) following directions to act
c) done, made, or given freely; of own volition or will
d) the letters a, e, i, o, or u

Word expansion:

a) Swinging a leg while sitting in a chair is a *voluntary* movement. (adjective)
b) A *volunteer* is a person who helps without expecting compensation. (noun)
c) Many people give *voluntarily* of their time to help others. (adverb)
d) Mary can't go to the party Saturday. She *is volunteering* at a fund-raiser for the Canadian Cancer Society. (verb, present continuous)

3. Grasp *(verb)*

In context:

a) A newborn baby will reach out and grasp your finger.
b) After a stroke, the patient may need to re-learn how to grasp a spoon.

Meaning: The word *grasp* can best be described as meaning

a) to pick up, take, or seize firmly
b) extend your fingers
c) breathe in quickly
d) none of the above

Word expansion:

a) The elderly lady was grasping my hand as she passed away. (verb, past tense continuous)
b) The baby grasped her father's finger and smiled. (verb, past tense)

4. Manipulate *(verb)*

In context:

a) A small child must learn to manipulate a button so that he may button up his shirt.
b) A surgeon must be able to manipulate small and large instruments in the operating room.

Meaning: The word *manipulate* can best be described as

a) change
b) to treat, use, or operate manually (by hand) or mechanically
c) coordinate
d) manual

Word expansion:

a) *Manipulation* of the shoulder joint can be done by the physiotherapist after the patient has a motor vehicle accident. (noun)
b) Psychologically, a person is said to be *manipulative* if he/she is good at convincing others to do what he/she wants. (adjective)
c) A person who operates machinery or a person who convinces other people can be called a *manipulator*. (noun)

5. Comprises *(verb, present tense)*

In context:

a) The musculoskeletal system comprises only one part of the entire body.
b) The sense of smell comprises only one part of the senses. There are five.

Meaning: *Comprises* can best be described as meaning
a) made up of or contains
b) settle differences by mutual agreement
c) bands on a CD
d) a bandage-like dressing for a wound that requires pressure

Word expansion:
a) Holistic health care is *comprised* of the biological, psychological, sociological, spiritual, and environmental aspects of the human experience. (verb)
b) Canada is a very large country *comprised* of 10 provinces and 3 territories. (verb)

6. Involuntary *(adjective)*

In context:
a) I cannot stop the hiccups; they are involuntary.
b) Blinking the eye can be voluntary and involuntary.

Meaning: The word *involuntary* can be described as meaning
a) under free will to act
b) instinctual
c) slow
d) not under control; not under free will to act or not act

Word expansion:
a) A patient who is admitted to a psychiatric unit is sometimes brought there *involuntarily*. (adverb)
b) When Anne had a severe asthma attack, she *voluntarily* admitted herself to the hospital. (adverb)

Applying What You Know to Further Expand Vocabulary. You probably know the names of many of the major bones of the body—by either their common names or their anatomical names. Use your knowledge to label the diagram of the human skeleton shown below.

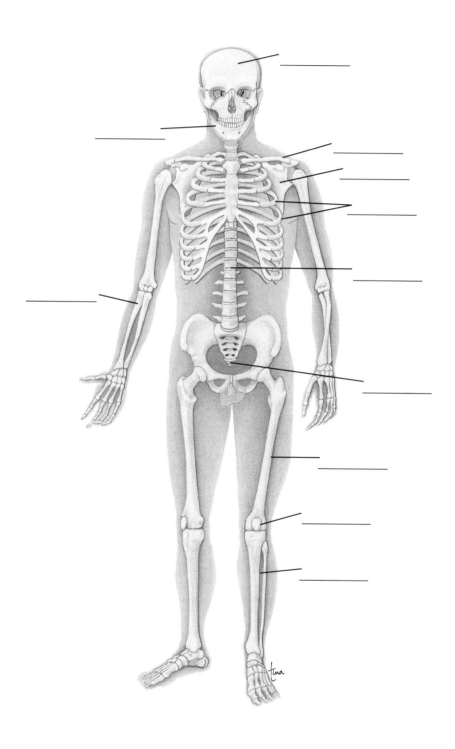

Mix and Match. Again, you might be surprised at how much vocabulary you already know. Use the following mix-and-match exercise in Box 2-4 to test yourself.

SPEAKING EXERCISE

Read the following completed sentences aloud. Ask a peer or teacher to help you with pronunciation. Proceed to the Pronunciation Hints section following. This will also help.

Blinking is an involuntary response to any object that suddenly comes toward your eye.

Winking is not blinking. Winking is voluntary. Blinking is not.

PRONUNCIATION HINTS

muscle – **mŭs'**ĕl

muscular – **mŭs'**kū-lăr

skeletar – **skĕl'**ĕ-tăr

skeleton – **skĕl'**ĕ-tŏn

compromise – **kŏm**-prŏ-mīz

musculoskeletal – **mŭs"**-kū-lō-**skĕl'**ĕ-tăl

BOX 2-4 Mix and Match: Anatomical and Common Names of Major Bones

Connect the common name of bones of the skeleton with their proper anatomical name. Here's a suggestion: Match the ones you know first and then proceed to the ones you do not know. This way you will feel more successful. You will be surprised at how much vocabulary you actually know.

COMMON NAME	ANATOMICAL NAME
backbone	femur
thighbone	clavicle
shin	cranium
rib	spine
collarbone	calcaneus
skull	scapula
shoulder blade	patella
knee cap	tibia
tailbone	coccyx
jawbone	rib
lower arm bone	mandible
heel	radius

The Musculoskeletal System

LISTENING EXERCISE

If you would like to hear more native English speakers from Canada and the United States, search the Internet for radio stations located here. Many radio stations have programs dedicated to the topic of sports. In some of these, the musculoskeletal injuries of athletes may be discussed. Try to find one. Listen carefully by Internet or radio to hear many of the words you have just learned.

WRITING EXERCISE

1) Use your new vocabulary. Write a sentence or two by combining these words in a meaningful way.

| men | muscles | injury | lifting pain |
| relief | ice | heavy | back |

_____

_____

2) Use a key word from the previous exercise to complete a new sentence.
   a) Tisha's arm hurts today. She may have strained a _____ playing baseball yesterday.
   b) The human arm is _____ of a number of muscles, not just one.
   c) Physiotherapists help clients _____ their joints after joint surgery.

SECTION TWO Body Movement, Posture, Gait, Ambulation, and Position

In this section, the context remains that of the musculoskeletal system and we begin to use vocabulary and grammar in a more meaningful way. Now there are opportunities to use language to describe and name parts of the musculoskeletal system. Procedures, explanations, and information reporting are explored. Exercises also include naming anatomical sites or landmarks and building a verb repertoire for working with clients.

Reading Selection 2-3

While you read the following paragraph, try to discover its social purpose. Why has it been written?

BONES AND MORE

As you know, the skeleton is comprised of bones. The spine is an example. The spine is sometimes referred to as the backbone. It consists of bones called vertebrae and of cartilage. It functions to keep the body upright and allows bending and twisting. In humans, bones continue to grow until we reach the age of 25. Bones can break for a variety of reasons: nutritional deficits, aging, injury, trauma, or disease. A broken bone is called a fractured bone. Every bone of the skeleton can potentially be broken. The place where two bones meet is called a joint. In conclusion, the human skeleton is the reason we are able to stand, sit, walk, and move in various ways.

READING EXERCISES

The following exercises will help you master information reports while building vocabulary.

Understanding the General Meaning

The paragraph you have just read is written to provide information. The genre of an information report has the social purpose of telling the reader something. Health professionals are very often required to give verbal and written information reports. This exercise will help you learn the structure of this genre.

1) What is the main subject of the paragraph?

_____

2) What is the main function or social purpose of the paragraph?

_____

3) Complete the following table by writing in the appropriate sentences to match this genre's format. The information report genre includes the grammatical elements of

- an introduction
- background information on the topic
- discussion of the main subject
- conclusion

Building Vocabulary

Take a moment now to review the reading Bones. Can you see vocabulary from previous exercises? In this section on movement, identify all the movement words you have just read. Jot them down here. In subsequent exercises, you may discover more opportunities to use these to tell or describe. Keep them here as a reference for yourself.

_____

_____

_____

Table 2-1 Elements of an Information Report	
Write in the appropriate sentences from the reading selection to match this genre's format.	
ELEMENT	EXAMPLE FROM READING SELECTION
Introduction	
Background Information	
Discussion of Main Topic	
Conclusion	

Sentence Completion. To build vocabulary, complete the following fill-in exercises. Use the Word Bank below to help.

WORD BANK

flexible

aging

tibia

cartilage

joint

move

fractured

hardens

fracture

1) Bob says he broke his leg below the knee. Nurses and doctors would say that he _____ his _____ or fibula.

2) Mathilde is 95 years old and at risk for a hip _____. Her bones are more fragile simply due to the _____ process.

3) As we grow older, the _____ in our spines _____ making us less and less _____.

4) _____ are located where bones meet and help us _____.

Multiple Choice. Continue to expand your new vocabulary by completing the following multiple-choice questions. You may not recognize all of the words, but feel confident that you do have enough skill now to be able to find the correct answers.

1) There are several aspects worth mentioning in the study of the musculoskeletal system. For example, there are the bones, diseases, and injuries. In this context, *aspects* can be described as
   a) attributes.
   b) conditions.
   c) parts making up a whole based on how it looks to the mind or to the eye.
   d) sections.

2) Choose the **best** answer to describe the function of the musculoskeletal system. It
   a) helps you stand up.
   b) allows you to walk.
   c) supports the skeleton.
   d) allows you to stretch.

3) *Pathologic* fractures occur as a result of
   a) diseases or conditions that cause bones to break spontaneously without an injury or trauma.
   b) brain disease.
   c) old age.
   d) sickness.

Deduction derives from the act of deducing. It is the conclusion you reach after using logic and reasoning, and after examining the evidence at hand.

Sentence Completion. The goal of the following is to acquire medical vocabulary used to identify types of bone fractures. To complete the exercise, read the descriptions. Try to match them with the name of the fracture found in the Word Bank below. To be successful, read through the entire exercise first. Then go back and through deduction, make the matches. Your own personal knowledge and experience in health care will help you with this exercise.

compound

closed oblique

compression

incomplete
longitudinal

pathologic

comminuted

1) When the bone is broken by being pressed or squeezed by very great force, we call it a _____ fracture.

2) Franklin's ulnar bone is broken to the degree that it protrudes out through his skin. You can actually see it. This is called a _____ fracture.

3) Brenda is going to need some surgery to repair her shin bone. It splintered into about 10 pieces in the car accident. This type of fracture is called a _____ one.

4) Shylo wasn't sure he broke a bone. He had a lot of pain, but when he looked at his arm, he couldn't see the typical swelling of a broken bone. Still, he could not use his arm to lean on without a lot of pain. The x-ray shows it is broken at an angle, sideways along the bone. This is a _____ type of fracture.

5) Engenoo has had brittle bone disease all of his life. He is 8 years old now and his bones are very fragile. He must be careful because with this condition one of his bones can break even without an injury. When this occurs, the doctor says he has a _____ fracture.

6) Reka thought she had a sprained ankle. She walked on her broken ankle for a couple of days. She shouldn't have done this. When she finally got it x-rayed, the doctor told her she had a long crack running down the bone. The nurse explained this was actually called a _____ fracture.

SPEAKING EXERCISE

Return to the previous exercise. Read it out loud to yourself or to a friend who is also studying *Medical English Clear and Simple.* Help each other with pronunciation or ask a native English speaker. Check the Pronunciation Hints box below, too.

PRONUNCIATION HINTS

comminuted – kŏm'ĭ-**nūt**-ĕd

compression – kŏm-**prĕsh**'ŭn

longitudinal – lŏn"jĭ-**tū**'dĭ-năl

pathologic – păth-ō-**lŏj**'ĭk

oblique – ō-**blēk**

compound – **kŏmp**'ownd

LISTENING EXERCISE

At this point you again have some homework. You are encouraged to speak to a native English-speaking health professional if you know one or watch an English language video clip about broken bones. Try this: on the browser on your computer type in "video clip, broken bones" or "video clip, fractures." You will be surprised what you can see and hear.

WRITING EXERCISE—CREATIVE WRITING

As a health professional or student in health studies, it is important to know how to write in a variety of genres. So far, you have looked at reporting the facts in the information report genre. Now you have an opportunity to be more creative. You are going to write a short story in the essay genre. In preparation for doing this writing, study the format of a short story/essay given in Box 2-5. Be sure to follow this format.

Write a short story using the 5-paragraph essay format. Use the following topic.

Fractures. When a bone is broken, it will either be splinted or casted to immobilize it. Using this vocabulary and words you have learned throughout this unit, write a short story about yourself or someone you know who has had a broken bone. Tell the reader a little bit about how the fracture happened and what the results were. Write in the past tense, but use your verbs correctly. Here are some pictures to help inspire you.

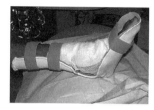 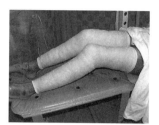 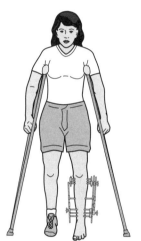 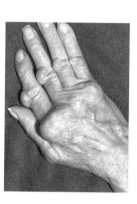

A standard form of essay writing is the 5-paragraph essay. This includes:

■ An introductory paragraph—Clearly identify what you will talk about in the essay.
■ Body
  ● first paragraph—The first sentence should make a very brief link to the introduction. This prepares the reader for the focus of the first paragraph. Next, identify the main topic of the paragraph—the point you would like to talk about.
  ● second paragraph—The first sentence or two should link to the previous paragraph in some way. It should also reflect the thesis or main topic that was identified in the introductory paragraph. Other sentences must make a new point or points related to that topic.
  ● third paragraph—This paragraph follows the same format as the previous two. It must also have its own clear point that relates to the main thesis (topic) of the essay. This paragraph should also provide a signal to the reader that the end of the essay is approaching.
■ Conclusion—The last paragraph must restate the original thesis or topic of your essay; it must reflect the introductory statement. Reflection means the sentence will contain similar information but will not be an exact copy of the original thesis statement. Next, summarize three main points, one from each paragraph of the body of the essay. Finally, include a statement that clearly shows the reader that the essay has come to an end.

Reading Selection 2-4

Read the following in preparation for exercises that talk about healthy joints and joint disorders. While you do so, notice that the joints are being labeled using common speech. The correct anatomical term appears in parentheses just after each common name.

JOINTS

A joint is the place in your body where two or more bones come together. Joints are movable. They articulate. In the human body, there are six types of movable joints. They are the hinge (ginglymus), pivot (trochoid), gliding (arthrodia), ball-and-socket (enarthrosis), condyloid, and saddle joints. Hinge joints only bend one way. Try to think of them like the hinge on a door. The knee is an example of a hinge joint; so are the knuckles in your fingers. Pivot joints allow you to turn a part of your body. This is referred to as rotation. In this case, the bone moves around a central axis without moving away from it. The neck is an example of a pivot joint. You can pivot your neck. A gliding joint, on the other hand, is one in which a connecting bone is able to swing back and forth as it passes smoothly over the other bone. Your ankle and wrist can do this. A ball-and-socket joint is one in which a rounded bone head moves within the cavity of another bone. An example of this is your shoulder and hip joint. The movement is called circumduction. A condyloid (ellipsoidal) joint allows movement in an elliptical, pivotal manner. It can also flex, extend, abduct, and adduct. The wrist is an example of a condyloid joint. A saddle joint has the same movements of a condyloid joint—flexion, extension, abduction, and adduction—but it cannot pivot or rotate. Thumbs are the only saddle joints in the human body.

Joints are under a lot of pressure and are quite prone to stress, injuries, and inflammation. The main diseases affecting them are gout, osteoarthritis, and rheumatoid arthritis. These usually cause inflammation. Injuries to the joint include contusions, dislocations, sprains, and penetrating wounds. Stress on a joint can come from heavy lifting or playing rigorous sports.

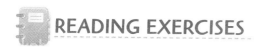
Understanding the General Meaning

Read the text again. Think about it.

1) What genre is this reading written in?

_____

2) What does the phrase "on the other hand" mean in the context of this reading?

_____

Building Vocabulary

Take a moment now to review what you have just read. List the anatomical names for joints here.

_____

_____

_____

Multiple Choice.   To promote acquisition of new words through context, complete the following multiple-choice questions. Please refer back to the reading for help at any time.

1) I can actually rotate my head. It must be a
   a) hinge joint.
   b) pivot joint.
   c) ball-and-socket joint.
   d) saddle joint.

2) When two things are joined together to allow motion between the parts, they
   a) articulate.
   b) meld.
   c) fuse.
   d) connect.

3) Gliding joints are also known as synovial joints. They allow two flat bones to come very close together without touching. The bones glide past one another as the movement occurs. This action is also known as
   a) swinging or sliding.
   b) circumduction.
   c) circulation.
   d) pivoting.

4) A sample of joint stress is
   a) jogging.
   b) sleeping.
   c) worrying too much.
   d) none of the above

5) An example of inflammation of a joint would be
   a) fever.
   b) bruising.
   c) arthritis.
   d) myocarditis.

6) Dislocation means
   a) moving to another town.
   b) changing color.
   c) displacement of a bone from its normal position in a joint.
   d) finding a new location.

Mix and Match.   Now that you have read about joints, locate them correctly in the body by doing the exercise in Box 2-6. In the previous exercises you have studied anatomy and that vocabulary will help you now.

Multiple Choice.   Begin to become familiar with proper terminology for assessing body movement. Study the pictures. Remember them. Take notes about them, if you like. Then answer the multiple-choice questions that follow. Note: the questions will not be about the pictures. They are questions that ask you to think about the topic and use the language in other ways. Answer the questions by choosing the best answer.

BOX 2-6 Mix and Match: Locating Joints

Draw a line to link the type of joint and where it is located.

JOINT	LOCATION
ball-and-socket	wrist and head
hinge	thumb
pivot	wrist
gliding	metacarpals, metatarsals, ribs
condyloid	shoulder and hip
saddle	finger, elbow, knee

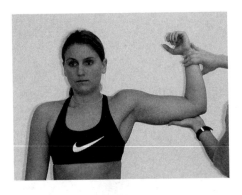

1) If I move my entire arm out, away from my body at the side, what am I doing?
   a) flexing
   b) extending
   c) rotating
   d) abducting

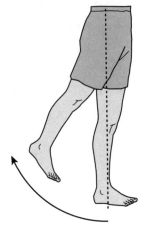

2) Stand up. Raise your right leg. Keep it straight. What movement are you doing?
   a) flexion of the hip
   b) extension
   c) inversion
   d) none of the above

The Musculoskeletal System

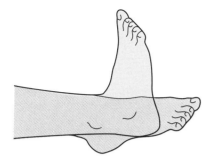

3) Put your feet flat on the ground. Keep your heels down. Raise your toes and feet without taking your heels off the ground. What is this called?
   a) silly
   b) impossible
   c) dorsal flexion
   d) extension

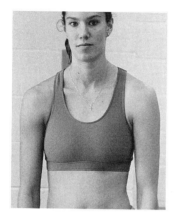

4) Put your arm down, straight at your side. What is this action?
   a) extension
   b) flexion
   c) adduction
   d) eversion

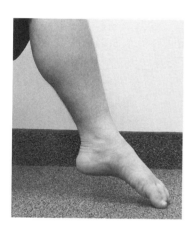

5) Sit down. Lift your heels and point your toes. What are you doing?
   a) plantar flexion
   b) standing up
   c) extending my feet
   d) opposing my feet

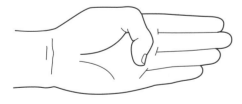

6) Hold up your hand. Open it, and then fold your thumb in, over the palm. What is this called?
   a) opposition of the thumb
   b) not possible
   c) extension of the thumb
   d) extension of the hand

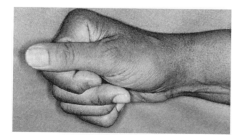

7) Hold up your hand. Open it. Curl the fingers down into the palm. What are you doing?
   a) nothing
   b) flexing my fingers
   c) opposing my fingers
   d) adducting my fingers

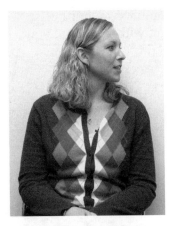

8) Sit up straight. Turn your head from left to right. What is this called?
   a) gliding
   b) adduction
   c) rotation
   d) nodding

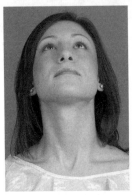

9) Sit up straight, again. Tip your head backwards. What is this called?
   a) painful
   b) flexion
   c) impossible at my age
   d) neck extension

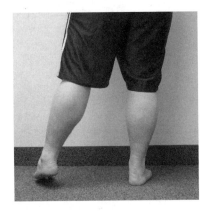

10) Stand up with your legs together. Now take your left leg away from your body, out to the side. Now bring it back in. What is this last action?
   a) opposition
   b) abduction
   c) inversion
   d) adduction

SPEAKING EXERCISE

Go back and read the last 10 questions and answers aloud. Ask a peer or teacher to help you with pronunciation. Proceed to the following Pronunciation Hints section for some guidance.

PRONUNCIATION HINTS

condyloid – **kŏn'**dĭ-loyd

inversion – ĭn-**vĕr'**zhŭn

adduction – ă-**dŭk'**shŭn

abduction – ăb-**dŭk'**shŭn

flexion – **flĕk'**shŭn

The Musculoskeletal System

LISTENING EXERCISE

You have just acquired some very difficult terminology. If you have the opportunity, record yourself pronouncing the words you found most difficult in this section. Ask an English-speaking person or an English language teacher to listen, if you can. Ask for some pronunciation guidance.

WRITING EXERCISE

This exercise asks you to conjugate verbs. It is extremely important for health professionals to be able to describe their patient and his or her activities precisely. Before you begin the exercise, review the Grammar Alert box.

> **GRAMMAR ALERT: VERBS ENDING WITH –ING** Present, continuous tense verbs are sometimes referred to as the –ing participle form of the verbs. They are found in combination with the verb "to be." Their basic function is to describe an action still in progress. Example: *He is working today.*
>
> **Adjectives ending with –ing**
> Adjectives of this type can describe the effect that something has on a person's feelings (emotions), while others can describe a process or state that continues over a period of time. Example: *A career as a surgeon is very appealing.*
>
> **Nouns ending with –ing**
> These types of nouns, technically called gerunds, may function as the subject of a sentence or as the object of a sentence or of a prepositions. They may or may not have an article before them.
>
> Example: *Smiling is good for your health.*
> *She is very proud of winning that contest.*
> *That patient won't object to eating solid food tomorrow.*

Now we will begin to look at gait and posture: the ways we walk, stand, and sit. You are given a verb that describes less than optimal functioning of gait or posture. Use the correct form of the verb to provide a full answer. Hint: Pay very close attention to the verb form in the question.

Example: **step**
What is he doing?
He is <u>stepping</u>.

1) **shuffle**
Rafe drags his feet on the ground when he walks. What is he doing?
He _____.

2) **stoop**
Edna is 88 years old. When she stands, her back is bowed and she looks toward the ground. How is she standing?
She _____.

3) **slouch**
Brenda never sits up straight when she watches TV. She's doing it now. How is she sitting?
She _____.

4) **limp**
Denzel sprained his ankle yesterday. How is he walking, today?
He is _____.

5) **lean**
Janice has been standing on her feet for a long time. She is putting stress now on her left hip only. How is she standing?
She is _____ on her left hip.

Treatments, Interventions, and Assistance

Musculoskeletal injuries are very common, and as a health professional, it is likely you will assess and treat them on a daily basis. This section introduces language for that purpose, from a patient call for an appointment, to the basic interview that gathers assessment data, to medical/nursing interventions. The sociocultural contexts of the doctor's office and the emergency department at hospitals acquaint the reader with health-care resources and customs in the United States and Canada. Before we begin, take note of this particular terminology.

Reading Selection 2-5

Read the following article. To help you understand the vocabulary, complete the exercises that follow.

WORD ALERT In the context of health care, it is important to distinguish the difference between treatment, intervention, and assistance.

Treatment refers to the medical actions employed to fight diseases and disorders, as well as to relieve symptoms of illness or injury.

Intervention includes assessing, monitoring, observing, referring, and providing direct patient care actions.

Assistance refers to all of those caring activities that health-care professionals engage in to educate, help, guide, or direct patient activities. Examples are assisting the patient with a bath and helping the patient get in or out of a chair.

USE OF EMERGENCY ROOMS

Across Canada and the United States of America, patients have a tendency to use emergency rooms at hospitals for nonemergency conditions. Rather than taking the time to make an appointment with a doctor or seek out a medical clinic, it has become the norm to simply pop into the nearest hospital emergency department. The result of this has been an ever-increasing demand on nurses and doctors to triage the patients they see. They must identify care priorities while sifting through the large numbers of people still waiting to be seen. In actuality, the waiting room is often filled with people who do not fit the definition of a patient suitable for emergency care.

Some of the complaints that people bring to the emergency rooms are simply minor in nature. They may be complaining of a fever or flu-like symptoms. They may have a simple rash or headache, perhaps even a sore stomach. They appear with their own subjective reports of their conditions and request what they believe is appropriate treatment. In many cases, it is simply that people want an antibiotic, analgesic, or a note for work that states they should take the next few days off.

The problem with the inappropriate use of emergency rooms is that it overburdens the staff and the facility. There is a shortage of nurses and doctors in some locales. Additionally, there can be a shortage of hospital beds and accommodations for the ill. As a result, it is unwise to tie up the system with less urgent cases. Walk-in clinics have sprung up around the continent to provide easier access to health care and treatment, with no appointment necessary. The intent is to encourage the public to use the walk-in clinics rather than the emergency departments at hospitals, saving the emergency rooms for what they were originally designed for—emergency care. Progress in changing this pattern of behavior has been slow over the past 20 years, but walk-in clinics are gaining in popularity. They are being utilized more and more as the public becomes more familiar with and comfortable using them.

READING EXERCISES

It is important not only to understand the general meaning of a passage, but also to remember and understand the specifics given. Remember, health professions need specific details when interviewing and assessing a patient. As you yourself recognize specifics, you will continue to build your language skills.

Understanding the General Meaning

Read the text again. Think about it. In short paragraph form, write a summary of no more than three sentences to demonstrate your understanding. Include the main point (thesis) of the reading.

_____

_____

_____

Learning Specifics

Take a moment now to review what you have just read.

1) What is the difference between the purpose of an emergency room and a medical clinic?

_____

_____

2) What term is used to explain the process of identifying cases that take priority over others for treatment?

_____

3) Who does the assessments in the emergency department?

_____

4) Which countries are being referred to in this article?

_____

5) Why is the emergency room at a hospital so busy?

_____

6) What is the purpose of a walk-in clinic?

_____

7) What is the main difference between a walk-in clinic and a doctor's office or clinic?

_____

8) Has public attitude changed about the use of emergency rooms yet? Explain.

_____

Building Vocabulary

To build vocabulary, study the following words or terms taken from the reading selection. Discover all you can about them by looking at them in context.

Multiple Choice.   Choose the correct meaning.

1) A non-emergency situation is not life threatening.
   Life threatening means it is
   a) critical.
   b) serious.
   c) valid.

2) Hospital staff must set care priorities and assess which patient should be treated first and why.
   In this context, the term *care priorities* means
   a) assigning a duty doctor to the case.
   b) understanding which case needs immediate attention.
   c) giving assistance in an orderly fashion for everyone.

3) In disasters and emergencies, a triage team assesses who will be treated first.
   In this context, *triage* can best be described as
   a) a system of dealing with patients according to highest need first.
   b) professionals who only deal with emergency cases.
   c) another word for emergency.

4) If you have an appointment with a doctor or even a banker, you likely have to sit and wait in his or her waiting room before being seen.
   In this context, *waiting room* can be described as
   a) the lobby.
   b) a sitting area specifically for patients or clients.
   c) a place to buy coffee and wait while your mom sees the doctor.

5) In health care, we need to obtain both objective and subjective reports. The first come from lab reports, x-rays, etc. The second come from the patients themselves.
   In this context, *subjective* reports means
   a) the patient's personal opinion of his or her own situation.
   b) the topic of the visit.
   c) another way to complain.

6) When too many people use the emergency room for reasons that are not urgent, they tie up the doctors and nurses. They prevent them from doing the best work that they possibly can because staff members are pressed for time to see so many patients. In this way, these people are tying up the system.
   In this context, *tying up* the system means
   a) interfering.
   b) making unreasonable demands.
   c) putting a rope around the staff and not letting them work.

   VOCABULARY ALERT The reason a patient comes to see a doctor or other health professional is because he or she has a health concern. These concerns are called *patient complaints.* In this context, patient complaints can be described as meaning a subjective report of signs and symptoms of health or illness.

Identifying Common Medical Complaints of the Musculoskeletal System.   Use a word from the Word Bank below to offer a possible diagnosis for the following signs and symptoms.

WORD BANK

sprain

fracture

osteoarthritis

arthritis

muscle tension

joint dysfunction
or disease

muscle strain from
overuse

1) Swollen and red; limited movement _____

2) Painful to swing arm or play tennis _____

3) Feels tight along the back of neck _____

4) Can't move wrist _____

5) Finger knuckles (joints) are swollen and disfigured _____

6) Pain and stiffness when trying to bend _____

7) Swollen, no movement possible _____

Using New Vocabulary in Sentences. Use your new vocabulary for the musculoskeletal system to talk about the following pictures of the types of equipment or devices a person might need for assistance. Use the equipment named for you in your sentences.

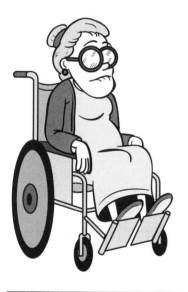

1) wheelchair

_____

_____

_____

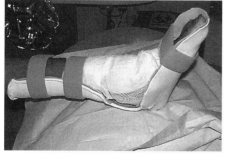

2) splint

_____

_____

_____

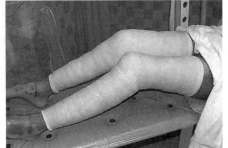

3) cast

_____

_____

_____

4) cane

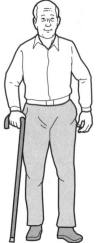

_____

_____

_____

5) walker

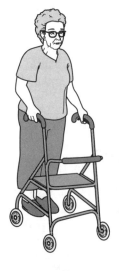

_____

_____

_____

6) scooter

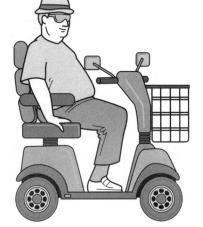

_____

_____

_____

SPEAKING EXERCISE

Read aloud the Use of Emergency Rooms, again. Ask a peer or teacher to help you with pronunciation. Proceed to the following Pronunciation Hints section. This will also help.

> **PRONUNCIATION HINTS**
>
> triage – **trē**-ăzh'
>
> analgesic – ăn"ăl-**jē**'sĭk

LISTENING EXERCISE

If you would like to hear more native English speakers from Canada and the United States, search the Internet for radio stations located here. Many radio stations have programs dedicated to the subject of health and wellness. Try to find one that talks about fitness or physiotherapy and exercise. Listen carefully by Internet or radio to hear many of the words you have just learned.

WRITING EXERCISE

Use your new vocabulary. Write two or three sentences by combining these words and names in a meaningful way.

grandmother	knit	hobby	arthritic
talented disfigured	hands	fingers	

Reading Selection 2-6

Read the following dialogue of an interview between the nurse, a doctor, and a patient. Notice how data is being gathered and a health assessment of the patient's condition is being made. Imagine the scene: A patient hops into the clinic on one foot, supported by her friend.

A VISIT TO THE WALK-IN CLINIC

Anna: Hi! I'd like to see a doctor.

Nurse: Uh-huh. What seems to be the matter?

Anna: I was running and playing with my dog. I twisted my ankle and fell. Now I can't walk on it.

Nurse: Sorry? You say you can't put weight on your foot?

Anna: Yes, my foot. My right foot. It really hurts and it's all swollen. I wrapped it up because I think it's sprained.

Nurse: OK. Do you have medical insurance?

Anna: Yes. Here it is.

Nurse: Thank you. Please, have a seat. I'll tell the doctor you're here.

***

Nurse: Anna? Here's your insurance card back. Dr. Smith will see you now. Come this way. Can you walk or would you like me to get you the wheelchair?

Anna: A wheelchair, please.

***

Nurse: OK, here we are. Please sit up on this table. Here, let me help you. Now, let's take that bandage off. There. OK, the doctor will be right with you.

Anna: Thank you.

***

Doctor: Hello, I'm Dr. Smith and you are Anna?

Anna: Yes, hello.

Doctor: So, you think you may have sprained your ankle—your right ankle, I see. When did you do that?

Anna: This morning.

Doctor: Uh-huh. And how did you do that?

Anna: I was running with my dog in the park and stepped on a pebble or something and bang. The next thing I knew I was on the ground and my ankle was killing me.

Doctor: No shoes?

Anna: No.

Doctor: In the dog park?

Anna: Yes. I know, I know . . . I should have had some shoes on, but it was hot and I just wanted to have some fun.

Doctor: Well, let's take a look. Have you been able to walk on it at all since this morning?

Anna: No. I tried, but it hurts a lot. Then my friend told me I should get to the hospital to get an x-ray. But I knew this walk-in clinic was closer and that you have an x-ray lab in the building, so I came here.

Doctor: Good. That was the best thing to do. Although I can see you have injured your ankle, it's not an emergency and you wouldn't want to tie up the ER at the hospital for this. Good thinking. Now, tell me some more about your ankle while I examine it. Have you applied any ice to it? Taken any pain medication?

Anna: No, I didn't put any ice on it, but I propped it up on the sofa. I know that you are supposed to elevate a sprain. But I don't think it helped very much. Look at how swollen it is. And it's turning red, don't you think?

Doctor: Yes, I can certainly see that it's swollen and discolored. Wiggle your toes for me, Anna. Good. Now, I am going to assist you to move your ankle in a clockwise rotation ever so gently. Ready?

Anna: OK, but that's going to hurt.

Doctor: We'll go slowly and gently. Just tell me when it hurts and when to stop.

Anna: OK.

Doctor: How's this?

Anna: Oh, oh, stop, stop! That hurts. Honestly, my ankle doesn't want to do that.

Doctor: Well, Anna I am quite certain you have sprained that ankle. Your self-diagnosis was correct. However, I think an x-ray would be a good idea just to rule out any fine, hairline fracture of the ankle or foot. What do you think?

Anna: Do I have to? Is it covered by my insurance plan? Who would have to pay for that?

Doctor: Yes, I believe your medical insurance pays for it. X-ray is right next door. Why don't you go there and bring the films back to me? You can take the wheelchair.

Anna: Thanks. And what happens if it is just sprained?

Doctor: Well, I'll have the nurse wrap it in the tensor bandage you brought and she can set you up with a pair of crutches for a couple of days. How would that be?

Anna: Great.

Doctor: Come and see me after the x-ray and we'll set up an appointment with the MOA for about 3 days from now. You can return the crutches then and I can have a look at your ankle. In the meantime, do NOT walk on it. Use those crutches. Elevate your sore leg intermittently throughout the day. An ice pack will help reduce swelling if you want to use one once in awhile. Finally, take some mild pain and anti-inflammatory medication if you wish. You can buy it over the counter in the drugstore.

Anna: OK, thanks, Doctor. I'll take your advice and I'll see you later. Bye.

Understanding the General Meaning

Read the text again. Think about it as you answer these questions.

1) Anna had an accident. What was it?

_____

2) Where did Anna go for treatment?

_____

3) What are her signs and symptoms?

_____

4) Anna has a musculoskeletal injury. Name it.

_____

5) What is the common treatment for this type of injury?

_____

6) Did Anna need an appointment at the walk-in clinic?

_____

7) Who works at this clinic?

_____

8) Why does the doctor ask her about not wearing shoes in the dog park? What is his intended meaning?

_____

9) Why didn't Anna go to the emergency room at the nearest hospital?

_____

Building Vocabulary

To build vocabulary, you will again try to learn the meaning of words from their context. You will also work with prepositions. A mix-and-match exercise will help you through some common idioms.

Determining Meaning from Context. Study the following words or terms taken from this text. Discover all you can about them by looking at them in context. Choose the correct meaning. Finally, take a look at how these words or terms expand in English.

1. Matter *(noun)*

In context:

a) The Department of Immigration handles matters of immigration while the Department of Revenue and Taxation handles matters of tax.

b) Something must be the matter with me. I have been sneezing all day.

Meaning: The noun *matters* can best be described as meaning

a) subject of interest or problem

b) error

c) conditions

Word expansion:

a) As a *matter of fact,* I do know all the answers. (expression meaning "point of fact")

b) If that exam really *mattered,* I would stay up all night and study for it, but it doesn't, so I won't. (verb, past tense)

2. Wrapped *(verb, past tense)*

In context:

a) I sprained my ankle so I wrapped a tensor bandage around it.

b) It's Martha's birthday. We wrapped her gift in colorful paper.

Meaning: The verb *wrapped* can best be described as

a) uncovered

b) dressing

c) covered or enclosed

Word expansion:

a) Please *wrap* the patient's knee in Room 141. It's beginning to swell. (verb, present tense)

b) I *was wrapping* the patient's wrist when I had to run to an emergency. (past progressive tense)

3. Bandage *(noun)*

In context:

a) Joshua fell and scraped his knee. He cried. His mom cleaned it and put a bandage on it.

b) If you put a bandage on your cut, you won't get an infection.

Meaning: A bandage can best be described as:

a) a dressing for a wound

b) something you wrap round and round an injury

c) anything sticky

Word expansion:

a) Excuse me while I *bandage* that patient's hand. (verb, present tense)

b) That wound is going to require stitches and *bandaging.* (noun, a gerund)

c) Your cut will need to be *bandaged.* Please wait here. (verb in past tense to show a completed action plus future auxiliary verb of "to be" to indicate that this action has to be started and completed)

Another way of saying a wound needs to be *bandaged* is to say it needs to be *dressed*. (verb in past tense to show a completed action plus future auxiliary verb of "to be" to indicate that this action has to be started and completed.)

Sentence Completion—Learning to Use Prepositions of Place. English language learners often have difficulty locating where they are. This is particularly challenging in medical English. For example, we are not "in" a ward of the hospital, we are "on" the ward. However, we are not "on" the Emergency Department, we are either "in" the ER or "at" it.

Complete the following sentences by filling in the blanks with the proper preposition of place.

1) If I have a serious injury, I must go _____ the Emergency Department at the nearest hospital.

   a) at   b) by

   c) in   d) to

2) The doctor works _____ the clinic.

   a) in   b) at

   c) for   d) within

3) We work _____ the Emergency Department. We are nurses.

   a) in   b) for

   c) at   d) to

4) What unit is my uncle _____ at the hospital? South? Thank you.

   a) at   b) in

   c) on   d) within

5) Where is the nearest hospital? Oh, is that _____ the shopping mall?

   a) nearby to   b) near

   c) far   d) located

6) Did you say the nearest hospital was _____ the shopping mall?

   a) at   b) close

   c) by   d) far away

7) Is the x-ray department _____ the hospital or next door?

   a) close   b) located

   c) in   d) along

SPEAKING EXERCISE

Read the following completed sentences aloud. Ask a peer or teacher to help you with pronunciation. Proceed to the Pronunciation Hints section following. This will also help.

Another way of saying a wound needs to be bandaged is to say it needs to be dressed.

I sprained my ankle so I wrapped a tensor bandage around it.

I was wrapping the patient's wrist when I had to run to an emergency.

PRONUNCIATION HINTS

bandage – **băn′dăj**

sprain – **sprān**

LISTENING EXERCISE

Record yourself and some friends reading the dialogue. Then play it back and listen to your pronunciation and everyone else's, too. Help each other perfect it.

WRITING EXERCISE

Use your new vocabulary. Write a few sentences by combining these words and names in a meaningful way. Use complete sentences.

doctor	nurse	patient	
shoelace	injury	walk	limping

_____

_____

_____

ANSWER KEY

Anatomy and Physiology

READING SELECTION 1—ORGANIZATION OF THE BODY

Understanding the General Meaning

Sample answer: The general meaning or focus of the reading selection is that cells, tissues, and organs are organized into body systems with specific functions.

Building Vocabulary

Determining Meaning from Context

1) d, 2) a, 3) a, 4) b, 5) a

Mix and Match

BOX 2-1 Types of Tissues: Answers	
CELL	**FUNCTION**
epithelial	external/internal surfaces of body skin and membranes
connective	anchors, connects, and supports other tissue, tendons, ligaments; highly vascular
muscle	stretches, contracts; allows movement
nerve	receives and carries impulses to and from the brain

BOX 2-2 Mix and Match: Body Cavities: Answers	
CAVITY	**ORGANS**
abdominal cavity	intestines, liver, stomach, kidneys
thoracic cavity	heart, lungs
cranial cavity	brain
oral cavity	tongue
pelvic cavity	bowels, reproductive organs

BOX 2-3 Mix and Match: Common Names for Body Cavities: Answers

ANATOMICAL NAME FOR BODY CAVITY	COMMON NAME
abdominal	belly
thoracic	chest
cranial	head
oral	mouth, chest
pelvic	pelvis

 # READING SELECTION 2—THE MUSCULOSKELETAL SYSTEM

Understanding the General Meaning

Sample answer: The purpose of this reading is to provide information about the musculoskeletal system. It highlights the functions of the two systems—the skeletal system and the muscular system—and how they work together as one larger, whole system.

Building Vocabulary

Determining Meaning from Context

1) a, 2) c, 3) a, 4) b, 5) a, 6) d

Mix and Match

BOX 2-4 Mix and Match: Anatomical and Common Names of Major Bones: Answers

COMMON NAME	ANATOMICAL NAME
backbone	spine
thighbone	femur
shin	tibia
rib	rib
collarbone	clavicle
skull	cranium
shoulder blade	scapula
knee cap	patella
tailbone	coccyx
jawbone	mandible

The Musculoskeletal System

Applying What You Know to Further Expand Vocabulary

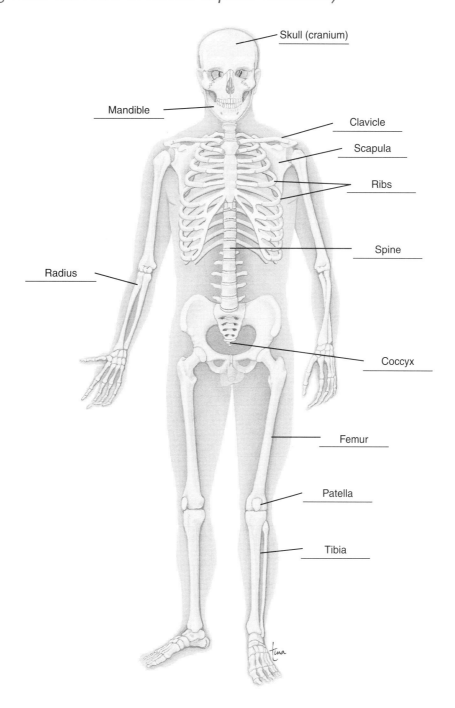

WRITING EXERCISE

1) Sample answer:
   Many men suffer back injuries from heavy lifting at work. This causes back pain and sore back muscles. Relief from the pain and soreness can be found by applying ice to the area.

2) a) muscle, b) comprised, c) manipulate

Body Movement, Posture, Gait, Ambulation, and Position

 READING SELECTION 3—BONES AND MORE

Understanding the General Meaning

1) The main subject of the paragraph is bones.

2) The main function or purpose of the reading selection is to inform the reader about bones.

Building Vocabulary

Sentence Completion

1) fractured, tibia

2) fracture, aging

3) cartilage, hardens, flexible (bend and twist)

4) joints, move

Multiple Choice

1) a, 2) c, 3) a

Sentence Completion

1) compression

2) compound

3) comminuted

4) closed oblique

5) pathologic

6) incomplete longitudinal

Table 2-1 Elements of an Information Report with Examples	
ELEMENT	EXAMPLE FROM THE READING SELECTION ON BONES
Introduction	A skeleton is comprised of bones.
Background Information	They are not all of the same type of consistency.
Discussion of the Main Subject	The spine is an example. The spine is sometimes referred to as the backbone. It consists of bones called vertebrae and of cartilage. It functions to keep the body upright and allows bending and twisting. In humans, bones continue to grow until we reach the age of 25. Bones can break for a variety of reasons: nutritional deficits, aging, injury, trauma, or disease. A broken bone is called a fractured bone. Every bone of the skeleton can potentially be broken. The place where two bones meet is called a joint.
Conclusion	In conclusion, the human skeleton is the reason we are able to stand, sit, walk, and move in various ways.

READING SELECTION 4—JOINTS

Understanding the General Meaning

1) The paragraph is written in the genre of an information report.

2) The phrase "on the other hand" means an opposite way to think about the same problem or situation.

Building Vocabulary

Anatomical names of joints: ginglymus, trochoid, arthrodia, enarthrosis, condyloid, saddle joint

Multiple Choice

1) b, 2) a, 3) a, 4) a, 5) c, 6) c

Mix and Match

BOX 2-6 Mix and Match: Locating Joints: Answers

Draw a line to link the type of joint with its location in the body.

JOINT	LOCATION
ball-and-socket	shoulder and hip
hinge	finger, elbow, knee
pivot	wrist and head
gliding	metacarpals and metatarsals, ribs
condyloid	wrist
saddle	thumb

Multiple Choice

1) d, 2) a, 3) c, 4) c, 5) a, 6) a, 7) b, 8) c, 9) d, 10) d

Writing Exercise

1) He is shuffling.

2) She is stooping.

3) She is slouching

4) He is limping.

5) She is leaning on one hip.

Treatment, Interventions, and Assistance

 ## READING SELECTION 5—USE OF EMERGENCY ROOMS

Understanding the General Meaning

Example: The main points are (1) emergency departments are often not used the way they are intended to be used, (2) hospital staff are overburdened because there is a shortage of nurses and sometimes doctors, and (3) walk-in clinics are one way to ease the burden on emergency departments at hospitals if more people would use them.

Sample paragraph: In many areas, emergency departments in hospitals are not used as they were intended to be used. People with minor illnesses use them when they should instead use walk-in clinics or make an appointment to see a doctor. The growing use of walk-in clinics may improve the situation and relieve the burden on frequently understaffed emergency rooms and hospitals.

Learning Specifics

1) The emergency room is for emergencies, while a walk-in clinic is for all other health problems.

2) The term used to explain the process of identifying cases that take priority is *triage*.

3) Doctors and nurses do assessments in the emergency room.

4) The United States and Canada are referred to in the article.

5) The emergency room in a hospital is typically very busy because it is overused by people who do not have true medical emergencies.

6) The purpose of a walk-in clinic is to provide easy access to care—assessment and treatment—for people with non-emergency medical complaints.

7) The main difference between a walk-in clinic and a doctor's office or non-walk-in clinic is that the client needs an appointment at a doctor's office but not at the walk-in clinic

8) Yes. People are beginning to use walk-in clinics more often.

Building Vocabulary

Multiple Choice

1) a, 2) b, 3) a, 4) b, 5) a, 6) a

Identifying Common Medical Complaints of the Musculoskeletal System

1) sprain

2) muscle strain from overuse

3) muscle tension

4) joint dysfunction or disease

5) arthritis

6) osteoarthritis

7) fracture

Writing Exercise

Example: My grandmother is very talented and loves to knit. It's her hobby, but now she can't do it because she's arthritic. Her hands are sore and her fingers are disfigured.

 # READING SELECTION 6—A VISIT TO THE WALK-IN CLINIC

Understanding the General Meaning

1) The accident was that Anna stumbled and fell, hurting her ankle.

2) She went to the walk-in clinic.

3) Her ankle hurt, she couldn't walk on it, and it was swollen and becoming red.

4) Her injury is probably a sprain.

5) The common treatment for a sprain is to apply ice to minimize swelling, take an anti-inflammatory/analgesic to relieve symptoms, elevate the limb intermittently throughout the day, and wrap it in an elastic-type of bandage to provide some support and reduce swelling.

6) No, she did not need an appointment.

7) A doctor, a nurse, and a medical office assistant (MOA) work at this clinic.

8) A dog park is designed especially for dogs. It will be a place where many dogs urinate and defecate. It is very unhealthy to walk barefoot in such a place. The doctor is asking Anna if she was aware of this and, if so, why she walked barefoot. Had she said something different in response, the doctor would have had to take the time to teach her about this health issue. It would be his responsibility to do so. (Note the word "teach," not "tell." In the United States and Canada, all health professionals teach clients; we do not tell them how to live.)

9) Anna didn't go to the emergency department because this was not a serious, critical injury that required that degree of medical attention.

Building Vocabulary

Determining Meaning from Context

1) c, 2) c, 3) a

Sentence Completion

1) d, 2) b, 3) a, 4) c, 5) b, 6) c, 7) c

Writing Exercise

Example: The nurse told the doctor a patient wanted to see him. The patient had a musculoskeletal injury related to tripping over her untied shoelace. The patient can't walk fully on her foot and is now limping. She also has a tissue injury: a wound infection.

Throughout the three sections of Unit 3, there are multiple opportunities to acquire vocabulary and grammar as well as to practice communication within the health context of the cardiovascular system. The unit progresses from a review of basic anatomy and physiology to identification, naming, and describing the normal functions of the systems and the failures/disorders that can affect them. There is an introduction to the language of diagnostics and assessments related to cardiovascular health and disease. Finally, the language of treatments, interventions, and assistance are explored through a case study of a patient with chest pain.

SECTION ONE | Anatomy and Physiology

In preparation for language studies of the anatomy and physiology of the cardiovascular and circulatory systems, the context of heart health in the United States and Canada is introduced. Culture, cultural context, and language cannot be separated and are important considerations when providing health care. This section offers exercises in medical and common terminology as it reviews the anatomy and physiology of the systems and the epidemiology of diseases affecting the systems.

Reading Selection 3-1

Read the following aloud or silently to yourself in preparation for the questions that follow.

NORTH AMERICAN HEALTH CONCEPTS

Heart disease in North America is a leading cause of death for men and women. Heart disease was once thought to affect men much more often than women, but this has changed dramatically over the past 50 years, affected by the changing lifestyles of women.

Coronary artery disease, commonly known as "hardening of the arteries," is a common disease/disorder of the cardiovascular system. It often leads to angina (chest pain) and to myocardial infarction (heart attack).

Many cases of cardiovascular diseases can be prevented. To maintain a healthy heart, physicians recommend limiting salt intake, quitting smoking, and eating a healthy diet full of fruits, vegetables, grains, fish, meats, and dairy products that are low in fat. In addition, a healthy weight and lifestyle should be maintained through inclusion of a program of regular exercise. Personal health promotion activities should include stress reduction exercises that help us cope with the increasingly busy and stressful demands of life in the 21st century.

READING EXERCISES

Understanding the general meaning of a reading passage and using it to increase your vocabulary are important steps in improving your use of the English language in health-care settings.

Understanding the General Meaning

Read the text again. Think about it. When you are ready, answer the following questions to ensure you have understood.

1) A myocardial infarction is sometimes referred to as an MI. What else is it called?

_____

2) What is another name for heart disease? _____

3) Do women suffer from heart attacks? _____

Building Vocabulary

Take a moment now to review what you have just read. Circle any words that are new to you. Write them down here for your own reference. In a moment, you may see them again in exercises that will help you understand their meaning. If not, at the end of this section, feel free to use your dictionary.

_____

_____

_____

Determining Meaning from Context. To build vocabulary, study the following words or terms taken from this text. Discover all you can about them by looking at them in context. Next, choose the correct meaning. Finally, take a look at how these words or terms expand in English.

1. Demographic *(adjective, sometimes used as noun)*

In context:
a) The current national demographic for heart disease identifies women over age 50 as at increasing risk for this diagnosis.
b) Demographic data for health and illness in the United States can be found through a variety of governmental and public resources.

Meaning: The word *demographic* can best be explained as meaning
a) types
b) data based on population size, characteristics, and vital statistics
c) criteria for distinguishing abnormalities
d) none of the above

Word expansion:
a) *Demography* is the study of traits within a population. (noun)
b) *Demographically* speaking, there are more French language speakers in the province of Quebec than anywhere else in Canada. (adverb)
c) *Demographic* studies show that the birth rate among native Europeans is declining. (adjective)
d) What are the *demographics* of the people living on this small island? (noun)

2. Coronary *(adjective)*

a) The patient had a major coronary and was admitted to the cardiac care unit this morning.
b) Diets high in fats can lead to blockage of the coronary arteries.

Meaning: The best description for the word *coronary* is
a) circular; a symbol of the shape of an artery
b) circular-shaped, hollow vessel, not flat
c) description of the arteries that supply the heart
d) both (a) and (b)

Word expansion:

a) The word *corona* refers to a circular shape that encircles an object. Its synonym is the word crown. (noun)

b) A *coroner* is a specialized health professional who investigates sudden, unusual, and/or suspicious deaths. The modern term for this person is medical examiner. (noun)

3. Cases *(noun, plural)*

In context:

a) Each year there are multiple cases of coronary occlusion diagnosed in this country. Surgery is often performed to treat the condition.

b) Severe cases of cardiovascular disease put the patient at risk for heart attack.

Meaning: The word *cases* can best be described as

a) types
b) incidents
c) crates
d) portables

Word expansion:

a) Mr. Brown's blocked arteries are a good *case* study for the medical students. (adjective modifying noun "study," but the two words together—case study—function as a noun, a term)

b) In *case* the coronary bypass surgery is not successful, Mr. Smith will have to return to the cardiac unit on life support equipment. (noun, object of preposition)

Using New Words in Sentences.   Use a key word from the previous exercise to create a new sentence.

1) The acronym CAD stands for _____.

2) They proper medical terminology for an MI is _____.

3) To prevent coronary artery disease, people should get involved in _____ promoting activities.

4) People who sit around a lot and do not get any exercise live a sedentary lifestyle. They are candidates for _____.

5) What would you as a health professional recommend to a patient who is quite sedentary?
_____

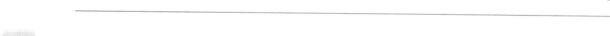

SPEAKING EXERCISE

Read the following completed sentences aloud. Ask a peer or teacher to help you with pronunciation. Proceed to the Pronunciation Hints section following. This will also help.

Coronary artery bypass surgery is sometimes called CABG. This abbreviation is pronounced "cabbage," just like the vegetable. The surgery is done to clear or re-route blood around blocked arteries.

PRONUNCIATION HINTS

coronary – **kor′**ō-nă-rē

myocardial – mī-ō-**kăr′**dē-ăl

angina – ăn-**jī′**nă

LISTENING EXERCISE

There are many American medical television shows. Some are fiction and others are documentaries. If you have access to these, please try to watch some. Invariably one of these shows will deal with heart disease. Listen closely to the vocabulary that describes the anatomy and physiology of the cardiovascular system.

WRITING EXERCISE—REFLECTIVE QUESTIONS

1) Use your new vocabulary. Write a sentence or two by combining new words and names (use the Word Bank below) in a meaningful way.

WORD BANK

coronary

myocardial infarction

cases

demographic

coronary artery disease

angina

2) The text talks about the changing lifestyles of women in North America over the past 50 years and suggests that this has caused a greater incidence of coronary artery disease. What are your thoughts about this? How does it compare with your country of origin? Write your reflections here.

Reading Selection 3-2

Read the following and answer the questions.

THE CARDIOVASCULAR SYSTEM OR CIRCULATORY SYSTEM?

The cardiovascular system is sometimes also referred to as the circulatory system, although they are not quite the same thing. The term cardiovascular speaks to the two parts of the system: *cardio* meaning heart and *vascular* meaning vessels. Anatomically, the major structures are the heart and blood vessels (arteries, veins, capillaries), but it is difficult to think of this system without including reference to the lungs (part of the respiratory system). The main function of the cardiovascular system is to distribute blood through blood vessels throughout the body. The main function of the heart is to pump the blood (to function as the engine of the cardiovascular system), beginning the process of circulation.

The heart consists of myocardial tissue and is divided into four chambers: two atria and two ventricles. The left and right atria are the two upper chambers of the heart, the left and right ventricles the two lower chambers. Blood that is high in oxygen (oxygenated) flows into the left atrium from the lungs through the pulmonary veins. The left atrium then contracts to pump a supply of blood to the left ventricle. The aorta is found in the left ventricle. It branches into a complex series of arteries that bring oxygenated blood to all of the organs of the body. When the blood reaches the capillaries, it delivers oxygen and in exchange picks up the waste product carbon dioxide to carry away through veins back to the heart. This blood in the veins empties first into the vena cava (the main vein in the human body), which then carries it to the right side of the heart. Next, this blood is pumped through the pulmonary artery to the lungs where it exchanges the carbon dioxide waste for a new supply of oxygen. The cycle then repeats. This cycle is powered by the contraction of the heart, which is caused by electrical impulses within the heart. The contraction of the heart is known as the heartbeat.

The circulatory system is a subsystem of the cardiovascular system. It concerns itself with blood and the function of blood, but it is difficult to think of the circulatory system without thinking about the lymphatic system. They are essential to each other. Lymph cells assist in cleansing the blood of dead cells and bacteria. Blood is the mode of transport for lymph, nutrients, hormones, electrolytes, gases (oxygen and carbon dioxide), water, and wastes to and from cells. The capillaries are the site of this exchange between the blood and the tissues that surround them. Blood also helps stabilize body temperature and the natural pH balance.

In summary, the cardiovascular system is most often thought of in terms of the heart, blood vessels, and the lungs. The circulatory system is most often thought of as the blood vessels, blood, lymph, and the heart.

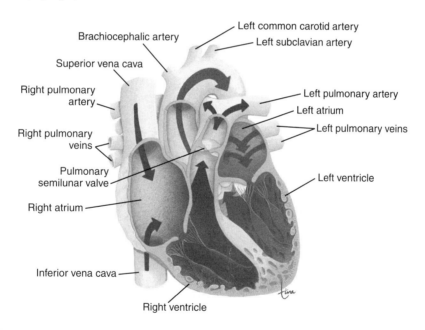

READING EXERCISES

Asking and answering specific questions about the reading selection will help you realize how much you have really understood as well as help you build your vocabulary.

Understanding the General Meaning

Read the text again. Think about it. Do you understand it? Try to answer the following questions to see if you do.

1) What does the heart do? _____

2) What is the function of the circulatory system? _____

3) What are the major structures of the cardiovascular system? _____

4) *Atria* is the plural form of this word. What is the singular form? _____

5) What is the genre or social purpose of this reading? _____

Building Vocabulary

The following exercises will help you in understanding the parts and functions of the circulatory system. Box 3-1 provides a mix-and-match exercise.

Mix and Match

BOX 3-1 Mix and Match: Parts of the Heart

To build vocabulary, study the following words or terms taken from this text. Choose the correct meaning by connecting each part of the heart with its function. Be careful. There is one word here you may not be familiar with. Match all of the vocabulary you can, first. When you have accomplished that, you will discover the meaning of the last one.

PART OF HEART	FUNCTION
right and left ventricles	wall dividing the heart down the middle
aorta	carries blood back to heart from the lungs
pulmonary vein	the body's main vein
septum	lower chambers of the heart
vena cava	the heart's main artery
left atrium	receives oxygenated blood from lungs

Sentence Completion.   Use a key word from the previous exercises to create a new sentence about the functions of the circulatory system.

1) An artery takes the blood _____.

2) The function of the heart is to _____.

3) The heart _____ to pump blood into the system.

4) Capillaries are very small blood vessels. They are located _____.

5) A vein functions to _____.

SPEAKING EXERCISE

Return to the last two exercises and read them aloud. Ask a peer or teacher to help you with pronunciation. Proceed to the Pronunciation Hints for help.

PRONUNCIATION HINTS

aorta – ā-**or**'tă

circulatory – **sĭr**"kū-lă-tōr'ē

cardiovascular – kăr"dē-ō-**văs**'kū-lăr

ventricle – **vĕn**'trĭk-l

pulmonary – **pŭl**'mō-nĕ-rē

atrium – **a**'trē-ŭm

vena cava – vē'nă -**kā**'vă

The Cardiovascular System

LISTENING EXERCISE

If you would like to hear a native English speaker talking about the circulatory system, try this online site: Oracle Think Quest Foundation, Library. Please note that this site is designed for school children. Audio references are limited, but they are helpful for the English language learner. Please also note the speakers may have British accents. http://library.thinkquest.org/28807/data/parofcir.htm

WRITING EXERCISE

Complete the simple diagrams related to the cardiovascular system shown below. Identify the process or path of each by naming each step as it occurs in a healthy human being. Fill in the blanks.

Your heart pumps in two ways:

a) Deoxygenated blood from your body moves into the vena cava and enters the heart this way . . .

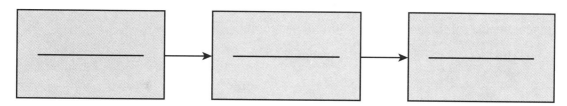

b) Oxygenated blood from the lungs enters the heart this way . . .

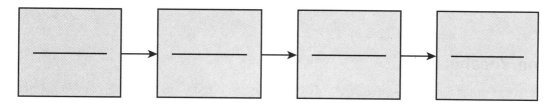

SECTION TWO # Assessing Function and Failure of the Cardiovascular/ Circulatory System

The health of the cardiovascular/circulatory system is critically important. In this section, assessment of the function and failure of the system is discussed using the language of measuring pulse and blood pressure. Assessment vocabulary includes an introduction to pathophysiological conditions with examples of congestive heart failure, angina, and myocardial infarction. There are opportunities for describing and reporting.

Reading Selection 3-3

Read the following aloud or silently.

PHYSIOLOGY OF THE PULSE

When the left ventricle of the heart contracts, it forces blood into the aorta and from there a wave of blood surges through the arteries. This wave is called a pulse. Pulse is measured in *beats per minute (bpm)*. The pulse can be palpated at various sites on the body where an artery crosses over a bony prominence. These include the radial (wrist), popliteal (knee), dorsal pedalis (foot), and carotid (neck) pulse sites. A rapid pulse (tachycardia) and a slow pulse (bradycardia) are examples of variations in rate. In each of these cases, the rhythm of the pulse is referred to as irregular, meaning the interval between each beat is not equal in length.

 # READING EXERCISES

The reading Physiology of the Pulse provides a clear example of the structure of the descriptive genre. This genre is actually a subset of the factual genre; it describes a person, place, or thing. Health professionals are expected to provide oral and written descriptions of a multitude of assessments throughout their work day. These descriptions must be succinct and clearly stated. An informative descriptive style is used. To write an informative description of the pulse in one paragraph, certain grammatical elements must be included. These are detailed in Box 3-2.

Understanding the General Meaning

Read the text again. Think about it. Do you understand it?

1) Who is the intended audience of this reading?

_____

2) What is the function or social purpose of the reading?

_____

3) What is the main theme or thesis of this reading?

_____

Building Vocabulary

As you learn to discern the meaning of words from their context, you increase your vocabulary and ability to use the proper and commonly used, terminology in health-care settings.

Determining Meaning from Context.   To build vocabulary, study the following words taken from the reading. Discover all you can about them by looking at them in context. Then, choose the correct meaning. Finally, take a look at how these words expand in English.

1. Surges *(verb, singular)*

In context:
a) Once the tourniquet is released, blood surges back out through the wound.
b) The blood of kings surges through Prince William's veins.

BOX 3-2 A Descriptive Report

a) The first sentence or phrase should inform the reader of the topic that is about to be described. It should also try to engage the reader's interest.

b) A series of sentences that each provides some detail or details about different aspects of the topic. Adjectives and medical descriptors are required.

c) The present tense is used.

Note: Opinions should not be included in an informative description.

The Cardiovascular System

Meaning: The verb *surges* is best described as meaning
a) to move very, very slowly
b) to rise and fall as if in waves
c) to thin out
d) both (a) and (c)

Word expansion:
a) There have been heavy rains this spring. The river *is surging* over its banks. (verb, present continuous)
b) After the candidate's speech, the crowd *surged* forward to congratulate him. (verb, past tense)
c) The *surge* in voter registration surprised all the candidates and their advisers. (noun)

2. Pulse *(noun)*

In context:
a) The patient's pulse is 120 and bounding.
b) I'm worried about Joaquim. I can barely feel his pulse.

Meaning: The word *pulse* can best be described as
a) a pressure wave that travels through the arteries
b) plural for pills
c) something babies don't have
d) slang for "please"

Word expansion:
a) The nurse could feel the patient's artery *pulsating* very quickly. (gerund, used as adjective)

3. Palpated *(verb, past tense)*

In context:
a) I palpated the pulse at the wrist.
b) The doctor palpated the liver when the patient was lying down.

Meaning: The word *palpate* can best be described as
a) to sound out
b) to run
c) to examine by touch/to feel
d) to draw a diagram

Word expansion:
a) The doctor uses the technique of *palpation* on the external surface of the body to assess the internal organs. (noun)
b) The carotid pulse is easily felt by hand. It is *palpable*. (adjective)
c) Today in nursing school I learned *to palpate* a pedal pulse. (verb, infinitive)

4. Site *(noun)*

In context:
a) There was a fire at the site of the accident.
b) There is a lot of bleeding at the site of the wound.

Meaning: The word *site* can best be described as
a) location or position
b) vision
c) giving a reason
d) a symbol

Word expansion:
a) I accurately *sited* the deltoid muscle before giving the injection. (verb, past tense)
b) Accurate *siting* for all injections is essential to good medication administration. (gerund, used as noun)

5. Prominence *(noun)*

In context:

a) A pulse can be taken where an artery is near a bone or bony prominence.

b) The ankle is a bony prominence.

Meaning: The word *prominence* can best be described as meaning

a) very famous

b) an organ that can be palpated

c) a projection or point

d) a broken bone

Word expansion:

a) David got an ulcer under his cast where the bony *prominence* of his ankle was rubbing it. (noun)

b) The Adam's apple is also known as the *prominentia laryngea.* (noun)

c) A promontory is a piece of land that juts out into the sea. (noun)

d) He is a *prominent* political leader. (adjective)

e) She was featured *prominently* in the news report. (adverb)

6. Tachycardia *(noun)*

In context:

a) Just prior to his heart attack, Mr. Hussein experienced tachycardia and shortness of breath.

b) If I run up a hill, I sometimes get tachycardia.

Meaning: *Tachycardia* is best described as

a) slow heart beat

b) rapid heart rate of over 100 beats/min even at rest

c) lack of oxygen

d) pulse under 50 beats/min

Word expansion:

a) The heart rate has been up for 20 minutes. The patient is tachycardic. (adjective)

7. Bradycardia *(noun)*

In context:

a) This patient's heart rate is 60/min. He has bradycardia.

b) Sometimes the elderly suffer from bradycardia.

Meaning: The term *bradycardia* is best described as

a) a slow heart or pulse rate under 60/min

b) racing heart rate over 100/min

c) a broken, irregular heart beat

d) none of the above

Word expansion:

a) Mrs. Anderson, 84 years old, has had a heart rate of <50/min for 2 days now. She is *bradycardic.* (adjective)

Mix and Match.   The mix-and-match exercises provided in Box 3-3 and Box 3-4 will help you learn the terms used to describe pulse sites and pulse characteristics.

SPEAKING EXERCISE

As health professionals, you will be familiar with the data in this box. However, you may not be familiar with how to write the information in a patient's chart. Study that here in Table 3-1.

BOX 3-3 Mix and Match: Terminology for Pulse Sites

This exercise asks you to name where pulses are taken using the proper medical terminology. Draw a line from the term on the right to its description on the left.

LOCATION (SITE)	PROPER TERM FOR SITE
behind the knee	apical
at the wrist along the thumb side	dorsal pedalis
under the nipple on the left side of chest	carotid
on the top of the foot	radial
under the jaw	popliteal

BOX 3-4 Mix and Match: Pulse Descriptors

Complete this exercise by matching the descriptive medical term with its description.

DESCRIPTIVE TERM	DESCRIPTION
thready	racing very quickly
pulse	rate, rhythm; rhythmic beat of the heart and blood vessels
faint	rhythm is erratic
slow	rhythm is not as quick as it should be; often found in the elderly
rapid	fine; scarcely perceptible
irregular	very hard to hear; weak
bounding	normal rhythm and rate; equal force and frequency of pulse wave
regular	jumping or bouncing; big beats

Read each of the normal pulse ranges aloud in full sentences. The Pronunciation Hints below will help. Follow this example:

The normal pulse rate for a baby ranges from 120 to 140 beats per minute. My patient is a baby. His pulse is 122 beats per minute (bpm).

Table 3-1 Normal Pulse Rates and How to Chart Them		
AGE RANGE	NORMAL PULSE	SAMPLE OF HOW TO CHART PULSE
Babies (1–11 months)	12–140 beats per minute (bpm)	P = 122/min*
Toddlers (2–5 years)	100–110 bpm	P = 110/min
Children	95–110 bpm	P = 108/min
Adults	80–100 bpm	P = 88/min
Elderly	60–80 bpm	P = 76/min

* Equals symbol (=) may be omitted.

LISTENING EXERCISE

At this point in *Medical English Clear and Simple* you have some homework again. You are encouraged to speak to a native English-speaking health professional if you know one or to watch an English language television show or film set in an American health-care setting. Listen.

WRITING EXERCISE

Here is a script that you can use with a patient. It uses the proper question-and-answer format for the United States and Canada. Fill in the blanks.

Student A: Hi, my name is _____. I'd like to_____ your pulse. Please _____ me your arm. Thank you.

Student B: Here it is . . . . OK, what is my pulse, please, nurse?

Student A: It's 88. That's 88 _____ per minute.

Student B: _____ that normal?

Student A: Let me think. Your chart says you _____ 33 years old._____ that right?

Student B: Yes.

Student A: Right. Thank you. Your pulse _____ normal.

Reading Selection 3-4

Read the following aloud or silently to yourself.

BLOOD PRESSURE

Blood pressure refers to the pressure of the blood within the arteries. When the left ventricle of the heart contracts, blood is forced out into the aorta and travels through the large arteries to the smaller arteries, arterioles, and capillaries. When the left ventricle contracts and pumps blood into the aorta, force is exerted on the arterial wall. This force is referred to as systolic pressure. When the heart is in the process of filling, the ventricle relaxes. The change in arterial pressure that results as the ventricle relaxes is called the diastolic pressure.

Blood pressure is assessed using a sphygmomanometer. This piece of equipment is commonly called a blood pressure cuff or cuff. Blood pressure is measured in millimeters of mercury (Hg). It is usually stated as a fraction—systolic over diastolic—as in 110 over 70. It is also written in fraction form, 110/70.

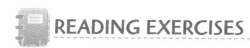

READING EXERCISES

As you increase your English vocabulary of both medical and common terms used in the health-care setting, you will increase your ability to answer specific questions as well as to have a general understanding of the meaning of a reading passage or conversation.

Understanding the General Meaning

Read the text again. Think about it. Do you understand it?
   What is the topic of the text?

_____

_____

Building Vocabulary

Take a moment now to review what you have just read. Jot down any words that you do not yet understand. Refer to this list throughout the section to see if you can discover the meaning from the exercises.

_____

_____

Determining Meaning from Context.   To build your vocabulary of medical terms, study the following words or terms taken from this text. Notice that seemingly common words are being used slightly differently in the medical context. Study this and then choose the correct meaning. Finally, take a look at how these words or terms expand in English.

1. Pressure *(noun)*

In context:
a) Physical activity causes the heart to work under pressure.
b) Blood moving through the arteries flows under pressure.

Meaning:
The term *pressure* is best described as
a) stress or force exerted on a body by tension, weight, or pulling
b) pulse is running too fast
c) circulation
d) congestive heart failure

Word expansion:
a) The nurse *pressed* down on the wound to help stop the bleeding. (verb, past tense)
b) After scuba diving in very deep waters, the swimmer had to be *depressurized* in a special tank. (verb)
c) Atmospheric *pressure* is the weight of the atmosphere. (noun)
d) Diastolic *pressure* is arterial pressure during dilatation of the heart chambers. (noun; used with adjective "diastolic," it is a term identifying a specific variable)
e) The air *was pressurized* in the cabin of the spacecraft. (verb, past tense)

2. Reflects *(verb)*

In context:
a) The mirror reflects my lovely image.

Meaning: The word *reflects* means

a) turning back on itself

b) bending your knee

c) having your eyes examined

d) massage therapy

Word expansion:

a) The *reflection* I see in the mirror in the morning isn't pretty. (noun)

b) Water is *reflected* off the skin. (verb, past tense)

3. Force *(noun)*

In context:

a) I must exert some force to move this table.

b) He punched the other man with a great deal of force.

Meaning: The word *force* can best be described as

a) lack of strength

b) pincers for holding things in surgery

c) use of a certain amount of strength and energy

d) a part of your skin

Word expansion:

a) Dr. Jacobs is very *forceful* when he gives orders. (adjective)

b) *Forcing* the elbow to bend will only injure it. (gerund, used as noun, subject of sentence)

c) He *forced* his way into the house with the intent of robbery. (verb, past tense)

4. Relaxation *(noun)*

In context

a) The muscle is no longer in contraction, it is in relaxation.

b) I am so glad I don't have a cramp and the muscle finally relaxed.

Meaning: *Relaxation* means

a) a lessening of tension or activity of a part

b) sleeping all day

c) abduction

d) painful

Word expansion:

a) If I think about it, I *can relax* the muscles in my shoulders. (verb, present tense)

b) Having a foot massage is very *relaxing*. (adjective)

c) You may need physiotherapy *to relax* the muscle in your arm and open up the elbow. (verb, infinitive)

Using New Words to Answer Questions.   Use vocabulary in the readings about the anatomy and physiology of the cardiovascular system and blood pressure to answer these questions. Use full sentences.

1) What must contract before blood can flow into the blood vessels?

_____

_____

2) How is blood forced out of the heart and into circulation?

_____

3) To take a pulse, palpate the veins. To take a blood pressure, locate and listen to what?

_____

The Cardiovascular System

SPEAKING EXERCISE

Read the following completed sentences aloud. Ask a peer or teacher to help you with pronunciation. Proceed to the Pronunciation Hints section following. This will also help.

High blood pressure can be caused by extreme emotional stress and by excessive sodium intake.

Postural hypotension (a drop in blood pressure) can occur when someone stands up too quickly.

PRONUNCIATION HINTS

diastolic – **dī**-ăs-tŏl'ĭk

systolic – sĭs-**tŏl'**ĭk

arterial – ăr-**tē'**rē-ăl

LISTENING EXERCISE

Find an opportunity to take someone's blood pressure. Listen. Then try to name what you hear using new vocabulary.

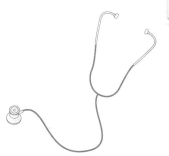

WRITING EXERCISE

Use these pictures to write one or two sentences explaining what is happening. Use full complete sentences and punctuation. Use proper medical terminology whenever possible. You may want to use the names of equipment.

_____

_____

_____

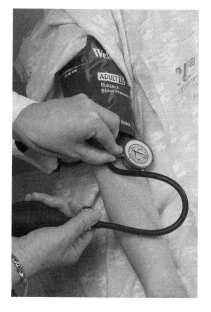

Reading Selection 3-5

Read the following aloud or silently.

CONGESTIVE HEART FAILURE

In common terms, *failure* means an inability to do something, to succeed at something, or to produce something. This meaning of the word is somewhat different in medicine. In medical terms, *failure* means a state of insufficiency or an inability of an organ or other body part to function the way it should at its expected level. It is very important for health professionals to recognize the inclusion of the word "insufficiency" here when they prepare to work with clients or patients who have had a diagnosis of congestive heart failure, kidney failure, or something similar. Failure does not simply mean that function ceases. A person can live with organ failure, but, for example, when a machine fails its life may very well be finished.

Congestive heart failure (CHF) is the inability of the heart to supply adequate amounts of blood, oxygen, and nutrients to the body. Blood backs up in the heart and then into the lungs. Once the lungs become swollen with fluid, the normal exchange of oxygen and carbon dioxide that takes place within them is affected. The patient may appear short of breath. The lungs may sound like they gurgle when you listen to them.

READING EXERCISES

It is important for health professionals to understand and be able to use not only medical terms but also the terms commonly used by patients.

Understanding the General Meaning

Read the text again. Have you understood it? It was written in quite normal, everyday English. Now read about congestive heart failure again, but this time the reading selection is written in a form that uses proper medical terminology.

CONGESTIVE HEART FAILURE

Heart failure is a term used in medicine to reflect the inability of the heart to pump blood with normal efficiency to meet the demands of the body to function normally or under exertion. A myocardial infarction, or heart attack, often decreases the strength of contraction of the left ventricle of the heart so that the heart fails to pump effectively. The etiology, or cause, of a myocardial infarction (MI) may include coronary artery disease (CAD), heart valve disease, hypertension, or a combination of these factors. When the left ventricle of the heart is damaged and not able to pump blood efficiently, the vessels in the lungs become edematous (swollen with blood). This leads to pulmonary congestion. A plasma leak into the alveoli and bronchial walls results when excessive back pressure in the capillaries of the lungs co-occurs. This is the condition of pulmonary edema. It interferes with normal oxygen and carbon dioxide exchange. A diagnosis of congestive heart failure is made in the presence of pulmonary congestion and pulmonary edema associated with heart-related causes.

1) Reflection: Compare your ability to comprehend the first reading with this one. What was your experience with both written texts? What does this tell you about your level of skill and competency with English for medical purposes? Take a moment to self-reflect and self-evaluate.

_____

_____

2) When the heart stops beating, what is this condition called?

_____

3) When the heart stops beating efficiently, what is this condition called?

_____

4) Congestive heart failure involves two major organs in the body. What are they?

_____

5) Pulmonary edema and pulmonary congestion associated with heart insufficiency leads to which diagnosis?

_____

6) If you have a diagnosis of congestive heart failure, has your heart stopped?

_____

Building Vocabulary

Vocabulary can be built by determining the meaning of a word from its context and from deduction using your previous professional knowledge.

Determining Meaning from Context. To build vocabulary, study the following words or terms taken from this text. Discover all you can about them by looking at them in context. Choose the correct meaning. Finally, take a look at how these words or terms expand in English.

1. Contraction *(noun)*

In context:
a) When the muscle of the heart is shortening or tightening, it is in contraction.
b) A contraction occurs when a muscle tightens.

Meaning: The word *contraction* can best be described as
a) a condition or process
b) an illness
c) painful
d) not normal

Word expansion
a) My hand *contracts* to hold an orange. (verb, present tense)
b) After Mr. Smith's stroke, his left hand *contracted*. Now he cannot open it. (verb, past tense)
c) Mr. Smith has a *contracture* in his left hand because he had a cerebral vascular accident. (noun)

2. Pump *(verb)*

In context:
a) The heart pumps blood through the body.
b) The heart is a pump. It fills up with blood and then releases it.

Meaning: The word *pump* can best be explained as
a) something that compresses fluids or moves them in and out of an area
b) the action of a hand on a lever
c) a motor
d) both (a) and (b)

Word expansion:
a) When the heart stops *pumping*, the patient will die. (gerund used as a noun)

3. Damaged *(verb, past tense)*

In context:
a) He had a severe heart attack. He's lucky he lived. Now his heart is damaged.
b) I damaged my wristwatch. I wore it in the water. It's very slow now.

Meaning: The word *damaged* can best be explained as
a) destroyed
b) harm caused by injury
c) useless
d) recovered

Word expansion:
a) Be careful not *to damage* your eyesight. Read with the lights on. (verb, infinitive)
b) There was serious *damage* to the car after the head-on collision. (noun)

4. Swollen *(past participle of "swell," adjective)*

In context:

a) After a long day, my ankles are swollen.

b) The vessel is swollen because it is occluded. It is full of fluid.

Meaning:

The word *swollen* can best be described as meaning

a) enlarged or full

b) broken

c) painful

d) discolored

Word expansion:

a) If you sprain your ankle, you will probably see it start *to swell* quickly. (verb, infinitive)

b) Applying ice to a sprained or strained muscle will reduce the *swelling*. (gerund used as noun)

c) Your feet *swell* when you have poor circulation. (verb, present tense)

d) Jack is allergic to lobster. When he eats it, his throat *swells* shut. (verb, present tense)

5. Back pressure *(noun; term)*

In context:

a) A vein is blocked and blood is appearing in the intravenous line because of the back pressure.

b) The garden hose has a knot in it. The water cannot get through. Back pressure builds behind the knot, causing the hose to move by itself.

Meaning: The term *back pressure* can best be explained as

a) seepage

b) pressure building up because fluids cannot continue to circulate

c) pain in the thoracic-lumbar area due to back injury

6. Plasma *(noun)*

In context:

a) Quickly! Let's get that patient started on some plasma. She's going into shock.

b) The patient has lost a lot of blood. He needs plasma quickly.

Meaning: *Plasma* can best be described as

a) blood

b) watery part of the blood that carries blood cells and nutrients and removes the waste products of metabolism

c) a type of food that can save your life

d) glucose in the blood

Word expansion:

a) A *plasmacyte* is a plasma cell found in connective tissue. (noun)

b) We will begin *plasmatherapy* immediately because the patient is going into shock. (noun)

c) Patients with certain disorders may be treated with *plasmapheresis*, a procedure in which cellular and other components of the blood are removed and the plasma returned to the body. (noun)

7. Alveoli *(noun, plural)*

In context:

a) Pulmonary alveoli are found in the lungs.

b) Inflammation of the alveoli can lead to a cough.

Meaning: *Alveoli* can best be described as
a) the air cells of the lungs
b) viruses
c) airborne droplets
d) organs in the chest

Word expansion:
a) An *alveolus* is a small hollow, cavity, or pocket. (noun, singular)
b) When the bronchioles and pulmonary *alveoli* are inflamed, you have bronchopneumonia or *alveobronchitis* (noun, plural; noun, singular)
c) *Alveolitis* is an inflammation of the *alveoli*. (noun, singular; noun, plural)
d) The *alveolar* duct is a branch of a bronchiole that leads to the alveoli of the lungs. (adjective, modifying "duct," but the two words together function as a noun, a term for a body part)

8. Bronchial *(adjective)*

In context:
a) Can you hear that? She has a real bronchial cough.
b) The bronchial tree contains bronchi and bronchial tubes.

Meaning:
The word *bronchial* can best be explained as
a) part of the urinary system
b) coughing
c) a description of part of the air passage into the lungs
d) asthma

Word expansion:
a) Do you have *bronchitis*? (noun)
b) The patient coughs, has difficulty breathing, and expectorates secretions in the morning. He has *bronchiectasis*. (noun)

> **VOCABULARY ALERT** Note the difference between a sign and a symptom in medicine.
> A *sign* is something you see. You can observe it.
> A *symptom* is something you experience. It can be identified through the patient's subjective report or through objective reports from laboratory tests and may meet criteria for illnesses, disorders, or diseases.

Mix and Match. Based on your own professional knowledge as a nurse, doctor, or other health professional, try to match the visible signs of an acute, immediate incident of CHF with its symptoms in Box 3-5. You will have gathered much of this vocabulary from this and previous chapters in this book.

SPEAKING EXERCISE

Read the following completed sentences aloud. Ask a peer or teacher to help you with pronunciation. Proceed to the Pronunciation Hints section following. This will also help.

Bob is 35 years old and is diagnosed with chronic alcoholism. He also has congestive heart failure. He was admitted to your unit in the hospital today with difficulty breathing. You notice he has audible breath sounds. He is wheezing. You notice he is mouth breathing. This is a sign that he is having difficulty filling his lungs. When he breathes, you also hear some gurgling sounds. This tells you that there is

BOX 3-5 Mix and Match: Signs and Symptoms of Congestive Heart Failure

Complete this exercise by matching the sign with its symptom.

SIGN	SYMPTOM
confusion	a raspy sound made when breathing
pallor	ashen color to skin
cyanosis	lack of oxygen in blood; symptoms such as blue lips
panic	not clear about time, place, person, activity
frothy sputum	rapid, shallow respirations
altered breathing pattern	unable to sit still
wheezing	extreme state of fear and desperation (for air and survival)
air hunger	behavior or gulping or seeming to try to eat the air: result of lack of O_2
restless	bubbly: white or pink with bubbles
mouth breathing and gasping	inability to get sufficient oxygen through normal breathing through nose

fluid on his lungs. You know these are signs of an acute episode of congestive heart failure.

PRONUNCIATION HINTS

congestive – kŏn-**jĕs′tĭ**v

wheezing – **hwēz**-ĭng

breath – **brĕth**

breathe – **brēth**

breathing – **brēth**-ĭng

frothy – **frawth**-ē

sputum – **spū′tŭm**

bronchial – **brŏng′kē**-ăl

alveoli – ăl-vē′**ō**-lī

LISTENING EXERCISE

Go online to the Cardiovascular Multimedia Information Network. Listen to the doctors talking about the heart and heart disease. Click on the menus on the left and right side of the page for audio clips. Listen carefully for pronunciation. Find this site at http://www.cvmd.org/

WRITING EXERCISE

Use your new vocabulary. Complete the following sentences. Use medical terminology whenever possible.

1) Heart failure is _____.

2) Gas exchange occurs when _____
_____.

3) Congestion is _____
_____.

4) When the heart pumps, it _____
_____.

5) Another way of saying the heart is damaged is to say _____
_____.

6) Another term for myocardial infarction is _____.

7) The word pulmonary refers to _____.

Reading Selection 3-6

Read the following description of angina and myocardial infarction. You will see much of the vocabulary you have acquired throughout Unit 3. You will also see the two new terms defined and described.

ANGINA AND MYOCARDIAL INFARCTION

Angina is a type of chest pain. It is caused by a narrowing of the arteries. Sometimes when the heart is asked to pump harder in response to physical or emotional stress, the coronary arteries cannot supply enough oxygen to the heart muscle. The result can be chest pain or angina pectoris.

When the heart is deprived of oxygen for too long, a myocardial infarction occurs. Oxygen-deprived cells die. Again, chest pain is experienced. An MI (heart attack) is usually caused by a progressive narrowing of the coronary arteries. Blockage or occlusion of an artery can occur suddenly. It may be the result of a thrombus (blood clot) or an embolus (a plug of organic or foreign matter, air, bacteria, or a dislodged thrombus).

READING EXERCISES

Understanding the General Meaning

Read the text again. Think about it. Do you understand it? What is the general purpose of the text?

_____

_____

Comprehending Specifics

1) What is the etiology (cause) of angina?

_____

2) Angina is actually a symptom. Describe the symptom using only two words.

_____

3) What is the etiology of a myocardial infarction?

_____

Building Vocabulary

Demonstrate that you really understand the meaning of new words you have learned. Try these exercises.

Determining Meaning from Context. To build vocabulary, study the following words or terms taken from this text. Discover all you can about them by looking at them in context, then choose the correct meaning. Finally, take a look at how these words or terms expand in English.

1. Arteries *(noun, plural)*

In context:
a) Hardening of the arteries is also known as atheriosclerosis.
b) An artery carries oxygenated blood from the heart to tissues of the body.

Meaning: The word *arteries* can best be described as
a) tubes
b) vessels of transportation
c) veins

Word expansion:
a) A word that begins with the prefix "arterio-" signifies a relationship to an *artery*. (Greek suffix; noun)
b) *Artheriopathy* is any disease of the arteries. (noun)
c) If your arteries begin to narrow, this is called *arteriostenosis*. (noun)

2. Oxygen *(noun)*

In context:
a) We breathe oxygen.
b) Plants breathe carbon dioxide and release oxygen.

Meaning: The word *oxygen* can best be described as
a) a gas essential for respiration by plants and animals
b) a toxic chemical
c) a pituitary hormone

Word expansion:
a) Newborn babies need to be *oxygenated*. (verb)
b) *Oxyhemoglobin* is found in arterial blood and is the compound that carries oxygen to the cells of the body. (noun)
c) *Oxygenated* blood is carried from the heart to the organs of the body via the arteries. (adjective)
d) *Deoxygenated* blood is carried through veins from the body cells back to the heart. (adjective)

3. Deprived *(verb, past tense)*

In context:
a) A baby who is deprived of oxygen at birth may be cognitively impaired.
b) Do you ever feel deprived of love and affection?

Meaning: The verb *deprived* can be described as meaning
a) missing
b) taken away or being kept away from something
c) forgotten

Word expansion:
a) Oxygen *deprivation* can lead to brain damage. (noun)
b) *Depriving* your pet dog of food is cruel. (gerund used as noun, continuous)

Using New Words in Sentences. Use the words in parentheses plus a few of your own to create a new sentence.

1) Cassandra has an _____ (beat, disease, irregular)

2) Devon has suffered two minor _____. He has _____ and is on the _____. (heart, cardiac care unit, attacks, atherosclerosis)

SPEAKING EXERCISE

Go back to the reading entitled Angina and Myocardial Infarction. Read it aloud to yourself first slowly and then again and again with increasing speed. This exercise will help with fluency as well as help you overcome any hesitation you may have with speaking new vocabulary aloud. The Pronunciation Hints section below will help.

> **PRONUNCIATION HINTS**
>
> infarction – ĭn-**fǎrk**'shŭn
>
> angina – ăn-**jī**'nă

LISTENING EXERCISE

If you would like to hear more native English speakers from the United States talking about the aspects of the cardiovascular and circulatory systems, pulses, and blood pressure, search the television networks. There are many news and documentary shows dealing with this subject, as well as whole television series based on situations in hospitals that often reflect this subject matter. Listen carefully to hear many of the words you have just learned as well as the context of when, where, and how they are spoken. Listen for content, context, and structure of speech.

WRITING EXERCISE: A SHORT PERSONAL NARRATIVE

Use new vocabulary to write a short story about the last time you had your pulse and blood pressure taken. Where were you (the context) and who did the assessment?

_____

_____

_____

_____

_____

SECTION THREE Treatments, Interventions, and Assistance

Unit 3 has introduced the language of the cardiovascular/circulatory system and included vocabulary, grammar, and information on structure and function to assist health professionals in assessing signs and symptoms of healthy and unhealthy systems. In this section, that theme continues while it moves the reader into the language of care for an emergency cardiac case. Critical reflection reinforces a holistic perspective of care. Through a case study, language skills including reading comprehension; identifying salient features in assessment data; word expansion; vocabulary building; adjectives, adverbs, and descriptors for the patient chart; answering (short, specific, and long answer); and reporting clearly, concisely, and specifically are addressed. The process of assessment is introduced when the patient is admitted to hospital.

Reading Selection 3-7

Read the following in preparation for the exercises that follow. If possible, have a friend or classmate read one role while you read the other.

CALLING 911 FOR HELP

Operator: 911. What is your emergency?

Patient: Hello . . . I . . . um . . . I . . . uh . . . I'm having some bad pain in my chest.

Operator: Describe your chest pain to me, sir.

Patient: Oh . . . it's awful. Oh, it hurts . . . it's like . . . uh . . .

Operator: Are you having trouble breathing, sir?

Patient: Yes . . . oh, I'm sick. Help me.

Operator: Yes sir, I will. Have you been diagnosed with a heart problem?

Patient: No. Oh, please . . . help me!

Operator: Where are you calling from, sir?

Patient: I . . . um . . . uh . . . I'm at home at . . . um . . . 6565-188 Street.

Operator: 6565-188 Street? Is that correct, sir?

Patient: Yes.

Operator: All right. I'm going to send an ambulance right now. It's on its way. Try to remain calm.

Patient: Please . . . hurry . . . please!

Operator: Do you have any other symptoms, sir?

Patient: My arm . . . it's going numb.

Operator: Which arm, sir?

Patient: My left arm . . . oh . . . it's hard to catch my breath.

Operator: Try to remain calm. The ambulance will be there in a couple of minutes.

Patient: Yes, I'm trying . . . sick. . . . I feel sick. Hurts.

Operator: Are you alone, sir? Is there anyone there who can help you?

Patient: No. My wife is out.

Operator: Is the door unlocked? Is your front door unlocked so the paramedics can get in?

Patient: No . . . um . . . I don't know . . . um . . . I can't remember. I can't think straight! Oh. . . . please hurry!

Operator: Listen carefully, sir. Are you listening?

Patient: Yes, oh . . . yes. . . .

Operator: I want you to go to the front door and open it. Leave it open. Then come right back to me. Don't hang up the phone. Do you understand?

Patient: Oh . . . I don't know. I'm dizzy . . . it's hard.

Operator: Sir? Bear with me, sir. You've got to open the front door so the paramedics can get to you. Do you understand?

Patient: Uh, yes . . . paramedics . . . the door . . .

Operator: Yes, sir. Put the phone down and do that now. Open the door. Don't hang up. Come back and tell me.

Patient: Uh . . . oh. . . . OK. . . . um.................I did it . . . oh, the pain. I think I'm going to pass out . . . oh . . . they're here! Oh, thank God!

 # READING EXERCISES

While understanding the general meaning of a reading passage or conversation is important, it is also essential to be able to ask specific pertinent questions and respond appropriately to the answers given. These exercises will help you to do so.

Understanding the General Meaning

Read the text again. Think about it. Do you understand it? What is the general theme or subject of the text?

Answering Closed Questions

Understanding questions and the answers provided by patients and other health-care professionals is a very important part of effective communication. Table 3-2 summarizes the structure and function of questions. After looking at the table, take a moment to review the reading selection and answer the following questions.

> **GRAMMAR ALERT: CLOSED QUESTIONS** Closed questions are those that ask for a *yes, no, I don't know,* or *sometimes* response only.

1) Who is having chest pain? _____

2) What does the 911 operator do for a living? _____

Table 3-2 Structure and Function of Questions			
QUESTION WORD	AUXILIARY VERB	SUBJECT	MAIN VERB
who	did	he/she/it	call
where	does	he/she/it	live
why	has	he/she/it	called?
when	will	he/she/it	arrive?

3) The patient has numbness. Where? _____

4) Who is on the way to the house? _____

5) What is on the way to the house? _____

6) Who can't think clearly? _____

7) What does the operator want the patient to do to help himself? _____

8) What number do you call for fire, police, or medical emergencies? _____

9) Where is the patient's wife? _____

10) How is the 911 operator? _____

11) How is the patient when he is on the phone? _____

12) What sex is the patient? _____

13) Has the patient been diagnosed with a heart condition? _____

14) Does the patient get rescued? _____

Building Vocabulary

To build vocabulary, study the words or terms taken from this text. It is important to understand different words that may have the same meaning or a very similar meaning. It is also important to understand the difference between words that may seem similar (because of spelling or pronunciation). The following exercises will help you learn about similarities and distinctions between words.

Mix and Match. The mix-and-match exercise in Box 3-6 will help you learn about synonyms, or words with similar meanings.

BOX 3-6 Mix and Match: Synonyms

Find the synonym or description for the following words. Draw a line to connect them.

TERM FROM TEXT	SYNONYM OR DESCRIPTION
paramedic	pain
911	operator
difficulty breathing	shortness of breath
numbness	emergency telephone line
relax	ambulance attendant
telephone operator	no feeling
hurt	calm

Recognizing Related Words. Find three words that relate to the word printed in boldface. Be careful. Not all words belong.

1) **chest** thoracic breast deltoid dorsal
   upper body

2) **pain** ouch sleepy hurt throbs aches badly

3)	**operator**	construction worker	telephone employee	switchboard person	phone attendant	
4)	**right now**	tomorrow	sooner	later immediately	right away stat	
5)	**anyone**	everyone	someone	somebody	whomever	any person
6)	**numb**	paresthesia	dull	ache	frozen no feeling	no sensation
7)	**dizzy**	crazy	vertigo	unbalanced	sense of spinning	
8)	**hurry**	go quickly move quickly	be happy congratulations	proceed rapidly		
9)	**short of breath**	can't catch my breath	apnea	no oxygen	running	rapid, shallow breathing
10)	**bear with me**	please be patient and wait	stand by	hold this with me	lean on me	be patient a moment

Recognizing Word Distinctions. Accuracy in reading and writing is essential for health-care professionals. Do you know the difference between these words that look or sound very similar? Explain the following. Try to do so without the aid of a dictionary. Test yourself.

1) What is the difference between sweet and sweat?

_____

2) What is the difference between palpation and palpitation?

_____

3) What is the difference between pallor and cyanosis?

_____

4) Grammatically, what is the difference between breathe and breath?

_____

5) What is the difference between numbness and tingling?

_____

6) What is the difference between nausea and vomiting?

_____

7) What is the difference between an ache and a pain?

_____

8) What is the difference between anxiety and apprehension?

_____

SPEAKING EXERCISE

Go back over the eight sentences you have just been working on. Read them aloud, paying strict attention to your pronunciation. Use the Pronunciation Hints below to help.

PRONUNCIATION HINTS

anxiety – āng-**zī'**ě-tē

sweat – **swĕt**

pallor – **pălʼ**or

numbness – **nŭm**-něs

LISTENING EXERCISE

Go back and record yourself doing the last exercise, then listen. Do not let the written words be your guide. Close your book while you listen. Evaluate yourself.

- What do you notice about your open pronunciation? _____
- Are you speaking clearly? _____
- Are you speaking at a normal rhythm and rate? _____

If you have not recorded yourself, ask a peer to read any part of this section aloud to you. Do NOT read along with them. Listen only. What do you notice about the way he or she speaks? What lesson do you learn from listening to another?

WRITING EXERCISE

Use words from the previous exercises to create new sentences.

1) The gentleman is experiencing _____.
2) Because the man is frightened, he cannot _____.
3) Paramedics don't work in hospitals; they _____.

Reading Selection 3-8

The following reading is a continuation of the last dialogue. Now, it is written as a case study in narrative form. Follow the story of the patient with chest pain.

ANGINA

On Friday, October 5th, Mr. Moore, a 56-year-old married man, was experiencing a great deal of pain in his chest. He was afraid he was having a heart attack. He was not sure. He knew that he had never been diagnosed nor treated for cardiovascular disease.

Mr. Moore knew enough to call 911 for emergency help. He gave his address as 6565-188 Street, Surrey, BC. While speaking with the operator, he was able to tell her he had numbness and tingling down his left arm, tightness and pain in his chest, and was having difficulty breathing. Mr. Moore reported that he was alone in the home, with no one to help him. The 911 operator advised him to put down the phone but not to hang it up. She directed him to unlock the door so the paramedics could get into the house without breaking the door down. He complied. The patient also mentioned that he was confused and unable to think clearly. He thought he was going to pass out. Luckily, the ambulance arrived in time to take him to the hospital.

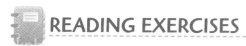

READING EXERCISES

The following exercises will help you understand the narrative genre.

Understanding the General Meaning

A narrative tells a story. It is usually written in chronological order and tells about something that has happened, is happening, or will happen. A central feature of the narrative is that it has a plot that engages the reader and makes them want to read on to find out how the story concludes.

1) What is the purpose of this narrative? What is the plot?

_____

2) How does the plot conclude in this narrative?

_____

3) In which tense is this narrative written?

_____

Understanding Specific Facts in a Reading

Take a moment now to review what you have just read. Answer the following questions.

1) What is the patient's name?_____

2) Was the patient able to provide his address?_____

3) Was the patient coherent? _____

4) Who was the operator speaking to?_____

5) Who might break down the front door? _____

6) Why might they break down the door? _____

7) Where was Mr. Moore going to be going? _____

8) How was the patient going to get to where he was going? _____

9) What were the patient's acute signs and symptoms? _____

10) Has Mr. Moore ever had a heart attack? _____

11) Mr. Moore was thinking clearly enough to do something. What was that?

_____

Building Vocabulary

It is important to learn not only new vocabulary words, but also to become familiar with commonly used terms and expressions.

Determining Meaning from Context. To build vocabulary, study the following words or expressions taken from this text. Discover all you can about them by looking at them in context. Next, choose the correct meaning of the word. Notice how many words expand but most expressions do not.

1. A great deal *(idiom/expression)*

In context:
a) The Queen of England has a great deal of money.
b) The patient with the broken hip is in a great deal of pain.

Meaning: The expression *a great deal* can best be described as
a) a large quantity
b) a large amount
c) severe
d) both (a) and (b)

2. Knew enough *(idiom/expression, past tense)*

In context:
a) My children knew enough to put their boots on in the rain.
b) If I knew enough about the stock market, I would invest in it.

Meaning:
The expression *knew enough* can best be described as meaning
a) was too stupid
b) had enough information
c) appropriate risk taking behavior
d) too much knowledge

3. Directed *(verb, past tense)*

In context:
a) The doctor directed me to start an intravenous.
b) The visitors were lost in the hospital. I directed them to the ward.

Meaning: The verb *directed* can best be described as
a) guided, shown the way
b) guided, instructed, or shown the way
c) required to show
d) supervised or used authority

Word expansion:
a) As nurses and doctors, we are often in *direct* contact with communicable diseases. (adjective)
b) Many academic courses today are *self-directed* study. That means you must do it on your own, without a teacher present. (adjective)
c) My boss spoke to me *indirectly* about my absences from work. I got a memo instead of seeing her in person. (adverb)
d) I prefer to be spoken to *directly* by my colleagues, rather than hear gossip. (adverb)
e) I gave you a firm *directive* to get that intravenous started stat! (noun, meaning "order")

4. Breaking it down

In context:
a) The gastric secretions of the stomach are responsible for breaking down the foods.
b) Remember the Berlin Wall? Do you remember seeing people breaking it down on television?

Meaning: The term *breaking it down* can be best described as
a) violently taking something apart
b) reducing something to pieces or parts
c) stopping a chain reaction
d) a chaotic response to something
e) both (a) and (b)

Word expansion:

a) On the way to work this morning, my car *broke down*. I was late. (verb, past tense)

b) Give me a good mathematical problem and I will find someone else *to break it down* for you. I am terrible at math. (verb, infinitive)

c) That couple fights all the time. Their communication *is breaking down*. (verb, present continuous)

5. Complied *(verb, past tense)*

In context:

a) I complied with the requirements of nursing school and was able to complete the program.

b) The patient complied with taking antibiotics for 7 days and is now feeling recovered.

Meaning: The verb *complied* can best be described as meaning

a) hoped for

b) conformed; followed through with required tasks

c) followed up

d) committed

Word expansion:

a) I *will comply* with your demands to work overtime, only if you pay me double-time. (verb, future conditional)

b) When Mary *complies* with her husband's wishes, she does so because she wants to, not because she has to. (verb, present tense)

c) To get *compliance* with a prescribed medication, you must teach the patient about the importance of taking it correctly. (noun)

6. Think clearly *(expression)*

In context:

a) George can think clearly now. His fever is gone.

b) Sometimes I need silence in order to think clearly.

Meaning: The expression *think clearly* can best be described as meaning

a) ability to problem solve

b) ability to put thoughts in logical order

c) thought processing

d) cognition

Word expansion:

a) Fred *was thinking clearly* when he bought his car. He paid cash instead of credit. (verb, past progressive)

b) *Try to think clearly*. Where did you put your house keys? (verb, infinitive)

7. Going to pass out *(idiom/expression; verb)*

In context:

a) Uh-oh, Paulo drank too much beer. He is going to pass out.

b) The pain is so severe that the patient is going to pass out.

Meaning: The term *to pass out* can best be described as meaning

a) faint or fall unconscious

b) get dizzy

c) suffer vertigo

d) go into a coma

Word expansion:

a) Monica *passed out* when she saw the dead body. (verb, past tense)

b) Please open a window. I think Mrs. Hill *is going to pass out*. (verb infinitive)

8. Arrived in time *(idiom)*

In context:

a) The ambulance arrived in time to save Mr. Moore's life.

b) The baby arrived in time. It was born exactly when the doctor predicted.

Meaning: The expression *arrived in time* can best be described as meaning

a) occurred on schedule

b) occurred spontaneously

c) was serendipitous

d) all of the above

Word expansion:

a) I hope the midwife *arrives on time*. They baby is ready. (verb, present)

Sentence Completion.   Refer to the words in the previous exercise to complete these fill-in-the-blank sentences.

1) The hospital has a *do not resuscitate* _____ available if patients do not wish to be saved in the event of a life-threatening situation.

2) When Mr. Moore arrived at the hospital, he tried to stand up but he almost _____.

3) After the Emergency Response Team _____ the door, they were able to rescue the elderly lady who had fallen and broken her hip.

4) After your door has _____ in an emergency, you will go to the hospital, but your house will remain open, unlocked, and unsecured.

SPEAKING EXERCISE

Read the narrative, again. Read it out loud. Try not to stop or hesitate as you do so. Repeat this until you can read the story at a normal pace, without hesitation. This exercise will help build confidence reading aloud. The Pronunciation Hints below will help.

> **PRONUNCIATION HINTS**
>
> tingling – **tĭng**′gl-ĭng
>
> resuscitate – rĭ-**sŭs**″ ĭ-tā′t

LISTENING EXERCISE

Emergency situations such as the one in this narrative are often the plot of American television shows. Try to find one on the TV or Internet. Or, you might like to search the Internet for an audio-visual clip. Try to find "How to Call 911 in an Emergency" by ExpertVillage.com (2006). If you visit their website, type the title into their Search bar. A series of short videos on this topic will appear, each narrated by a real 911 operator. Or, look for this same video on Google videos. Once again, type in the title. Listen for vocabulary related to this unit and section of *Medical English Clear and Simple*.

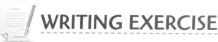

WRITING EXERCISE

Use your new vocabulary. Write a short story (narrative) about someone you know or have heard about who was at home and had to call an ambulance for help. Be sure to use the narrative format and check that you are using verbs in the proper tense to tell the story.

_____

_____

_____

_____

_____

_____

_____

Reading Selection 3-9

Once again, we are going to be considering the case of Mr. Moore after his arrival at the hospital. Read the following in preparation for this.

HEAD-TO-TOE ASSESSMENT

Head-to-toe assessment is the first priority of care when a patient arrives in the Emergency Department. This is a routine, expected method of data collection in American and Canadian health care. It provides an inclusive, logical, and systematic assessment of the patient in a short period of time. The data gathered forms a base line of health information that is necessary to know prior to administering care. It also provides information that will form the initial working diagnosis. The head-to-toe assessment works sequentially from a general survey that begins at the head and ends at the feet/toes. This includes a general inspection scan of the patient's physical appearance. It goes on to include an assessment of orientation to time, place, and person; vital signs; neck veins; heart sounds; pupils; skin; breath sounds; bowel sounds; and peripheral body parts (e.g., is edema present?).

READING EXERCISES

Understanding the General Meaning

Read the text again. Think about it. Do you understand it?

1) What is the general meaning of the text? What is its focus?

_____

2) What is the purpose of a head-to-toe assessment?

_____

_____

3) What is a head-to-toe assessment?

_____

Building Vocabulary

To build vocabulary, study the following words or terms taken from this text.

Multiple Choice. Use this multiple-choice exercise to fine tune your understanding of a head-to-toe assessment.

1) A complete head-to-toe assessment begins, of course, at the patient's head. It will include
   a) general appearance.
   b) level of consciousness.
   c) disorientation.
   d) both (a) and (b) are correct.
   e) all of the above.

2) The head-to-toe assessment is designed to
   a) systematically assess the patient's physical status.
   b) systematically observe the patient.
   c) systematically assess postoperative distress.
   d) none of the above.
   e) only (a) and (b).

3) For the head-to-toe assessment to be effective and accurate, the professional must
   a) recognize cues and make inferences.
   b) know anatomy and physiology.
   c) understand postoperative care.
   d) read the chart first.
   e) none of the above.

4) The head-to-toe assessment includes the following
   a) objective reports and data collected by nurses.
   b) objective and subjective assessments by nurse and patient.
   c) subjective reports from patient and family members.
   d) none of the above.

Defining New Words. In your own words, define the following terms.

1) systematic _____

2) sequential _____

3) orientation _____

4) peripheral _____

SPEAKING EXERCISE

Read the information about the head-to-toe assessment aloud now. Record yourself. The Pronunciation Hints below will help.

PRONUNCIATION HINTS

systematic – sĭs"tĕ-**măt**'ĭk

sequential – sē'**kwĕn**-shăl

orientation – or"ē-ĕn-**tā**'shŭn

peripheral – pĕr-**ĭf**'**ĕr**-ăl

The Cardiovascular System

LISTENING EXERCISE

Listen to the recording of yourself reading the information about the Head-to-Toe Assessment. Now consider that you are a nursing instructor. Listen again. How do you sound? Confident? Knowledgeable?

WRITING EXERCISE—PERSONAL REFLECTION

Take a moment or two to consider what you've just read. Does the head-to-toe assessment have the same name in your country of origin? Write some notes about that.

_____

_____

Reading Selection 3-10

Now we are going to assume that Mr. Moore is being admitted to the Emergency Department of your hospital. You are on duty. The following exercises will provide a very brief introduction to admission and treatment forms in English. There is also the opportunity to work with a laboratory requisition.

ADMISSION TO THE EMERGENCY DEPARTMENT

Mr. Moore has arrived by ambulance and the paramedics have verbally advised the admitting nurse and doctor of his signs and symptoms. His current status is stable, but he remains frightened. Both you and the doctor attend the patient. The doctor introduces you both to the patient and immediately asks if the patient has any allergies. The patient reports that he has no known allergies. The doctor completes the head-to-toe assessment while you assist. He asks about the patient's medical history, particularly related to cardiovascular disease. Mr. Moore is given a working diagnosis of angina, not myocardial infarction. However, he is to have lab work done and be monitored closely on cardiac monitors and by the nursing staff for the next few hours. He is started on an intravenous (IV) of normal saline to keep the vein open (2KVO) in case medication is needed quickly. Now that the patient has been seen and made comfortable, the admission charting and lab requisitions must be completed.

READING EXERCISES

This reading selection introduces several new words and some abbreviations. Use the following exercises to help you master this new vocabulary.

Understanding the General Meaning

Read the text again. Think about it. Do you understand it?

1) What has the doctor concluded from his examination of the patient?

_____

2) Who will observe the patient closely over the next few hours?

_____

3) What is an IV?

_____

4) Identify the steps in the admission procedure for this cardiac patient.

_____

_____

Building Vocabulary

To build vocabulary, study the following words or terms taken from this text. Discover all you can about them by looking at them in context of the reading selection.

Multiple Choice.   Answer the following questions by choosing the correct meaning.

1) *IV* is an abbreviation for
   a) intercellular.
   b) interpersonal.
   c) interlinear.
   d) intravenous.

2) The abbreviation *2KVO* often appears on the doctor's orders. This means
   a) two ketones per vein or orally.
   b) to keep vein open.
   c) to kaopectate the venous opening.
   d) to kidneys via oral hydration.

3) The term *working diagnosis* indicates
   a) the final diagnosis for the patient based on assessment data.
   b) the priority diagnosis for the patient.
   c) the suspected diagnosis for which the patient is being treated based on assessment data.
   d) the diagnosis has not yet been made and no treatment will be ordered until this occurs.

Answering Specific Questions.   The admission procedure is quite complex. It includes questions about the patient's past and present health history and emotional and even financial concerns so that the staff can treat the patient holistically. Answer the following questions. They are very similar to those found on an admission form at the hospital.

1) What is the purpose in asking about the patient's allergies?

2) How important is it to get a clear description of the patient's allergies?

3) Why is it important to get a clear description and document the patient's allergies?

4) What is the medical term for a severe allergic response that can be life threatening?

5) Why do medical personnel ask about a patient's medication use upon admission?

6) At the time of admission, no matter how old the patient is, he or she is asked about their potential contact with HIV/AIDS, tuberculosis, and hepatitis. Why is this?

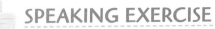

SPEAKING EXERCISE

Read the following script aloud. Find a partner to help you, if you can. Read it again and again until you are comfortable with it. The Pronunciation Hints section below the script will help.

Then try to "act" it with emotion and expression in your voice. Talk to each other afte... experience, about putting emotion into your speech. What value does this have?

Nurse: Well, Mr. Moore, the doctor says you are stable now and you can go home.

Mr. Moore: Home? Stable? What do you mean?

Nurse: I can hear from your voice that you are still a bit frightened by what has happened to you this evening, Mr. Moore. Let's talk about that.

Mr. Moore: Yes, yes . . . thanks. I'm worried, you know.

Nurse: Tell me more, Mr. Moore.

Mr. Moore: I'm worried I'm going to have a heart attack as soon as I leave the hospital.

Nurse: I can appreciate your concern, Mr. Moore. Dr. Johnson has given you a complete and thorough examination. We are very sure you are not going to have a heart attack. And, your lab tests and x-rays came back fine, too.

Mr. Moore: But, but. . . .

Nurse: Mr. Moore, you have been diagnosed with chest pain. We call that angina. There could be many reasons for that and that is why Dr. Johnson has referred you to Dr. Wong, our local cardiologist. Here's the referral form. Just call that number in the morning. Dr. Wong's office will be expecting you. In the meantime, here is your medication. Dr. Johnson has given you a couple of pills of nitroglycerine to alleviate any more chest pain should it occur. And here are a few tablets of an anti-anxiety medication to help reduce that fear and apprehension you are having.

Mr. Moore: Oh . . . I need medication?

Nurse: Yes. Just until you see Dr. Wong and he will decide what you might need, if anything after that.

Mr. Moore: OK. All right. Tell me about these medications again, please.

Nurse: All right, but first, why don't I get your wife from the waiting room and we can all sit together while I teach you about these meds and we talk about your discharge plans?

Mr. Moore: OK. That's a good idea.

PRONUNCIATION HINTS

nitroglycerine – nī″trō-glĭs′ĕr-ĭn

anaphylactic – ăn″ă-fĭ-lăk-tĭk

LISTENING EXERCISE

Try to watch an American TV show about an Emergency Room. You will see that the nurses speak with patients like this. Listen carefully.

...w vocabulary. Write a sentence or two by combining these words and names in a
...l way to talk about how nurses communicate with patients in your country of origin.
...same as it is in this last dialogue?

_____

_____

_____

Anatomy and Physiology

 READING SELECTION 3-1—NORTH AMERICAN HEALTH CONCEPTS

Understanding the General Meaning

1) heart attack

2) coronary artery disease

3) yes

Building Vocabulary

Determining Meaning from Context

1) b, 2) c, 3) b

Using New Words in Sentences

1) coronary artery disease

2) myocardial infarction

3) health

4) coronary artery disease or heart attack/MI

5) exercise

Writing Exercise

Sample answer: Many people with coronary artery disease experience angina and/or a myocardial infarction. Many of these cases can be controlled and/or prevented if people follow a healthy diet, limit salt intake, stop smoking, and exercise regularly.

 READING SELECTION 3-2—THE CARDIOVASCULAR SYSTEM OR CIRCULATORY SYSTEM?

Understanding the General Meaning

1) The heart pumps blood.

2) The circulatory system functions to transport nutrients, gases, antibodies, electrolytes, and wastes through the body via the blood.

3) The major structures of the circulatory system are the heart and the blood vessels (arteries, veins, capillaries).

4) The singular form is atrium.

5) The purpose or genre of this reading selection is explanation.

Building Vocabulary

Mix and Match

BOX 3-1 Mix and Match: Parts of the Heart: Answers

PART OF HEART	FUNCTION
right and left ventricles	lower chambers of the heart
aorta	the heart's main artery
pulmonary vein	carries blood back to heart from lungs
septum	wall dividing the heart down the middle
vena cava	the body's main vein
left atrium	receives oxygenated blood from lungs

Sentence Completion

1) An artery takes the blood away from the heart.

2) The function of the heart is to pump blood through the circulatory system.

3) The heart functions (contracts) to pump blood into the system.

4) Capillaries are very small blood vessels. They are located throughout the body.

5) A vein functions to move blood from tissues in the body to the heart.

WRITING EXERCISE

1) Deoxygenated blood from your body enters the heart from the vena cava this way.

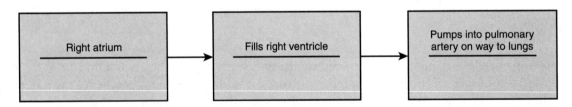

2) Oxygenated blood from the lungs enters the heart this way.

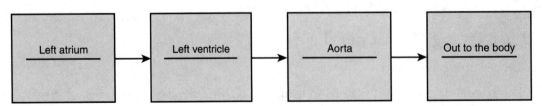

Assessing Function and Failure of the Cardiovascular/Circulatory System

 ## READING 3-3—PHYSIOLOGY OF THE PULSE

Understanding the General Meaning

1) The audience for this reading is most likely students in biology or health-related studies.

2) The function or social purpose of this reading is to describe the physiology of the pulse and how it is measured.

3) The main theme of this reading is the physiology of the pulse and how it can be palpated and measured.

Building Vocabulary

Determining Meaning from Context

1) b, 2) a, 3) c, 4) a, 5) c, 6) b, 7) a

Mix and Match

BOX 3-3 Mix and Match: Terminology for Pulse Sites: Answers	
LOCATION (SITE)	PROPER TERM FOR SITE
behind the knee	popliteal
at the wrist along the thumb side	radial
under the nipple on the left side of chest	apical
on the top of the foot	dorsal pedalis
under the jaw	carotid

BOX 3-4 Mix and Match: Pulse Descriptors: Answers	
thready	fine; scarcely perceptible
pulse	rate, rhythm; rhythmic beat of the heart and blood vessels
faint	very hard to hear; weak
slow	rhythm is not as quick as it should be; often found in the elderly
rapid	racing very quickly
irregular	rhythm is erratic
bounding	jumping or bouncing; big beats
regular	normal rhythm and rate; equal force and frequency of pulse wave

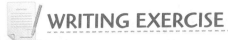

WRITING EXERCISE

Student A: Hi, my name is _____. I'd like to **take** your pulse. Please **give** me your arm. Thank you.

Student B: Here it is. . . . OK, what is my pulse, please, nurse?

Student A: It's 88. That's 88 **beats** per minute.

Student B: Is that normal?

Student A: Let me think. Your chart says you **are** 33 years old. **Is** that right?

Student B: Yes.

Student A: Right. Thank you. Your pulse **is** normal.

READING 3-4—BLOOD PRESSURE

Understanding the General Meaning

The topic of the reading selection is the physiology of blood pressure and how it is reported.

Building Vocabulary

Determining Meaning from Context

1) a, 2) a, 3) c, 4) a

Using New Words to Answer Questions

1) The left ventricle of the heart must contract before oxygen-rich blood can flow into the arteries of the body. The right ventricle of the heart must contract before deoxygenated blood can flow to the lungs to receive oxygen.

2) Blood is forced out of the heart and into circulation by contraction of the heart.

3) Blood pressure is measured by listening (with a sphygmomanometer and stethoscope) to the pressure in the arteries during both contraction (systolic blood pressure) and relaxation (diastolic blood pressure) of the ventricles of the heart.

WRITING EXERCISE

Sample Answers:

The nurse is using a stethoscope to listen to the heart rate of a patient.

The doctor is inflating a blood pressure cuff, or sphygmomanometer, and using a stethoscope to determine the blood pressure when the heart contracts and relaxes.

READING 3-5—CONGESTIVE HEART FAILURE

Understanding the General Meaning

1) personal reflection—no sample answer

2) heart failure

3) congestive heart failure

4) heart and lungs

The Cardiovascular System

5) congestive heart failure

6) no

Building Vocabulary

Determining Meaning from Context

1) a, 2) d, 3) b, 4) a, 5) b, 6) b, 7) a, 8) c

Mix and Match

Box 3-5 Mix and Match: Signs and Symptoms of Congestive Heart Failure: Answers

SIGN	SYMPTOM
confusion	not clear about time, place, person, activity
pallor	ashen color to skin
cyanosis	lack of oxygen in blood; symptoms such as blue lips
panic	extreme state of fear and desperation (for air and survival)
frothy sputum	bubbly: white or pink with bubbles
altered breathing pattern	rapid, shallow respirations
wheezing	a raspy sound made when breathing
air hunger	behavior or gulping or seeming to try to eat the air: result of lack of O_2
restless	unable to sit still
mouth breathing and gasping	inability to get sufficient oxygen through normal breathing through nose

 ## WRITING EXERCISE

1) Heart failure is cessation of the beat of the heart. The heart stops beating.

2) Gas exchange occurs when oxygen and carbon dioxide are traded one for the other via the circulatory system and the lungs. Nitrogen is released from the body.

3) Congestion is the presence of an excessive amount of blood or fluid in tissue of an organ . . . often causing the vessel or organ to be blocked, jammed, plugged, or occluded.

4) When the heart pumps, it contracts to push blood out into the body. It then relaxes to allow blood to re-enter the heart.

5) A damaged heart is a heart that has incurred an injury and no longer functions at full capacity.

6) A myocardial infarction (MI) is also known as a heart attack.

7) The word *pulmonary* refers to the lungs.

READING 3-6—ANGINA AND MYOCARDIAL INFARCTION

Understanding the General Meaning

The general purpose of the reading selection is to explain the nature, causes, and symptoms of angina and myocardial infarction.

Comprehending Specifics

1) Angina is caused by a narrowing of the arteries. The etiology of angina is a narrowing of the arteries.

2) Two words to describe angina are *chest pain*.

3) A myocardial infarction is caused by a progressive narrowing of the coronary arteries. Blocking of an artery or an occlusion usually occurs suddenly and may be the result of a thrombus/blood clot or embolus.

Building Vocabulary

Determining Meaning from Context

1) b, 2) a, 3) b

Using New Words in Sentences

Examples of possible answers:

1) Cassandra has an irregular heartbeat and a diagnosis of heart disease.

2) Devon has suffered two minor heart attacks. He has arteriosclerosis and is on the cardiac care unit now.

Treatments, Interventions, and Assistance

 ## READING 3-7—CALLING 911 FOR HELP

Understanding the General Meaning

The subject of the reading is a man who seems to be having a heart attack and calls for emergency help.

Answering Closed Questions

1) The man on the phone is having chest pain.

2) The 911 operator answers calls to the 911 emergency number.

3) The patient reports numbness in his left arm.

4) Paramedics are on the way to the man's home.

5) An ambulance is also on the way to the man's home.

6) The man on the phone—the patient—can't think clearly.

The Cardiovascular System

7) She wants him to calm down and unlock the front door so the paramedics can get into the house to help him.

8) 911 is the number to call for police, fire, or medical emergencies.

9) The patient's wife is not at home; she is out.

10) The 911 operator is calm, professional, and helpful. (Note: this question asks "how.")

11) The patient on the phone is confused, short of breath, afraid, and in pain.

12) The patient is male.

13) The patient has not been previously diagnosed with a heart condition.

14) Yes, the patient gets rescued.

Building Vocabulary

Mix and Match

BOX 3-6 Mix and Match: Synonyms: Answers

TERM FROM TEXT	SYNONYM OR DESCRIPTION
paramedic	ambulance attendant
911	emergency telephone line
difficulty breathing	shortness of breath
numbness	no feeling
relax	calm
telephone operator	operator
hurt	pain

Recognizing Related Words

1) **chest:** thoracic, breast, upper body

2) **pain:** ouch, hurt, aches badly

3) **operator:** telephone employee, switchboard person, phone attendant

4) **right now:** immediately, right away, stat

5) **anyone:** someone, somebody, any person

6) **numb:** paresthesia, no feeling, no sensation

7) **dizzy:** vertigo, unbalanced, sense of spinning

8) **hurry:** go quickly, move quickly, proceed rapidly

9) **short of breath:** can't catch my breath; apnca; rapid, shallow breathing

10) **bear with me:** please be patient and wait, stand by, be patient a moment

Recognizing Distinctions Between Words

1) Sweet is a taste; sweat is perspiration.

2) Palpation is assessment by touch; palpitation is an irregular or rapid beat of your heart.

3) Pallor is lack of color, a paleness of the skin; cyanosis is a condition of insufficient oxygen in the cells, often observed as bluish or grayish color of the skin.

4) Breathe is a verb meaning to take in air; breath is a noun.

5) Numbness is lack of sensation; tingling is a prickling sensation

6) Nausea is the feeling of being about to throw up; vomiting is the act of throwing up.

7) An ache is less hurtful than a pain.

8) Anxiety is a state of alertness and responsiveness that can feel good or bad; apprehension is fear of the unknown.

Writing Exercise

1) fear, anxiety, chest pain

2) think clearly

3) work with the ambulance service; in ambulances

READING SELECTION 3-8—ANGINA

Understanding the General Meaning

1) The purpose of the narrative is that the man is experiencing pain and discomfort, fears he may be having a heart attack, and calls for emergency help.

2) The plot concludes with the ambulance and paramedics arriving to take the man to the hospital.

3) The narrative is written in the past tense.

Understanding Specific Facts in a Reading

1) The patient's name is Mr. Moore.

2) Yes, the patient was able to provide his address.

3) Yes, the patient was coherent.

4) The operator was speaking to Mr. Moore.

5) The paramedics might have had to break down the door to Mr. Moore's house if he was not able to unlock it.

6) The paramedics might break down the door to reach Mr. Moore and provide him with assistance.

7) Mr. Moore was going to be going to the hospital.

8) Mr. Moore was going to get to the hospital via ambulance.

9) The patient's acute signs and symptoms were numbness and tingling in left arm, shortness of breath (SOB), confusion, and pain and tightness in his chest.

10) No, Mr. Moore has never had a heart attack before.

11) Mr. Moore was thinking clearly enough to call 911 for help.

Building Vocabulary

Determining Meaning from Context

1) d, 2) b, 3) b, 4) e, 5) b, 6) b, 7) a, 8) a

Sentence Completion

1) directive, 2) passed out, 3) broke down, 4) been broken down

READING SELECTION 3-9—HEAD-TO-TOE ASSESSMENT

Understanding the General Meaning

1) The general meaning or focus of the reading selection is to explain what a head-to-toe assessment is, what it includes, and why it is performed.

2) The purpose of a head-to-toe assessment is to gather data as a base line of health information and to help make a working diagnosis.

3) A head-to-toe assessment is a routine, expected method of data collection in American and Canadian health care. It provides an inclusive, logical, and systematic assessment in a short period of time.

Building Vocabulary

Multiple Choice

1) d, 2) a, 3) a, 4) b

Defining New Words

1) Systematic means to follow a system or procedure to achieve a certain goal. A head-to-toe assessment is a systematic way to collect health data.

2) Sequential means following a sequence. The head-to-toe assessment follows a sequence of steps starting with the head and neck, proceeding to vital signs, orientation, heart tones, breath sounds, bowel sounds, etc., to collect data.

3) Orientation means position or change of position of body parts OR general or lasting direction of thought, inclination, or interest.

4) Peripheral means relating to the outer or surface part of something, away from the center as in being in the outer, or peripheral, field of vision or the peripheral nervous system being outside of the central nervous system.

READING SELECTION 3-10—ADMISSION TO THE EMERGENCY DEPARTMENT

Understanding the General Meaning

1) The doctor has concluded that the patient has a working diagnosis of angina.

2) The nurses will observe the patient closely over the next few hours.

3) An IV is an intravenous infusion of fluids or medications into the body.

4) The steps in the admission procedure for this cardiac patient were: obtain information and status of the patient from the paramedics, complete a head-to-toe assessment, connect heart monitor, start an IV, observe closely, and complete documentation.

Building Vocabulary

Multiple Choice

1) d, 2) b, 3) c

Answering Specific Questions

1) The purpose in asking about a patient's allergies is to assess for and control any possible allergic reactions or prevent them from occurring.

2) It is extremely important and absolutely essential to get a clear description of a patient's allergies.

3) It is important to get a clear description of patient's allergies and document them because some allergic reactions can be life-threatening. In addition, health-care professions are legally liable if they do not ask the patients about allergies.

4) The medical term for a severe allergic response is anaphylactic shock.

5) Medical personnel ask about a patient's medication use upon admission to prevent mixing medications that are contraindicated or overmedicating patients.

6) Patients are asked about their potential contact with HIV/AIDS, tuberculosis, and hepatitis because these are all infectious diseases that may be spread in the hospital by the patient.

UNIT 4

Unit 4 explores vocabulary, medical terminology, and concepts related to the respiratory system. The goal of the unit is not only to build language skills and competencies, but also to enhance your ability to communicate with patients, peers, and other members of the multidisciplinary health-care team. The unit begins with both a knowledge and language review of basic anatomy and physiology. This is followed by an introduction to the language and processes used to identify, name, and describe the function of the system and the failures that may occur within it. The language of diagnostics and assessments related to respiratory system health and disease includes case studies and disease exemplars. Throughout each section, the focus is on improving communication through vocabulary acquisition and the use of grammar, structure, and form. The unit rounds itself out with exposure to and practice with the language of treatments, interventions, and assistance for patients challenged by respiratory illness or crisis.

SECTION ONE | Anatomy and Physiology

A review of the anatomy and physiology of the respiratory system for health professionals provides the context in which the medical terminology, vocabulary, and grammar related to the system are introduced and applied through practice exercises.

Reading Selection 4-1

Read the following short paragraph aloud or silently to yourself.

THE PURPOSE OF THE RESPIRATORY SYSTEM

The cells of the body require a continuous supply of oxygen (O_2) to function properly. As cells use oxygen, they release the waste product of carbon dioxide (CO_2), which must be expelled from the body. The respiratory system is responsible for this gas exchange, from the external world outside the body to the inner world of the body in a never-ending cycle.

 READING EXERCISES

Being able to understand the general meaning of a reading passage is important, as is the acquisition of new vocabulary.

Understanding the General Meaning

Read the text again. Think about it. Do you understand it?

1) What is the general theme or premise of the short paragraph you have just read?

_____

2) Is it healthy for the body to retain carbon dioxide?

_____

_____

Building Vocabulary

Take a moment now to review what you have just read. Jot down any words or phrases that are unfamiliar to you. Keep this list for a reference. Work through the rest of the chapter to discover their meaning. Refer back to this list from time to time and write down the definition.

_____

_____

Determining Meaning from Context. To build vocabulary, study the words or terms used in the following exercise and, based on the context of the sentence, explain their meaning.

1) When the two words *waste* and *product* are used together in a medical context they are referring to what?

_____

2) What does the word *exchange* mean in relation to the concept of gas exchange?

_____

3) Gas is exchanged from the internal world to the external one. In an anatomical context, what does this mean?

_____

Mix and Match. Use the exercise in Box 4-1 to learn about the structure of the respiratory system. Some of the words may be new to you. Start with the words you know from the context of the reading. There is one item that does not belong to the respiratory system, but its close proximity sometimes can lead to confusion about terminology. See if you can find that term.

BOX 4-1 Mix and Match: Parts of the Respiratory System

Connect each part or structure of the system with its description.

STRUCTURE OR PART	DESCRIPTION
esophagus	passage leading from pharynx to the lungs
diaphragm	passage leading from mouth and throat to stomach
trachea	creates suction in chest to draw in air to lungs
pharynx	guards entrance to trachea and closes when swallowing
epiglottis	sends incoming air from nose and mouth to trachea
larynx	moves air being breathed in and out and makes voice sounds

Sentence Completion. Use a key word from the previous exercise to create a new sentence. Fill in the blanks.

1) Too much _____ in the body can cause confusion, anxiety, and even unconsciousness.

2) An excess of _____ in the body can make a person feel very pleased, happy, and content for a short while.

3) Cell life depends on the health of the _____.

SPEAKING EXERCISE

Read the following short paragraph aloud. Ask a peer or teacher to help you with pronunciation. Proceed to the Pronunciation Hints section following. This will also help.

Many major substances are harmful to the respiratory system. These include indoor air contaminants such as environmental tobacco smoke, industrial chemicals such as dry cleaning fluids and paints, and biological compounds and allergens as well as combustion products, such as exhaust from vehicles.

PRONUNCIATION HINTS

substances – sŭb'stăns-ĕz

oxygen – ŏk'sĭ-jĕn

respiratory – Note: There are two common ways to pronounce this word:

rĕs-pīr'ă-tō-rē or rĕs'pĭ-ră-tō"rē

LISTENING EXERCISE

Repeat the speaking exercise and record your voice. Listen back. Are you able to speak fluently without hesitating? Are there particular sounds in some words that are difficult for you? Practice those now, or ask a native English speaker for some help.

WRITING EXERCISE

Use your new vocabulary. Write a sentence or two by combining these words in a meaningful way. Use as many words as possible.

oxygen	enough	supply	inadequate
air	hungry	nose	breathing
breathe	mouth		

_____

_____

_____

Reading Selection 4-2

Read the following aloud or silently to yourself.

ANATOMY AND PHYSIOLOGY OF THE LUNG

In the normal lung, air is inhaled, or taken in, from outside the body. It passes through the trachea and into the bronchial tree. From there it is dispersed (scattered) into the bronchiole tubes. At the end of those tubes the air reaches the alveoli sacs in the lungs. The alveoli expand (open) to pull fresh air in and then contract to push used air out. There are capillaries in the wall of each alveoli sac which relinquish carbon dioxide by exhalation and receive oxygen by inhalation. Inhalation and exhalation are the process of respiration.

 ## READING EXERCISES

Health-care professionals must be very specific in their understanding of anatomical terms. These exercises will help you gain that knowledge in English.

Understanding the General Meaning

Read the text again. Think about it. Do you understand it?

1) In which genre is this text written?

_____

2) While the reading provides information, it also describes a process. What is that process?

_____

Recognizing Specifics

Take a moment now to review what you have just read. Use that information to label the parts of the lung.

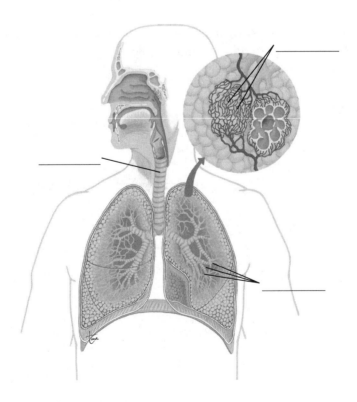

The Respiratory System

Building Vocabulary

Determining the meaning of words from the context in which they are used and then using the words in sentences increases your vocabulary and communication skills.

Determining Meaning from Context.   To build vocabulary, study the following words or terms taken from this text. Discover all you can about them by looking at them in context. Choose the correct meaning. Finally, take a look at how these words or terms expand in English.

1. Bronchial   *(adjective)*

In context:

a) The bronchial tree carries air from the trachea into the lungs.

b) Bronchial pneumonia can include blockage in the bronchi and bronchioles.

Meaning: The term *bronchial* can best be described as meaning

a) having to do with the lungs; describing parts of the lung

b) a tree and oxygen exchanges

c) an expanded process for gas exchanges

d) the respiratory system

Word expansion:

a) *Bronchium* is one of many small tubes in the lung designed for the passage of air. (noun, singular)

b) *Bronchiectasis* is a chronic dilation of the bronchial tubes. (noun)

c) The word for more than one brochium is *bronchi.* (noun)

d) *Bronchitis* is an inflammation of the *bronchi.* (noun, singular; noun, plural)

2. Alveoli   *(noun, plural)*

In context:

a) When the alveoli of the lung are congested or blocked, gas exchange is impeded.

b) The doctor suspects the child may have an infection in the alveoli. That is why the child is not getting enough oxygen and seems irritable and confused.

Meaning: The word *alveoli* means

a) vibration within the lung

b) extending from the jawbone

c) small sacs, cavities, or pits

Word expansion:

a) The singular form of alveoli is *alveolus.* (noun, singular)

b) *Alveolar* lung disease can be the result of pneumonia, emphysema, lupus, or tuberculosis. (adjective)

3. Inhalation   *(noun)*

In context:

a) Inhalation of toxic fumes can cause brain damage.

b) All public buildings have air ducts for inhalation of fresh air and air exchange.

Meaning: *Inhalation* can best be described as

a) blowing air out

b) respiration

c) inspiration

d) exhaustion

Word expansion:

a) Nurses are dealing with more and more young patients who sniff *inhalants.* (noun, plural)

b) Nasal *inhalers* are recommended for sinus congestion. (noun)

c) If you *inhale* paint fumes, you might get high but you might also get severe brain damage. (verb)

4. Exhalation (noun)

In context:

a) The nurse must listen closely sometimes to hear if there is any exhalation of breath from the elderly patient.

b) Exhalation can be observed by placing a small mirror close to the nostrils and waiting for a vapor-like print to appear on the glass.

Meaning: The word *exhalation* can be defined as

a) exalted happiness

b) inspirational respiration

c) respiration

d) expression of air or breath from the inside to the outside

Word expansion:

a) When a person smokes marijuana, they inhale and then hold the smoke inside their lungs for a moment or two before *exhaling*. (gerund, used as noun)

b) Breathe in, breathe out; inhale, *exhale*. (verb)

c) When I *exhale* on a cold day outdoors, I can see my breath. (verb, present tense)

5. Relinquishes (verb, present tense)

In context:

a) In the case of a national disaster, the local government often relinquishes its control to federal government agencies.

b) After trauma or an extreme shock, the nervous system often relinquishes control over organs such as the bladder and the person urinates involuntarily.

Meaning: The word *relinquishes* can be defined as

a) giving up or surrendering control

b) without a reasonable doubt

c) forcibly removed

d) inevitably

Word expansion:

a) In 2008, President Musharraf of Pakistan *relinquished* his control over the army when he stepped down from the presidential office. (verb, past tense)

b) When the patient who is dying asks that his medical treatment stop, he is relinquishing his life.(verb, present continuous)

c) Pulmonary function will be relinquished if the patient is taken off the artificial respirator. (verb, future perfect)

Using New Words in Sentences.   Practice: Use a key word from the previous exercise (items 1–5) to create a new sentence of your choice.

1) _____

2) _____

SPEAKING EXERCISE

Read the following short article aloud. Ask a peer or teacher to help you with pronunciation. Proceed to the Pronunciation Hints section following the article. This will also help.

It is now estimated that more than 22.9 million Americans have abused inhalants at least once in their lives and that this abuse started at an early age of 8 to 10 years old. Substances and products inhaled include aerosols, hairspray, spray paint, and household cleaners which provide a sense of euphoria and dreamlike state for the sniffer. Nail polish remover, gasoline, and glue are also sniffed. Whipped cream dispensers (spray-type canisters found in the dairy section of the grocery store) are also inhaled because they contain nitrous oxide, a form of laughing gas. Inhaling is accomplished by spraying or putting the product in a bag, holding the bag snuggly around your mouth and nose, and breathing in. Sometimes, a tiny hole is punched in the bottom of an aerosol container and the fluid that leaks from that is sniffed, or even sometimes, drunk.

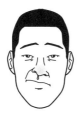

VOCABULARY ALERT What or who is a sniffer?
The verb *to sniff* or *sniff* identifies the action taken consciously to smell something. The verb can also be expanded to other situations. When a person has a cold, sinus infection, or reaction to airborne allergens, the person often *sniffles* (verb). When a person cries, they also get the *sniffles* (noun). In these two instances, we *sniffle* (verb) because of secretions that run down through our nose. (Casually, this is referred to as *post-nasal drip.*) The person doing the sniffing is the *sniffer* (noun).

PRONUNCIATION HINTS

inhalant – ĭn-**hā**'lănt

inhalation – ĭn"hă-**lā**'shŭn

LISTENING EXERCISE

If you would like to hear more native English speakers from the United States and Canada, search the Internet for radio stations located here. Many radio stations have programs dedicated to the subject of addictions such as "sniffing." Try to find one. Listen carefully by Internet or radio to hear many of the words you have just learned. If you would like to hear people speaking about inhalant abuse in the United States, search online for the video clip "The Dangers of Inhalants/Inhalant Abuse Educational Video." It is a combination of television news reports, medical commentaries, and stories of families whose children have died of inhalant abuse. This video is produced as a public service announcement (PSA) by the Alliance for Consumer Education (2006), Washington, DC.

WRITING EXERCISE—SELF-REFLECTION

Take a moment now to consider what you have just read or heard about inhalants. Is this a subject you are familiar with in your own work as a health-care professional? Write a few sentences here that highlight your reaction to the article and your thoughts about this health problem for young people in America and your country of origin.

SECTION TWO # Common Disorders and Diseases of the Respiratory System

In this section, terminology for common disorders and diseases of the respiratory system are introduced, including the language of pathophysiology. The concept of chronicity is introduced and language pertinent to the diagnosis and treatment of three respiratory system diseases—bronchitis, asthma, and chronic obstructive pulmonary disease (COPD)—is presented. Through these exemplars, linguistic opportunities arise for learning new vocabulary and understanding prefixes commonly used in medical terminology. There are also opportunities for improving speaking skills through the process of chaining and writing in the information report genre.

Reading Selection 4-3

CHRONIC OBSTRUCTIVE PULMONARY DISEASE

A chronic disease is one that lasts longer than three months. It may last throughout the individual's entire life. A chronic disease has phases of remission and acute exacerbation. When it is in remission, signs and symptoms are still present but they are manageable on a day-to-day basis. In an acute episode, however, the client's life is interrupted by the disease and both medical treatment and interventions are required to reduce and stabilize the symptoms. Chronic obstructive pulmonary disease (COPD) is an example of one such illness. COPD is a broad term representing disorders associated with chronic obstruction of the air flow into and out of the lungs. It includes the conditions of emphysema, asthma, and chronic bronchitis. A chronic disease leaves residual damage or alteration to the body or body systems. Clients living with chronic disease experience a diminished capacity to function directly related to that disease. This means they may need ongoing support, education, and training by a health-care provider to learn to adapt to their health challenge.

 # READING EXERCISES

This reading selection provides information about a specific disease and presents new vocabulary important to your knowledge and ability to discuss it.

Understanding the General Meaning

Read the text again. Think about it. Do you understand it?

1) What is the general theme of the text?

_____

2) What is the genre of this reading?

_____

3) Identify the structure of the genre to confirm your answer to question #2 above. (Hint: Refer back to Unit 1.)

_____

4) What is the purpose of an information report?

_____

Building Vocabulary

Once you have learned the meaning of a new word, often from its use in the context of a sentence, you should be able to use that word in your own sentences.

Determining Meaning from Context.   To build vocabulary, study the following words or terms taken from this text. Discover all you can about them by looking at them in context. Then, choose the correct meaning by answering the multiple-choice question. Finally, study how these words or terms expand in English.

1. Chronic *(adjective)*

In context:
a) Diabetes is a chronic illness.
b) Schizophrenia is a chronic disease that most often starts between the ages of 18 to 25 and continues throughout a lifetime.

Meaning: The word *chronic* can best be described as meaning
a) enduring over a long period of time
b) expanding over a long period of time
c) exacerbating over a long period of time
d) extenuating over a long period of time

Word expansion:
a) Addressing *chronicity* is a major focus in the delivery of health-care research and program delivery. (noun)
b) There are many different and varied types of *chronic* diseases, many of which can affect every body system, organ, and cell. (adjective)

2. Remission *(noun)*

In context:
a) After an acute episode of pneumonia complicated by COPD, Alfred's symptoms are in remission. He is off the oxygen and antibiotics and is now breathing on his own. He can be discharged from the hospital.
b) Chemotherapy treatments for cancer patients most often lead to remission of the acute signs and symptoms of the disease.

Meaning: The best way to explain the term *remission* is to say that it means
a) a return to the healthy, disease-free state
b) symptoms of the illness disappear
c) a slowing of the disease, an abatement, or a lessening of something
d) a slowing of the disease and an increasing in something

Word expansion:
a) Helga's pain is *unremitting*. (adjective)
b) Multiple sclerosis can be considered a *remissive* disorder. (adjective)
c) After treatment, the itchiness associated with Fred's psoriasis *is remitting.* (verb, present continuous)

3. Exacerbation *(noun)*

In context:
a) Now that it is spring time, many asthmatics are suffering an exacerbation of their symptoms due to the pollen in the air.

Meaning: *Exacerbation* can best be defined as
a) continuing
b) complicating
c) a worsened state
d) a life-threatening state

Word expansion:
a) Madeline *exacerbates* her emphysema by refusing to quit smoking cigarettes. (verb, present)
b) Denny's pneumonia *is exacerbated* by the fact he has chronic bronchitis. It is very, very painful for him to cough or expectorate. (verb, past participle verb)
c) The *exacerbating* factors in the patient's care are her age and her frailty. (adjective)

4. Diminished capacity *(term, consisting of adjective + noun)*

In context:

a) Paul had a severe workplace accident. He fell from a 10-foot structure at a construction site. He had numerous musculoskeletal injuries. Now he has diminished capacity for motor movement. He needs a lot of physiotherapy to recover.

b) Phil has had asthma since he was born. He is now 44 years old. These years of the illness have led to diminished aerobic capacity for him and he is no longer able to play a lot of sports.

c) In court, a client who has been deemed unable to understand the crime he or she is accused of due to a mental disease or disorder is referred to as having diminished mental capacity.

Meaning: The best choice to describe the term *diminished capacity* is

a) lessened opportunity

b) capability

c) ability

d) lessened ability

Sentence Completion. Use a key word from the previous exercise and the reading. Fill in the blanks.

1) In the aging population, _____ is increasingly more common than in the younger population.

2) Some hospitals and office buildings are now identified as "scent-free" zones. This is a health promotion regulation to prevent the _____ of respiratory diseases or disorders.

3) The full name for COPD is _____ disease.

4) The types of COPD mentioned in the reading are _____ and asthma.

SPEAKING EXERCISE— CHUNKS AND CHAINS OF SPOKEN LANGUAGE

This exercise starts with reading "chunks" of language. Read each chunk of the following aloud, over and over, until you can say it fluently and without hesitation. Then move to the next chunk. Repeat the process until all "chunks" have been completed. The exercise is designed to help you break longer sentences up into manageable pieces, practice saying them aloud, and then finally, connect this chain of phrases into one long sentence. When you reach that final sentence, say the entire thing without stopping. The Pronunciation Hints section that follows the exercise will help.

1) The term chronic obstructive pulmonary disease →

2) represents a cluster of respiratory illnesses →

3) that adversely affects air flow into and out of the lungs. →

4) The term chronic obstructive pulmonary disease represents a cluster of respiratory illnesses that adversely affect air flow into and out of the lungs.

PRONUNCIATION HINTS

chronic – **krŏn'ĭ**k

obstructive – ŏb-**strŭk'**t ĭv

pulmonary – **pŭl'**mō-nĕ-rē

exacerbation – ĕks-ăs"ĕr-**bā'**shŭn

remission – rĭ-**mĭsh'**ŭn

asthma – **ăz'**mă

emphysema – ĕm"fĭ-**sē'**mă

LISTENING EXERCISE

At this point in *Medical English Clear and Simple,* you have some homework. You are encouraged to speak to a native English-speaking health professional if you know one or watch an English language television show or film set in an American health-care setting. Listen. The purpose of this exercise is simply to begin to familiarize yourself with how English is spoken in the context of health care.

WRITING EXERCISE

Reassess the reading on chronic obstructive pulmonary disease. Fill in Table 4-1 with phrases or words that match the proper category (genre highlights). Prove to yourself that the reading is written in the information report genre.

Table 4-1 Information Report	
GENRE HIGHLIGHTS	EXAMPLES FROM THE READING SELECTION
Structure	
topic identified	
at least 1 or 2 facts given	
Grammar	
adjectives used	
conjunctions used	
correct verb tenses used	
Writing Features	
a plan or theme	
sentences containing facts	
capital letters and full stops	
paragraph form used (no example required; just checkmark)	
spelling check (no example required; just checkmark)	

Reading Selection 4-4

ACUTE BRONCHITIS AND ASTHMA

A patient with an acute asthmatic attack will want to sit upright. He or she generally leans forward and gasps for breath, demonstrating air hunger. This person may cough, but it is nonproductive. There is no phlegm arising from the lungs. However, breathing is audible and the nurse or doctor can easily hear a wheezing or whistling sound on expiration of the breath. Expiration is prolonged, whereas inspirations are short. Assessment procedures will show that the patient has increased respiratory and pulse rates. This patient will also look very frightened and may be confused, not responding to questions or directions logically. The patient may be in panic mode.

On the other hand, the patient with a long history of chronic bronchitis may appear somewhat differently in the acute phase. He or she may show signs of impaired oxygenation in the form of cyanosis. While they, too, have audible wheezing with prolonged expiration, they also have a recurrent, productive cough. The nurse and doctor may see distended neck veins in this patient, increased respiratory rate, and tachycardia with a heart rate of greater than 100/min.

READING EXERCISES

It is important for the health professional to be able to distinguish between closely related diseases that may present with similar symptoms.

Understanding the General Meaning

Take a moment now to review what you have just read.

1) Identify the thesis or main topic of this reading.

_____

2) What is the difference between an acute asthmatic attack and an acute attack of chronic bronchitis?

_____

_____

3) What signs or symptoms do these two acute episodes of an illness share?

_____

Building Vocabulary

Determining Meaning from Context. To build vocabulary, study the following words or terms taken from this text. Discover all you can about them by looking at them in context. Choose the correct meaning. Finally, take a look at whether and how these words expand in English.

1. Audible *(noun)*

In context:
a) Some people, particularly some men, make an audible sound when they are sleeping. It is called snoring.
b) When a patient is very weak, their voice is often barely audible. You must stand very close to them to hear.

Meaning: The word *audible* can best be described as

a) the ear
b) listen
c) capable of being heard
d) incapable of being heard

2. Whistling *(present continuous form of verb)*

In context:

a) Sometimes when the person who snores exhales, he purses his lips and makes a whistling sound as the air is expelled from his lungs.

Meaning: The word *whistling* in the context of the respiratory system can best be described as meaning

a) producing a purely musical sound on air
b) the sound of a productive cough
c) producing a high-pitched sound by air forced quickly through an opening
d) exhalation

Word expansion:

a) When Bob is awake, he likes *to whistle* his favorite tunes. When Bob is asleep he still *whistles*, but it is part of the way in which he snores. (verb, infinite; verb, present)

3. Wheezing *(verb, present continuous)*

In context:

a) His chest was crushed by the steering wheel in his car. He is able to breathe, but he is wheezing. It sounds difficult.

Meaning: The word *wheezing* can best be described in the context of respiratory signs and symptoms as

a) a whistling, squeaking, or puffing sound made by the passage of air
b) a squeaking or musical sound made by pumping air in and out
c) plucking small hairs to make an area smooth
d) none of the above

Word expansion:

a) If you have a seafood allergy and accidentally eat some seafood, you might begin *to wheeze* as one of the body's first negative reactions to it. (verb, infinitive)

4. Expiration *(noun)*

In context:

a) Inspiration of air is usually much quieter than expiration.

Meaning: In this context, the term *expiration* can best be defined as meaning

a) death
b) blowing
c) exhalation
d) inspiration

Word expansion:

a) *Expiratory* reserve volume is a measure of the maximum amount of air a person can expel from their lungs. (adjective)

Sentence Completion.   Match the medical terms in the Word Bank below to the pathologic conditions described in the following sentences. You will notice that some of the words have the same root (-pnea) and have a prefix added to make the meaning more specific. For example, apnea means temporary cessation of breathing, dyspnea means labored or troubled breathing, and eupnea means normal breathing. The use of prefixes like this is common in medical terminology.

WORD BANK

apnea

asthma

emphysema

dyspnea

eupnea

tachypnea

1) _____ means a lack of or cessation of breathing.

2) _____ is a condition in which air flow in and out of the lungs is not smooth or normal.

3) _____ signifies normal breathing by rate and depth.

4) _____ is a medical term that may be used to describe "air hunger" and/or labored, difficult breathing.

5) A person who snores when they sleep sometimes stops breathing temporarily. This condition is known as sleep _____.

6) The child is very frightened about getting an injection. Her eyes are wide and she is breathing rapidly. She is showing signs of _____.

 ## SPEAKING EXERCISE

Return to the last exercise. Read each of the completed sentences aloud. Ask a peer or teacher to help you with pronunciation. Proceed to the following Pronunciation Hints section. This will also help.

PRONUNCIATION HINTS

mucous – **mū′kŭs**

eupnea – **ū′p-nē′ă**

dyspnea – **dĭsp-nē′ă**

apnea – **ăp-nē′ă**

 ## LISTENING EXERCISE— THE SOUNDS FOR "P," "B," AND "V"

It is important to distinguish between these three consonants when you are speaking to your colleagues and patients. Try this exercise using the words in the Pronunciation Hints box above.

1) Smile. Continue to smile and put your two lips together. Breathe out through your mouth and teeth and say the letter "p." It should make a sound like "puh." At no time should your smile disappear. Do not move your jaw.

2) Next, continue to smile with your lips together. Repeat the exercise, but this time you will say the letter "b." Push the air out through your mouth, but this time make an audible sound and say "buh." This is how to pronounce the letter "b." Do not move your jaw. Notice that "p" has almost no sound—it is air; but "b" is a definite sound and you must forcibly and consciously make it.

3) Now, continue to smile, but this time place a pen or pencil horizontally between your lips. Hold it there. Blow the air out of your mouth again, but this time say the letter "v." Do not move your lips or your jaw. Notice that as "v" escapes the mouth it makes an audible vibration. This distinguishes it from the letters "b" and "p."

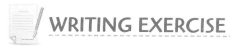

WRITING EXERCISE

Use your new vocabulary. Write a sentence or two identifying what has been salient to you in this section so far. In other words, what learning has been new, important, or significant for you?

_____

_____

_____

Reading Selection 4-5

*Read the following aloud or silently to yourself. This is a long text with many medical terms. Read it through once entirely before stopping to study individual words, **then re-read it**. Notice how many of the medical terms are derived from vocabulary previously studied in this book. Congratulate yourself for recognizing them.*

MORE ABOUT THE LUNGS AND RESPIRATORY SYSTEM

Breathing patterns are altered when there is infection, disease, blockage, or injury to the respiratory system. The ability of the lung to accommodate a sufficient intake of air is known as pulmonary capacity. This is measured in terms of volume. Several types of lung volumes are used to assess and diagnose the health or illness of the lungs. These include inspiratory volume, functional residual volume, vital capacity, and total capacity. The rate at which the lungs inflate and deflate (the ventilation rate) can be affected by infection or other disease and by various other stimuli. Factors that may increase the rate and depth of ventilation include increased or decreased levels of arterial blood gases, an increase in prolonged pain, and a decrease in blood pressure. Factors that can decrease or inhibit the rate and depth of ventilation include severe pain causing apnea, decreased body temperature, increased blood pressure, and increased levels of arterial blood gases.

Health professionals recognize the importance of assessing for and ensuring adequate oxygenation for health and healing. Any impairment in the respiratory system, particularly the lungs, adversely affects every other organ and cell of the body. Disease of any part of the lung can affect the pH balance of the body. The term pH stands for the potential hydrogen in the body. Human blood is rated at 7.4 on the pH scale. A reading of less than 7 (<7) indicates an acidic imbalance called acidosis; while a reading of greater than 7 (> 7) indicates alkalinity.

The respiratory system has its own capacity to protect itself from toxins, viruses, bacteria, and other disease-causing agents. This is accomplished through the system's ability to secrete mucous. It is the system's most significant protective mechanism. Mucous traps toxins and attempts to isolate or expel them. It is then expelled from the body by the process of sneezing and coughing. Phlegm, on the other hand, is a sticky secretion of mucous that originates only in the lungs. When expelled by a cough, it is referred to as sputum.

READING EXERCISES

While understanding the general meaning of a reading selection is important, it is essential that all health professionals be very specific; exact in reporting or explaining something.

Understanding the General Meaning

Read the text again. Think about it as you answer the next questions.

1) What is the general meaning of the text? Its focus?

_____

2) What is the purpose of this text and who is it written for?

Learning Specific Facts

Take a moment now to review what you have just read. Have you understood it?

1) What can cause a change in normal breathing patterns?

2) What is pulmonary capacity?

3) What are secretions?

4) Give an example of a secretion in the context of the respiratory system.

Building Vocabulary

Many of the very technical terms in this reading have been derived from words used in previous chapters in this textbook. Box 4-2 will help you recognize some of them. Once you recognize these words and their meaning you should be able to use them in sentences and to answer specific questions.

Using New Words in Sentences. Use the words given in Box 4-2, in any form, to write a full and complete sentence. Use the sentence given as inspiration for your sentence.

1) Gwen has emphysema. ————————————————————————

2) The respiratory technician at the hospital has a piece of equipment called a spirometer and one end of this goes in the mouth. ————————————————————

3) Frieda is suffering from shortness of breath and the nurse has inserted nasal prongs for her.

4) Cheryl needs an oxygen mask. ——————————————————

Using New Words to Answer Specific Questions. Use new vocabulary in new and meaningful ways by completing this exercise.

1) When the lungs expand with air, so do the intercostal ribs and the diaphragm.
   In this context, *diaphragm* means ——————————————————

BOX 4–2 Word Expansion	
FIRST EXPOSURE TO THE WORD	CURRENT USE OF THE WORD
capacity	capacities
inspiration (inhalation)	inspiratory
function	functional
oxygen	oxygenation

2) The trachea is also known as the windpipe. This is because

_____

3) Aspiration occurs when an object goes down the windpipe instead of the esophagus.
   a) Where does the esophagus lead? _____
   b) Where does the windpipe lead?_____
4) Is aspiration of an object into the lungs potentially deadly?

_____

Fill in the Blanks.   Fill in the blanks in this script to help a patient breathe correctly and attain healthy respirations or in preparation to clear his lungs.

"Hello, _____ (patient's name). I'm your _____ (nurse, doctor, respiratory therapist). I'm going to help you breathe more efficiently. Watch me and do as I say. Take a deep _____ in then _____ it. Count to three and then _____ the air. Good. _____ in. Hold. _____ out. Good. Now we're going to _____ deeply. Put your _____ on your _____ so that you can feel where the air should be going. _____ your mouth and breathe only _____ your _____. OK. _____ deeply again, with your hands on your _____. 1-2-3, begin. Breathe _____. Good."

VOCABULARY ALERT Be very careful to distinguish the difference between the verb **breathe** and the noun **breath,** both in writing and in speaking. This is an expectation of clarity for a health professional.

SPEAKING EXERCISE

Read the short script you wrote in the fill-in-the-blank exercise aloud. Stand in front of a mirror and do the physical, nonverbal activities described as well as speak the words. Communication requires the use of both in English.

PRONUNCIATION HINTS

diaphragm – **dī′ă-frăm**

phlegm – **flĕm**

sputum – **spū′tŭm**

LISTENING EXERCISE

You have just been through a very complicated reading. When you are ready, try to record your voice as you read it again aloud. Listen to yourself when you play back the recording. Are some words becoming more familiar to you and therefore easier to pronounce?

WRITING EXERCISE

Many terms in the reading include their definition. Write them here.

1) pulmonary capacities _____

2) ventilation rate _____

3) pH _____

4) mucous _____

5) congestion _____

6) phlegm _____

7) sputum _____

Reading Selection 4-6

Read the following aloud or silently to yourself.

LUNG CANCER AND DEMOGRAPHICS

Lung cancer is a pathological disease of abnormal cell growth in the tissues of the lungs. In 2004 in the United States 196,252 people were diagnosed with lung cancer; 158,006 died of it. During that same year in the United Kingdom, 38,313 people were diagnosed with the disease. In 2005, China reported that rates of lung cancer are the highest of all types of cancer in that country, particularly for men who also have the highest death rate from it. More recently, in 2008, it is expected that more than 27,000 Canadians will be diagnosed with lung cancer and approximately 20,000 will die from it.

In the Western world, men and women are being diagnosed with this horrific disease at equal rates. While the vast majority of cases of lung cancer are related to cigarette smoking, other causes are air pollution, exposure to asbestos or radon, and exposure to cigarette smoke. Early diagnosis and detection are essential if lives are to be saved.

The proper medical terminology for cancer is carcinoma. Small-cell carcinoma is the most frequent type of lung cancer diagnosed. Cancer cells are assessed to determine if they are malignant (harmful, likely to spread or be fatal) or benign (harmless and not life-threatening). A diagnosis of lung cancer is not a death sentence. Progress in treating the disease with surgery, chemotherapy, and radiation have saved and prolonged lives. As yet, however there is no guaranteed cure.

READING EXERCISES

Understanding the General Meaning

Read the text again. Think about it. Do you understand it?

1) What is the topic of this text?

_____

2) In which country is lung cancer for men on the rise?

_____

3) In the Western world, who has more chance of getting lung cancer, men or women?

_____

Building Vocabulary

Increasing your vocabulary will assist you in answering specific questions and determining if a statement is true or not.

Determining Meaning from Context.   To build vocabulary, study the following words or terms taken from this text. Discover all you can about them by looking at them in context, then choose the correct meaning. Finally, take a look at how these words or terms expand in English.

1. Pathological *(adjective)*

In context:

a) Cancer is a pathological disease related to the growth of abnormal cells in the body.

b) A person who does not tell the truth even when it is safe and appropriate to do so is called a pathological liar. This may be a symptom of his or her psychiatric diagnosis.

Meaning: The adjective *pathological* can best be described as meaning

a) ill

b) bad

c) description of a disease

d) diseased state

Word expansion:

a) The laboratory technician examines specimens for *pathology.* (noun)

b) In an autopsy, the coroner examines the body for signs of *pathology* that may have caused the patient's death. (noun)

c) A good number of *pathologists* are employed at the Centers for Disease Control and Prevention (CDC) in Atlanta, Georgia, and in Vancouver, Canada. (noun, title)

2. Chemotherapy *(noun)*

In context:

a) The cancer patient has chemotherapy treatments once per week for the next month. She doesn't like it. They make her feel very ill.

b) Chemotherapy is prescribed by doctors to treat a variety of diseases.

Meaning: The true meaning of the word *chemotherapy* is

a) chemical therapy

b) medication therapy

c) chemist's therapy

d) all of the above

3. Radiation *(noun)*

In context:

a) X-ray technicians must be wary of exposure to radiation. They wear lead aprons and stand behind a protective wall when taking a patient's x-ray.

b) Radiation is part of the treatment regime for cancer patients. It does not cause them to lose their hair. The chemotherapy agents do that.

Meaning: The word *radiation* can best be described as meaning

a) shiny and brilliant

b) the ability to turn around or in a circular motion

c) the process of transmitting radioactive rays

d) a device for determining distance and direction

Word expansion:

a) Specially trained medical technicians *radiate* cancer cells with highly specialized equipment and technology. (verb)

b) Radium is a *radioactive* metal used as a radiation source for cancer treatment. (adjective)

c) *Radioactivity* is the term used to describe the process of nuclear disintegration through the emission of energy. (noun)

4. Malignant *(adjective)*

In context:

a) A diagnosis of a malignant form of cancer means the patient will not survive.

b) Malignant hypertension is a severe form of hypertension that rapidly causes serious damage and cell death to arteriolar walls in the kidney and retina.

Meaning: The term *malignant* can best be described as meaning

a) potential for death

b) resistant to treatment, progressive

c) leads to death

d) both (b) and (c)

Word expansion:

a) *Malignancy* is a worry for all patients when they are scheduled for a tissue or bone biopsy. (noun)

5. Benign *(adjective)*

In context:

a) The results of the tissue biopsy show the patient's lesion is benign. It has ruled out malignant melanoma.

b) A benign tumor is one that does not metastasize or spread and does not require radiation therapy.

Meaning: The word *benign* can best be described as meaning

a) potentially fatal

b) treatment resistant after 3 months

c) nonmalignant, mild character

Word expansion:

a) He smiled *benignly* at his granddaughter. (adverb)

True or False.   Answer the following true-or-false questions about lung cancer based on the reading and your own knowledge of the subject. Observe how vocabulary is used within sentences. Circle your choice.

1) Lung cancer is the most commonly diagnosed form of cancer.
   True   False

2) Smoking increases a person's risk of getting lung cancer 20 times.
   True   False

3) A known risk factor for cancer is smoking marijuana.
   True   False

4) If a doctor suspects lung cancer, the first diagnostic step is to get an x-ray.
   True   False

 ## SPEAKING EXERCISE

Once again, you have had the opportunity read a complicated text with advanced vocabulary as well as some very large numbers. Practice re-reading it aloud until you feel comfortable doing so. Practice, practice, practice. This will help familiarize your tongue and mouth with any new sounds and pronunciation. It will improve your ease and confidence with career-specific language. The Pronunciation Hints box below will help.

PRONUNCIATION HINTS

malignant – mă-**lĭg'**nănt

carcinoma – kăr"sĭ-**nō'**mă

pathological – pă-thŏl'**ō-jĭ**-kăl

LISTENING EXERCISE

If you would like to hear more native English speakers from the United States and Canada, search the Internet for radio stations located here. Many radio stations have programs dedicated to the subject of health and wellness. Try to find one. Listen carefully by Internet or radio to hear many of the words you have just learned.

WRITING EXERCISE

Use your new vocabulary to write a few sentences reflecting on the lung cancer situation in your own country of origin. You might want to compare and contrast that with what you have just read here.

_____

_____

_____

SECTION THREE Treatments, Interventions, and Assistance

This section provides the English language learner with the ability to talk about respiratory illnesses, symptoms, and diseases in the context of medical treatment, interventions, and assistance given by both health-care professionals as well as members of the public.

Reading Selection 4-7

RESPIRATORY SYMPTOMS

Viruses, bacteria, and toxins most often enter the body through the nose or mouth. Most respiratory symptoms, such as post-nasal drip, coughing, and sneezing, are the result of sinus infection, bronchitis, rhinitis, the common cold, or influenza (flu). Left untreated, respiratory symptoms can develop into inflammation and congestion of the airways, nose, throat, trachea, and bronchi.

The immune system mobilizes to respond to these disease-causing agents in an attempt to fight them by trying to expel, immobilize, or destroy them. Fever is one of the body's defense mechanisms used to kill viruses and other germs. It is a natural response to infection and should not always be treated with fever-reducing medication. (However, if a fever is prolonged, particularly in very small children, medication is necessary to prevent such adverse effects as swelling in the joints and pain.) The best method of protection against respiratory illness is to wash your hands frequently.

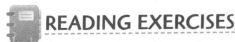

READING EXERCISES

Understanding the General Meaning

Read the text again. Think about it. Do you understand it?

1) What is the general message of this text?

_____

2) What process does this text describe?

_____

3) What is the general theme of this text?

_____

Building Vocabulary

It is important that you not only learn to determine the meaning of a word from its context, but that you also familiarize yourself with the use of the proper tense of verbs when speaking to another health professional or to a patient.

Determining Meaning from Context. Review the following words taken from the text. Try to discover their meaning from context, then study the word expansion, if one is available for the term.

1. Rhinitis *(noun, proper name)*

In context:
a) The patient presented in the clinic today with a complaint of inability to breathe through his nose and a general sense of malaise. He was diagnosed with rhinitis, likely due to recent exposure to paint fumes while re-painting his house.

Meaning: The term *rhinitis* can best be used to describe
a) an inflammation of the nasal mucous membrane
b) post-nasal drip
c) an infection of the lower respiratory tract
d) a form of cancer

Word expansion:
a) The root word of *rhinitis* is rhino, meaning the nose. (medical prefix)
b) *Rhinedema* is the term for a swelling of the mucous membrane of the nose. (noun)
c) A specialist in diseases of the nose is called a *rhinologist.* (noun)

2. Autoimmune *(adjective)*

In context:
a) Arthritis is thought to be a form of autoimmune disease in which the body actually fights against itself.

Meaning: The best way to define *autoimmune* is
a) active initiation of mucosal response
b) active initiation of immune responses against self
c) enzymatic digestion of cells
d) initiation of a cytotoxic antibody

Word expansion:
a) When the body's immune response is triggered to work against its own tissues, the condition is called *autoimmunity.* (noun)

Fill in the Blanks. Vocabulary related to the respiratory system is used here in the context of a fill-in-the-blank exercise that highlights the use of verbs. Use the Word Bank below to help with any verbs you are not familiar with.

WORD BANK

throbs

wheeze

smoke

caught

sneeze

breathe

congested

rises

choke

inhale

swells

make

hurts

1) How much tobacco do you _____ per day?

2) I want you to breathe deeply so I can watch you _____.

3) When food gets stuck in your throat, you _____.

4) I suffer from asthma. I _____ when I _____.

5) I _____ when I have something itchy in my nose.

6) My temperature _____ when I am sick.

7) My head _____ when I have a headache.

8) I _____ an appointment if I want to see a doctor.

9) I breathe through my mouth when my sinuses are

_____.

10) The throat _____ when it is infected.

11) I _____ flu on the airplane, I think.

12) It _____ when I cough. I have bronchitis.

SPEAKING EXERCISE

Go back to the reading. Work on fluency in oral speaking by reading it aloud. Pay very special attention this time to pronunciation of the letters "v," "b," and "p." The Pronunciation Hints box below will help.

PRONUNCIATION HINTS

viruses – **vī′**rŭs-ĕz

autoimmune – ăw-tō- ĭm-**ūn′**

toxins – **tŏks′**ĭnz

rhinitis – rī-**nī′**tĭs

bacteria – băk-**tē′**rē-ă

LISTENING EXERCISE

Ask a classmate, friend, or colleague who speaks English to read the reading selection for you aloud. Do not look at the text while he or she is reading. What difficulties did you have? Does it help that you have already worked through the reading and vocabulary prior to doing this exercise?

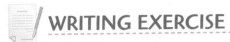

WRITING EXERCISE

Respiratory congestion often accompanies both flu and a cold. There are several distinguishing factors that separate the two. Your own years of experience in the health profession will make you familiar with the diagnostic criteria, and this exercise will now provide that vocabulary in English. This will improve your ability to discuss signs and symptoms with your patients.

Refer back to the reading and then use a sign or symptom listed in the Word Bank below to complete Table 4-2.

WORD BANK

nasal congestion

fever

mild fatigue

headache

sneezing

chest congestion

sore throat

cough

muscle and joint aches

scratchy throat

fatigue

Table 4-2 Differentiating Cold and Flu Symptoms	
Choose a sign or symptom from the Word Bank and place it in the correct table. Yes, some words may be used twice.	
COLD SYMPTOMS	FLU SYMPTOMS

Reading Selection 4-8

Read the following information in preparation for the dialogue reading.

PATIENT COMPLAINTS The term *patient complaints* is used widely in all health-care situations. It refers to the subjective report from the patient about his or her own perceived state of health. It is their report of their signs and symptoms of illness. As health professionals, we want to collect both subjective and objective reports before diagnosing and treating the individual.

A *subjective report* is what the patient tells you he or she is feeling or experiencing.

An *objective report* is what the doctor or nurse observes and assesses through tests and examination regarding the person's state of health.

Note: This exercise takes a very different approach to the reading in this unit. In this instance, YOU must participate in the construction of a dialogue between a patient and his doctor. To do so, use vocabulary from all previous units, but especially from this unit on the respiratory system to fill in the blanks. When you have completed that task, read the dialogue aloud or silently to yourself. Be sure that your responses create logical sentences.

The Respiratory System

MAKING A SIMPLE DIAGNOSIS

Scene: At Doctor Crabb's office.

Doctor: Hello, Mr. Johnson. My name is _____. I understand that you think you may have pneumonia. Does it hurt to _____?

Patient: No.

Doctor: Are you short of _____? Have a cough?

Patient: No, but I can't breathe through my nose.

Doctor: OK. Does your chest _____ when you breathe?

Patient: No, but I can hear it.

Doctor: Oh. At times do you _____ noisily?

Patient: Yeah.

Doctor: I can see you are breathing through your _____ now. Is your _____ plugged?

Patient: Yes. But sometimes it runs.

Doctor: When you blow your _____, do you have any discharge?

Patient: Yes. It hurts to _____ my _____.

Doctor: What color is that discharge? Brown, clear, or green?

Patient: It's actually kind of a yellowish-brown.

Doctor: I'm going to press my fingers around your eyes and nose. Tell me if it _____ at all.

Patient: Yes. Right there, behind my right eye . . . feels like a lot of pressure. And yes . . . there, too . . . underneath my left eye.

Doctor: Fine. I'm going to take your _____ now. Put this under your _____.

Thank you. Don't _____ for a minute.

* * *

Fine. All right. I see you have a slight temperature of 99°F (37.2°C) . . .

Patient: Is that OK? What do you think? Do I have pneumonia?

Doctor: Well, one last test. I'm going to listen to your chest. Please unbutton your _____ a little for me. OK. Breathe _____. Now _____. Again. Again.
OK. That's good. Well, I don't believe you have _____. It seems you are _____ and having difficulty _____. Your _____ are definitely blocked, but I don't think they are _____.

Patient: Do I need medication?

Doctor: Not really. But you might want to try some nonprescription _____
to alleviate some of that _____. It will make it easier to sleep. Get
some _____, take a day or two off work, and you'll be OK. Take
an _____ for signs of _____ or pains or an antipyretic
to reduce signs of a fever every 4–6 hours. You'll be OK.

Patient: Thanks, bye.

READING EXERCISES

Use what you have learned in constructing the dialogue above to ensure that you understand the
general meaning of the exchange, can describe specifics, and have built additional vocabulary.

Understanding the General Meaning

Read the text again. Think about it.

1) One of the characters has a specific purpose. Who is it?

_____

2) What is that specific purpose?

_____

Learning Specifics

1) What is the official diagnosis? In other words, what does this patient have?

_____

2) Give your rationale. Explain why you have decided upon this diagnosis.

_____

3) What is the doctor's name?

_____

4) What is the patient's name?

_____

Building Vocabulary

Determining Meaning from Context. To build vocabulary, study the following words
or terms taken from this text. Discover all you can about them by looking at them in context.
Choose the correct meaning. Finally, take a look at how these words or terms expand in
English.

1. **Congested** *(adjective)*

In context:
a) When people have very bad colds they cannot breathe through their mouths because
their sinuses are congested.
b) Every morning and every afternoon in a big city, the roads are congested with traffic
commuting to and from work.

Meaning: The word *congested* in the context of the respiratory system can best be described
as meaning
a) barrier
b) stopped

c) hampered

d) clogged or blocked

Word expansion:

a) Lung *congestion* makes it difficult to breathe and cough. (noun)

b) The man was diagnosed with *congestive* heart failure. (adjective)

2. Decongestant *(noun)*

In context:

a) A decongestant is a type of medicine that helps open the sinuses.

Meaning: The word *decongestant* can best be described as meaning

a) removal of injurious agents

b) expectorant

c) expulsive

d) something having the ability to reduce congestion

Sentence Completion. Cough and cold medications are used to treat the symptoms of these illnesses. Use the Word Bank below to complete the sentences. You may use a word more than once.

WORD BANK

antitussive

decongestant

expectorant

antibiotic

1) If you have congestion in your lungs (your lower respiratory tract), it is important to cough deeply and expectorate any phlegm. The type of medication needed for this is a/an

   _____

2) If you have congestion in your sinuses or nose (your upper respiratory tract), you may have to breathe through your mouth. To reduce these symptoms, the type of medication needed is a/an

   _____

3) If you have a respiratory infection that has spread to your throat, you may need this medication to reduce or alleviate the symptoms.

   _____

4) If you have pneumonia, you might be prescribed these two types of medication to alleviate the symptoms and promote recovery.

   _____

5) If you have a cold with a cough, and that cough keeps you awake at night, you might be wise to take this over-the-counter medication.

   _____

SPEAKING EXERCISE

Go back through the Sentence Completion exercise and read it aloud to someone. Ask a peer or teacher to count the number of times you had to stop to struggle with a word. Then, write those words down so that you may practice their pronunciation. The Pronunciation Hints box below will help.

PRONUNCIATION HINTS

expectorant – ĕk-**spĕk**′tō-rănt

decongestant – dē′kŏn-**jĕs**′t- ănt

pneumonia – nū-**mō**′nē-ă (note the silent letter "p")

LISTENING EXERCISE

If you have recorded yourself reading the exercises aloud, listen to your recording now without looking at the words in this book. Listen only. Do not let the written words be your guide. Evaluate yourself.

- What do you notice about your open pronunciation?

- Are you speaking clearly?

- Are you speaking at a normal rhythm and rate?

If you have not recorded yourself, ask a peer to read any part of this section aloud to you. Do NOT read along with them. Listen only. What do you notice about the way they speak? What lesson do you learn from listening to another?

WRITING EXERCISE

Use a key word from the previous exercises to create new sentences to describe some of the common treatments and medications for the illnesses described in this section of Unit 4.

_____

_____

_____

Reading Selection 4-9

Read the following short story about two people who rescued a child. Remember, we are still working within the context of the respiratory system.

LACK OF OXYGEN

Mary and Emmanuel were having a picnic at the lake. It was a hot, lazy August day and the beach was crowded with happy people. There were a lot of people in the water, playing and splashing, and generally just having fun. Mary noticed some children laughing and playing around a small inflatable raft. Inside the raft was a child of no more than 8 or 9 years old. She pointed this out to Emmanuel, commenting the child seemed young to be alone in the boat. He noticed the little girl was not wearing a life jacket, either. The other children were excitedly trying to turn the raft over. Everyone was laughing wildly.

Mary and Emmanuel drifted back to their own conversation and began to have lunch. Suddenly, there was a great commotion: children screaming and people running toward the beach! They jumped up and ran, too. The raft and the child had overturned. And the child was missing! Emmanuel charged through the crowd and out into the water. He lifted the little raft high and tossed it away. There was the little girl . . . floating with her face down in the water . . . lifeless. He flipped her over as fast as possible and headed for shore. Mary met him halfway out and they quickly brought the child to land. She yelled at the child and shook her, just a little. The girl was unconscious. Mary looked directly at Emmanuel. She instructed him to call an ambulance, tell them a little girl drowned, and then return to her on the beach. She checked for signs of breathing. None. She gave the little girl two short breaths and checked for breathing. Then she checked for a pulse. None.

Mary began CPR. She worked diligently and hard for 2 or 3 minutes until the little girl regained consciousness. The girl sputtered and coughed. Mary quickly rolled her on her side into the recovery position so the little girl could cough out the water from her lungs.

The ambulance arrived within minutes and the child was taken to the hospital. She survived.

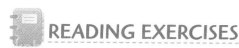

READING EXERCISES

Understanding the General Meaning

Take a moment now to review what you have just read. Read the text again. Think about it. Do you understand it? Explore the general meaning of the text by completing this exercise.

1) What is this story about?

_____

2) What happened to the little girl in the raft?

_____

3) Why were Mary and Emmanuel interested in the raft and the children playing around it?

_____

4) What were the little girl's signs and symptoms when they brought her to the beach?

_____

Applying What You Know and Have Learned to Answer Questions

Take a moment now to review what you have just read. Read the text again. As a health professional, you will be familiar with the concepts behind the questions.

1) Why did Mary use full cardiopulmonary resuscitation (CPR) instead of only mouth-to-mouth pulmonary resuscitation (artificial respiration)?

_____

2) What does CPR stand for?

_____

3) What are the ABCs of emergency first aid?

_____

_____

Building Vocabulary

Defining New Words.   In this exercise you are asked to create your own definition of the following words and expressions taken from the text. Do not use a dictionary. Try to define the term simply from reading and re-reading the story. Please note that while these words are written in common English, it is important for the health professional to be able to understand them. Each and every time a new patient is encountered, the health professional must listen actively to ascertain the details of the incident, accident, injury, or illness.

1) drowned _____

2) lifeless _____

3) sputtered _____

4) commotion _____

5) crowded _____

6) splashing _____

7) over-turned _____

8) floating _____

9) diligently _____

10) jumped up and ran _____

11) tossed it away _____

12) charged through the crowd _____

Mix and Match: Synonyms. Some words and phrases have very similar meanings. Use the exercise in Box 4-3 to see if you can recognize the similarities.

Improving Your Use of Medical Terminology. The following text is written in simple, basic English. Rewrite or summarize the selected sentences using medical terminology. Sometimes two sentences will fit together into one new sentence.

Example: *She checked for signs of breathing = She assessed for breathing.* Or you might write: *She assessed respiration.*

> She yelled at the child and shook her, just a little. The girl was unconscious. Mary looked directly at Emmanuel. She instructed him to call an ambulance, tell them a little girl drowned, and then return to her on the beach. She checked for signs of breathing. None. She gave the little girl two short breaths and checked for breathing again. None. Then, she checked for a pulse. None.
>
> Mary began CPR. She worked diligently and hard for 2 or 3 minutes until the little girl regained consciousness. The girl sputtered and coughed. Mary quickly rolled her on her side into the recovery position so the little girl could cough out the water from her lungs.

BOX 4-3 Mix and Match: Synonyms

Find the synonym for the following words. Draw a line to connect them.

TERM	SYNONYM
unconscious	call an ambulance
checked her	assessed her
call 911	not responding

---

1) She checked for signs of breathing. Then she checked for pulse.

   _____

2) She yelled at the child and shook her, just a little.

   _____

3) She instructed him to call an ambulance, tell them a little girl drowned, and then return to her on the beach.

   _____

4) Mary began CPR.

   _____

5) The girl sputtered and coughed.

   _____

6) Mary quickly rolled her on her side into the recovery position so the little girl could cough out the water from her lungs.

   _____

SPEAKING EXERCISE

Memorize the following information. Stand in front of a mirror or a friend and recite it aloud smoothly and with confidence. Practice your public speaking in this way.

> Artificial respiration is also known as mouth-to-mouth resuscitation. It is the procedure followed when an individual is unable to breathe on their own; in the procedure, air is forced in to and out of the lungs.
>
> Cardiopulmonary resuscitation is most commonly referred to as CPR. This is the accepted procedure for providing artificial ventilation and external cardiac compression when the patient is not breathing on his or her own AND a pulse cannot be found. CPR is never initiated on a person who has a pulse or heart beat.

PRONUNCIATION HINTS

initiate – ĭn-ĭsh′ ē- ā′t

unconscious – ŭn-kŏn′shŭs

ventilation – vĕn″tĭ-lā′shŭn

LISTENING EXERCISE

If you would like to listen to emergency medical professionals talk about and teach basic skills for dealing with respiratory emergencies, search the Internet. Type in the search words "respiratory, video" or "respiratory emergencies, video clips." Most video clips have an audio component.

WRITING EXERCISE—A SHORT STORY

In this exercise you are asked to write a short story. The short story genre has specific characteristics and requirements. See Box 4-4 to learn about the structure of the short story genre.

BOX 4-4 The Short Story Genre

The requirements of the short story genre include the following:

Plan—To compose a story, a plan is needed. Short stories require a plot or problem to be resolved.

Characters—Characters need to be identified and it is they who will work through the problem.

Setting—A story requires a setting. It is set in a specific time frame. It has a beginning, middle, and end. The beginning usually sets the scene within which the story will be told and introduces the main character or characters.

Voice—The writer must consider voice. Who is telling the story and what choice of language (i.e., formal or informal; adult or child; active or passive voice) will they use to communicate the story?

---

1) Write a short story entitled "An Incidence of Cardiopulmonary Resuscitation." Use the words provided in the Word Bank below and add words of your own. Be sure to use all of the words provided, but you may need to change the form or tense for logic. This is an exercise in sentence structure and story composition.

WORD BANK

man

fell

awoke

45 years old

ground

strangers

heart

unconscious

rescue

paramedics

was not

chest

_____

_____

_____

_____

_____

_____

_____

_____

_____

_____

2) Check your work. Complete Table 4-3 by copying your sentences or phrases into the format of a short story.

3) Use your new vocabulary again to express yourself in writing. Write a sentence or two to offer your own professional opinion on the following question. Share your answer with a colleague who is not from the same country as you. Are there any differences in the suggestions? Question: What follow-up care would you recommend for this child when she arrives at your hospital?

_____

_____

_____

Table 4-3 Applying the Format of a Short Story

STRUCTURE	EXAMPLE FROM MY STORY
Characters	
Setting or scene	
Plot or problem established	
Problem resolved	
Time frame: When does the story occur?	

ANSWER KEY

Anatomy and Physiology

 READING SELECTION 4-1—THE PURPOSE OF THE RESPIRATORY SYSTEM

Understanding the General Meaning

1) The premise of the short paragraph is that the respiratory system functions to exchange gas. This is the system's purpose.

2) No. It is not healthy for the body to retain carbon dioxide (CO_2). It must be expelled from the body.

Building Vocabulary

Determining Meaning from Context

1) When used together the words *waste* and *product* refer to an unusable or unwanted material or substance.

2) The word *exchange* in relation to gas exchange means to trade or swap or replace one for the other.

3) Gas is brought in as components of air from the environment. The body extracts or keeps the incoming gases that it needs to function; that is, oxygen and nitrogen. This displaces or pushes out/expels the internal gases that it does not want or need—that is, carbon dioxide. Some gases derive from physiological processes within the body and need the trigger of incoming gases to force them out of the body.

Mix and Match

BOX 4-1 Mix and Match: Parts of the Respiratory System: Answers	
PART OR STRUCTURE	**DESCRIPTION**
esophagus	passage leading from mouth and throat to stomach
diaphragm	creates suction in chest to draw in air to lungs
trachea	passage leading from pharynx to the lungs
pharynx	sends incoming air from nose and mouth to trachea
epiglottis	guards entrance to trachea and closes when swallowing
larynx	moves air being breathed in and out and makes voice sounds

Sentence Completion

1) carbon dioxide

2) oxygen

3) respiratory system

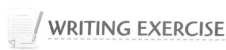

WRITING EXERCISE

Example:

If I can't get enough oxygen when I am breathing through my nose, I get hungry for air and breathe through my mouth.

READING SELECTION 4-2—ANATOMY AND PHYSIOLOGY OF THE LUNG

Understanding the General Meaning

1) The reading selection is in the genre of an information report.

2) The selection describes the process by which oxygen and carbon dioxide are exchanged.

Recognizing Specifics

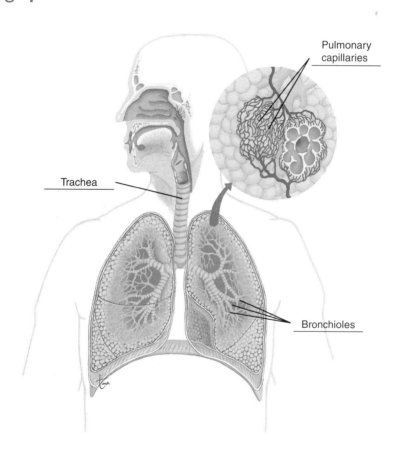

Pulmonary capillaries

Trachea

Bronchioles

Building Vocabulary

Determining Meaning from Context

1) a, 2) c, 3) c, 4) d, 5) a

Using New Words in Sentences

Sample Answers:

1) Capillaries in the alveoli of the lungs are the main agents of gas exchange, swapping carbon dioxide for oxygen.

2) Inhalation of adequate amounts of oxygen is very difficult for people with asthma or COPD.

Common Disorders and Diseases of the Respiratory System

 READING SELECTION 4-3—CHRONIC OBSTRUCTIVE PULMONARY DISEASE

Understanding the General Meaning

1) The general theme of the text is chronic illness.

2) The genre of this reading selection is that of an information report.

3) The components of an information report are structure, textual features, and grammatical features.

4) The purpose of an information report is to classify and/or describe something using clear and detailed information.

Building Vocabulary

Determining Meaning from Context

1) a, 2) c, 3) c, 4) d

Sentence Completion

1) chronicity

2) exacerbation

3) chronic obstructive pulmonary disease

4) chronic bronchitis, emphysema

 WRITING EXERCISE

The Information Report on the reading about COPD.

Table 4-1 Information Report: Answers	
GENRE HIGHLIGHTS	HIGHLIGHTS COPIED FROM READING SELECTION
Structure	
topic identified	
at least 1 or 2 facts given	A chronic disease is one . . .
	It has phases of remission and acute exacerbation
Grammar	
adjectives used	chronic, residual, diminished
conjunctions used	and, but, with
correct verb tenses used	all verbs are in present tense
Writing Features	
a plan or theme	COPD

Table 4-1 Information Report: Answers	
GENRE HIGHLIGHTS	HIGHLIGHTS COPIED FROM READING SELECTION
Writing Features	
factual sentences	all of the sentences are factual
capital letters and full stops	Yes, for beginning of sentences and ends of sentences. Also proper names and titles are capitalized.
paragraph form used	√
spelling check	√

READING SELECTION 4-4—ACUTE BRONCHITIS AND ASTHMA

Understanding the General Meaning

1) The thesis or main theme of this reading selection is the signs and symptoms of acute bronchitis and acute asthma.

2) The person with an attack of chronic bronchitis may look cyanotic and have a recurrent, productive cough. Visually, the nurse and doctor may see distended neck veins in this patient, increased respiratory rate, and tachycardia with a heart rate of greater than 100/min. The asthmatic patient leans forward to gasp for air, has a nonproductive cough, appears frightened, and has short inspirations, prolonged expirations, and increased respiratory and pulse rates.

3) Clients with chronic bronchitis and asthma share the symptoms of audible wheezing with prolonged expiration as well as a cough.

Building Vocabulary

Determining Meaning from Context

1) c, 2) c, 3) a, 4) c

Sentence Completion

1) apnea

2) dyspnea

3) eupnea

4) asthma

5) apnea

6) tachypnea

READING SELECTION 4-5—MORE ABOUT THE LUNGS AND RESPIRATORY SYSTEM

Understanding the General Meaning

1) The general meaning and focus of the reading selection is the physiology (function) of the respiratory system.

2) The purpose of the reading selection is to explain the function of parts of the respiratory system. It is likely written for students studying biology, medicine, nursing or other health-care subjects.

Learning Specific Facts

1) Infection, disease, blockage, or other injury to the respiratory system can cause a change in normal breathing patterns.

2) Pulmonary capacity is the ability of the lung to accommodate a sufficient intake of air. It is determined by a combination of specific lung volumes.

3) Secretions are fluid-like substances excreted in the respiratory system. They trap toxins in an attempt to isolate and expel them.

4) Examples of secretions in the respiratory system are mucous and phlegm.

Building Vocabulary

Using New Words in Sentences

Sample Answers:

1) Gwen has limited pulmonary capacity.

2) When the patient puts it in her mouth, she must inhale deeply in order to gain a measure of her capacity.

3) She receives oxygen through the prongs.

4) This improves her respiratory and cardiac function.

Using New Words to Answer Specific Questions

1) The diaphragm is an expanse of muscle between the abdominal and thoracic cavities.

2) The trachea is also known as the windpipe because it is shaped like a hollow tube or pipe and air (wind) travels down it.

3a) The esophagus leads to the stomach.

3b) The windpipe leads to the lungs.

4) Yes. If a particle blocks or inhibits the lung's ability to expand or contract, respiratory arrest may occur. If it doesn't fully block the airway passage, it may rest in the lung, decompose over time, and become the source of a major infection that could lead to death.

Fill in the Blanks

Sample Answer:

"Hello, **Florence.** I'm your **nurse.** I'm going to help you breathe more efficiently. Watch me and do as I say. Take a deep **breath** in then **hold** it. Count to three and then **release** the air. Good. **Breathe** in. Hold. **Breathe** out. Good. Now we're going to **breathe** deeply. Put your **hands** on your **diaphragm** so that you can feel where the air should be going. **Close** your mouth and breathe only **through** your **nose.** OK. **Breathe** deeply again, with your hands on your **diaphragm.** 1-2-3, begin. Breathe **deeply.** Good."

WRITING EXERCISE

1) Pulmonary capacities are combinations of specific lung volumes that signify the ability of the lung to accommodate a sufficient intake of air.

2) The ventilation rate is the rate at which the lungs inflate and deflate.

3) pH means potential hydrogen in the blood.

4) Mucous is the name for the secretions that trap toxins in an attempt to isolate and expel them.

5) Congestion is a blockage of the passage of air.

6) Phlegm is a sticky secretion of mucous that originates only in the lungs.

7) Sputum is expelled phlegm.

READING SELECTION 4-6 —LUNG CANCER AND DEMOGRAPHICS

Understanding the General Meaning

1) This reading selection reports lung cancer statistics and trends and incidents/demographics.

2) The incidence of lung cancer for men is on the rise in China.

3) In the Western world, men and woman have an equal chance of getting lung cancer.

Building Vocabulary

Determining Meaning from Context

1) c, 2) b, 3) c, 4) d, 5) c

True or False

1) True, 2) True, 3) False (there is not scientific proof of this), 4) True

Treatments, Interventions, and Assistance

READING SELECTION 4-7—RESPIRATORY SYMPTOMS

Understanding the General Meaning

1) The text tells how to prevent respiratory infection.

2) The text describes the process of autoimmune reaction to respiratory threats.

3) The general theme of the text is respiratory symptoms.

Building Vocabulary

Determining Meaning from Context

1) a, 2) b

Fill in the Blanks

1) smoke, 2) inhale, 3) choke, 4) wheeze, breathe, 5) sneeze, 6) rises, 7) throbs, 8) make, 9) congested, 10) swells, 11) caught, 12) hurts

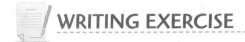

WRITING EXERCISE

COLD SYMPTOMS	FLU SYMPTOMS
nasal congestion	fever
sneezing	headache
mild fatigue	fatigue
sore throat	chest congestion
cough	cough
scratchy throat	muscle and joint aches and pains

READING SELECTION 4-8—MAKING A SIMPLE DIAGNOSIS

Scene: At Doctor Crabb's office.

Doctor: Hello, Mr. Johnson. My name is **Dr. Crabb.** I understand that you think you may have pneumonia. Does it hurt to **breathe**?

Patient: No.

Doctor: Are you short of **breath**? Have a cough?

Patient: No, but I can't breathe through my nose.

Doctor: OK. Does your chest **hurt** when you breathe?

Patient: No, but I can hear it.

Doctor: Oh. At times do you **breathe** noisily?

Patient: Yeah.

Doctor: I can see you are breathing through your **mouth** now. Is your **nose** plugged?

Patient: Yes. But sometimes it runs.

Doctor: When you blow your **nose,** do you have any discharge?

Patient: Yes. It hurts to **blow** my **nose.**

Doctor: What color is that discharge? Brown, clear, or green?

Patient: It's actually kind of a yellowish-brown.

Doctor: I'm going to press my fingers around your eyes and nose. Tell me if it **hurts** at all.

Patient: Yes. Right there, behind my right eye . . . feels like a lot of pressure. And yes . . . there, too . . . underneath my left eye.

Doctor: Fine. I'm going to take your **temperature** now. Put this under your **tongue.**

Thank you. Don't **speak** for a minute.

* * *

Fine. All right. I see you have a slight temperature of 99°F (37.2°C) . . .

Patient: Is that OK? What do you think? Do I have pneumonia?

Doctor: Well, one last test. I'm going to listen to your chest. Please unbutton your **shirt** a little for me. OK. Breathe **in.** Now **out.** Again. Again. OK. That's good. Well, I don't believe you have **pneumonia.** It seems you are **congested** and having difficulty **breathing.** Your **sinuses** are definitely blocked, but I don't think they are **infected.**

Patient: Do I need medication?

Doctor: Not really. But you might want to try some nonprescription **decongestant** to alleviate some of that **congestion.** It will make it easier to sleep. Get some **rest,** take a day or two off work, and you'll be OK. Take an **analgesic** for signs of **aches** or pains or an antipyretic to reduce signs of a fever every 4–6 hours. You'll be OK.

Patient: Thanks, bye.

Understanding the General Meaning

1) Mr. Johnson has a specific purpose.

2) Mr. Johnson's purpose is to get treated for his ailment.

Learning Specifics

1) The official diagnosis is congested sinuses which may be inflamed from exposure to an airborne toxin or allergen. His sinuses don't seem to be infected.

2) The patient's signs and symptoms—pain and pressure when his sinus cavities are pressed, nasal congestion, and runny nose—indicate congested sinuses. The patient's lungs are clear and he has no cough, ruling out pneumonia.

3) The doctor's name is Dr. Crabb.

4) The patient's name is Mr. Johnson.

Building Vocabulary

Determining Meaning from Context

1) d, 2) d

Sentence Completion

1) expectorant, 2) decongestant, 3) antibiotic, 4) expectorant and antibiotic, 5) cough medicine also known as antitussive medication

WRITING EXERCISE

Sample Answers:

The doctor recommended that the patient take an over-the-counter medication such as acetaminophen to reduce his fever and alleviate his aches and pains.

The patient complained of having difficulty breathing through his nose and feeling clogged up. He was told to take a decongestant.

Understanding the General Meaning

1) It is a story about a rescue from an incident of near-drowning.

2) She nearly drowned when she fell into the water.

3) Mary and Emmanuel were interested in the children playing around the raft because there were no adults nearby to supervise the children. It was an unsafe situation.

4) She had no pulse, wasn't breathing, and was unconscious.

Applying What You Know and Have Learned to Answer Questions

1) CPR is used in the absence of a heartbeat and absence of spontaneous breathing. Mouth-to-mouth resuscitation is used if the heart is beating.

2) CPR stands for cardiopulmonary resuscitation.

3) The ABCs of emergency first aid are airway, breathing, and circulation. In other words, the airway should first be checked to see if it is open, then breathing assessed, and then circulation (heartbeat) assessed.

Building Vocabulary

Defining New Words

1) drowned—suffocated in water

2) lifeless—not showing any signs of being alive

3) sputtered—made popping sounds while trying to make words or vocalize. People may sputter if they have fluids in their mouth at the same time they wish to talk or are suddenly surprised. A motorboat engine will sometimes sputter in the water when it is having difficulty starting. Little children like to sit in the bath tub and put their lips on the surface of the water and blow to make a sputtering sound.

4) commotion—a disturbance

5) crowded—many people in very close proximity. In the United States and Canada, the zone of proximity or area of personal space that is comfortable for people is the distance of one arm: approximately one arm's length between people.

6) splashing—the act of slapping or forcefully moving water

7) over-turned—turned upside down

8) floating—the act of resting atop the water rather than in it

9) diligently—done with great attention

10) jumped up and ran—a spontaneous movement of rising to one's feet and beginning to run almost all at the same time

11) tossed it away—threw it away or discarded it

12) charged through the crowd—ran through the crowd, disregarding people and bumping into them as he ran through them in a hurry.

Mix and Match: Synonyms

BOX 4–3 Mix and Match: Synonyms: Answers	
TERM	**SYNONYM**
unconscious	not responding
assessed her	checked her
call 911	call an ambulance

Improving Your Use of Medical Terminology

1) She checked vital signs or life signs.

2) She assessed for level of consciousness.

3) She followed the accepted procedure for calling for help.

4) Mary initiated cardiopulmonary resuscitation.

5) The child regained consciousness, struggled to breathe, and expelled lake water from her lungs.

6) Mary rolled the patient onto her side to prevent re-absorption of water into the lungs, promote expulsion of water from the respiratory system, and promote healthy ventilation.

WRITING EXERCISE

1) Individual short story using words in the Word Bank.

2) Table 4-3 completed using sentences from original story.

3) Your professional opinion.

4) Your suggestions concerning follow-up.

Unit 5 continues to use reading selections and exercises to help you acquire career–specific language and build competencies in communication. It explores language through the example of the gastrointestinal system.

SECTION ONE   Anatomy and Physiology

The unit begins with an overview of the anatomy and physiology of the gastrointestinal system to build vocabulary and context for the rest of the unit. It also provides an introduction to the language of nutrients and nutrition. Grammar exercises will help reinforce naming, describing, and explaining. There are opportunities for working with question words and parsing new verbs, all within the specific health context of the gastrointestinal system.

Reading Selection 5-1

Read the following in anticipation of the exercises that follow.

THE GASTROINTESTINAL SYSTEM

The gastrointestinal system, often abbreviated as the GI system, is also known as the digestive system. The terms are completely interchangeable. They refer to a system designed to ingest and transport food so that digestion can occur. The system's main function is to provide the body with healthy nutrients and provide a means to expel waste materials and toxins. This occurs through a series of processes: ingestion, digestion, metabolism, absorption, and elimination.

The alimentary canal forms the core of the system. A 28-foot long tract, it begins at the lips and proceeds through to the anus. It is composed of eight organs: the mouth, pharynx, esophagus, stomach, small intestine (and all associated glands), the large intestines (colon), rectum, and the anal canal and anus.

When an object or fluid is placed in the mouth, the first process, ingestion, begins. Ingestion means taking a fluid, material, or substance into the body and swallowing it. For solids and semi-solids, this is accomplished through the moistening of material in the mouth by saliva (a product of the salivary glands). Chewing (mastication) breaks larger pieces of solid materials into smaller pieces. Digestion also begins in the mouth when enzymes released by the salivary glands begin to break down sugars and other carbohydrates. The tongue then rolls the now moist and manageable-sized portions back toward the throat. Simply stated then, when oral ingestion occurs, passage of the material is facilitated through the response of the salivary glands and the processes of chewing and swallowing. The ingested material then passes the pharynx and enters the esophagus. Next, it travels downward through the alimentary canal to the stomach.

The stomach beings to process its contents within the first 20 minutes of receiving food, fluid, and any other matter/substance. That material is broken down, metabolized, and formed into new substances, which are then passed along to the small intestine. Accessory organs such as the liver and pancreas are located adjacent to (near to) the GI system. They supply enzymes and hormones that further facilitate digestion and metabolism of the ingested material.

It generally takes up to 6 hours for digestion to occur. During this process, solid products of digestion are transported into the small intestine. In the small intestine, the metabolized byproducts of digestion are absorbed for use by the body's cells, tissues, and organs. By the end of a 6–12 hour period, most of the ingested, digested material should have passed into the colon (large intestine). There water is absorbed and solid feces formed. Twenty-four hours from the time the material passed the lips and entered the gastrointestinal system, waste products will have arrived in the rectum to be defecated.

In summary, the main functions of the GI tract are ingestion, digestion, metabolism, absorption, and defecation.

 READING EXERCISES

Take a moment now to review what you have just read. While you are very likely quite knowledgeable about the process of digestion and the gastrointestinal system, it is less likely that you are familiar with the English terminology. These exercises will help you acquire that vocabulary.

Understanding the General Meaning

In your own words, describe the process of digestion from beginning to end.

_____

Learning Specific Facts

1) What is the difference between digestion and ingestion?

_____

2) What is the difference between nutrients and waste?

_____

3) How long does the entire process of digestion take?

_____

4) What is a synonym for the gastrointestinal system?

_____

5) What is meant by the word *tract* as in GI tract or digestive tract or even respiratory tract?

_____

6) How long is the alimentary canal?

_____

7) Another way to say that the body expels waste material is to say that it _____ it. Find a synonym.

Building Vocabulary

As your vocabulary grows, you will be able to label body parts, discern the meaning of new words from their context, become familiar with terms for accessory organs, and learn how certain verbs are used.

Labeling Anatomical Parts. Label the diagram of the digestive system shown below.

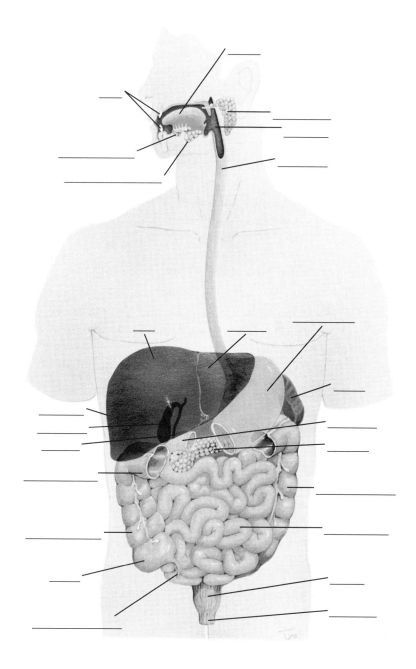

Determining Meaning from Context. To build vocabulary, study the following words taken from this text. Refer back to the reading and review them in context, then choose the correct meaning. Finally, take a look at how these words or terms expand in English.

1. Metabolism *(noun)*

In context:
a) The true function of the gastrointestinal system is metabolism.
b) Metabolism occurs when molecules are broken down to produce energy.

Meaning: The word *metabolism* can best be described as meaning
a) a process of intake and output
b) the GI tract
c) chemical reactions that break down and then build up complex molecules
d) all of the above

Word expansion:

a) In order *to metabolize* sugars, the pancreas must be able to secrete insulin. (verb, infinitive)

b) *Metabolic* acidosis is a disruption in the pH balance of the body that can result from gastrointestinal disorders. (adjective)

2. Digestion *(noun)*

In context:

a) Digestion is facilitated by the hunger response to smell.

b) To promote digestion, go for a walk after a large meal.

Meaning: The word *digestion* can best be described as meaning

a) the process by which food is converted, absorbed, and assimilated

b) the process of taking in foods

c) chewing and swallowing

d) the process of food breakdown in the stomach and small intestine

Word expansion:

a) *Digestive* disorders can include vomiting, diarrhea, and gas. (adjective)

b) When the autopsy was performed, the coroner found partially *digested* shrimp in the person's stomach. (adjective)

c) For the elderly, spicy foods can be difficult *to digest*. (verb, infinitive)

3. Defecate *(verb, infinitive to defecate)*

In context:

a) After the age of 2, our culture expects that a person will defecate only in the toilet.

Meaning: The word *defecate* can best be described as meaning

a) sitting

b) utilizing

c) voiding feces

d) voiding urine

Word expansion:

a) The elderly patient is highly embarrassed because for the first time in his adult life, he *defecated* in his bed. (verb, past tense)

b) *Defecation* is a normal body process for eliminating wastes. (noun)

4. Ingestion *(noun)*

In context:

a) The ingestion of large amounts of alcohol can lead to coma and death.

b) Ingestion of small toys, peas, marbles, and coins is not uncommon for very small children. Everything goes into their mouths.

Meaning: The word *ingestion* can best be described as meaning

a) swallowing

b) metabolism of nutrients

c) taking in, absorbing, eating

d) inhaling materials into the digestive tract

Word expansion:

a) The emergency room doctor believes the patient *ingested* 20 tranquillizers in an attempt at suicide. (verb, past tense)

b) The person next door in our apartment building has cerebral palsy. He *ingests* food through a tube leading to his small intestine, not his mouth. (verb, present tense)

5. Waste *(noun)*

In context:

a) Biological wastes originating in the body are generally excreted through the bowels.

b) Airborne waste can be excreted through the process of breathing, coughing, and sneezing.

Meaning: In the medical, biological context, the word *waste* can best be described as meaning

a) a process

b) a product

c) the function of eating and absorbing

d) the undigested residue of food that will be excreted from the body

Word expansion:

a) The patient has been unable to eat or take fluids for almost a week. She is frail and beginning *to waste away*. This means her body is not able to conserve any nutrients and she is beginning to weaken. Her health is declining. (verb, infinitive)

Recognizing Grammatical Structure and Meaning. The reading above refers to *accessory organs* as playing a role in the process of digestion and elimination. An accessory organ in this context refers to an organ that aids in digestion but is not part of the digestive tract. Accessory organs of the digestive system are the salivary glands, liver, gallbladder, and pancreas. The next two exercises provide vocabulary for naming, defining, locating, and describing those organs. Review the Grammar Alert and proceed to the first exercise.

> **GRAMMAR ALERT: LINKING VERBS** A word or word group that functions to describe, define, or locate the subject of the phrase is known as a *copula* and many of these are verbs. Also known as *linking verbs*, copulative verbs link or establish a relationship between the subject and its complement. They can also identify characteristics of an activity done by the subject or describe or rename a subject.
>
> Linking verbs include all forms of the verb *to be* as well as *look, feel, seem, appear, become, grow, remain, look, smell, sound,* and *taste*. They do not show action, but some of them can also be used as action verbs. For example, in "I feel angry," *feel* is a copulative/linking verb, but in the sentence "I feel pain in my arm," *feel* is an action verb. Interestingly, linking verbs also include occasions in which a non human subject is assigned an activity (a verb) that it cannot actually do. For example, "the blood felt sticky." Blood cannot feel. In this example, *felt* could easily be replaced with a more appropriate verb, such as *was*.
>
> Here is a little test to help you determine if a verb is a linking or copulative verb. Substitute the verb for some form of *to be* and determine if it makes sense. For example, "I feel tired" can be changed to "I am tired" so *feel* is being used as a linking/copulative verb. However, "I feel pain from the injury to my arm" cannot be changed to "I am pain from the injury . . ." so it is not a linking verb.

1) The pancreas is found in the abdomen. It sits just below the stomach. The pancreas is a gland that secretes digestive enzymes and hormones. The enzymes are secreted into the small intestines to affect the breakdown of carbohydrates, fats, and proteins.

   a) Identify the linking verb phrase. Explain the rationale for your choice.

   _____

   _____

   b) Replace the linking verb with a more appropriate one. Rewrite the sentence.

   _____

   _____

c) Glands *secrete*. Based on your own medical knowledge, explain the verb *secrete* in English.

_____

d) There are a number of copulas (linking verbs) in Question 1. Identify one that describes the subject of a phrase.

_____

2) Salivary glands are found in the mouth and throat. There are several of them and they secrete either digestive juices or mucus. Combined, they produce a substance called saliva. Saliva keeps the mouth moist and lubricates particles (materials) to aid in swallowing.

a) Identify one linking verb that locates the subject of a sentence.

_____

b) Identify a copular verb or copular verb phrase that identifies the characteristics of an activity done by the subject.

_____

3) The pancreas lies posterior to the stomach. It serves both the digestive and endocrine systems. It secretes digestive juices into the duodenum (beginning section of the small intestine) to facilitate the breakdown of carbohydrates, proteins, and fats into simpler compounds.

a) Identify the copular verb phrase. Explain the rationale for your choice.

_____

_____

b) Rewrite the first sentence using a more appropriate verb.

_____

4) The liver is a very large organ. It is also a gland. Located in the upper abdomen, just under the diaphragm, its function is the metabolism of carbohydrates, fats, and proteins in preparation for use or excretion. The liver also detoxifies a variety of substances as part of the process of digestion.

a) Identify one linking verb that describes the subject of a sentence.

_____

b) Identify one verb copula (linking verb) that describes the characteristics of an activity carried out by the subject.

_____

c) Based on your own medical knowledge of the liver, define the term *detoxify*.

_____

d) Based on your own medical knowledge, is there a difference between the terms *excretion* and *elimination?* If so, explain.

_____

5) The gallbladder is a gland found on the underside of the liver that stores bile which it receives from the liver. It secretes bile into the small intestine when it becomes aware of the presence of fats.

a) Identify one verb copula that describes the subject of a sentence.

_____

b) Based on your own medical knowledge, describe the color of bile.

_____

c) Rewrite the following sentence using a more commonly used descriptor to locate this organ: *It is found on the underside of the liver.*

_____

Using New Words to Identify Body Organs.
In previous units, the terms *function* and *responsibility* have been used in a medical context to describe the activity or purpose of various parts of the body. Use the Word Bank below and write the name of the organ described in the appropriate blank space. Your own knowledge of anatomy and physiology will aid you.

WORD BANK

stomach

salivary glands

rectum

pancreas

large intestine

liver and gallbladder

1) Absorbs water so that water is conserved and solid feces are produced. _____

2) Produce and release bile that helps digest fat. _____

3) Produces acid and enzymes that partially break down food.

_____

4) Receives and signals the need to eliminate stool. _____

5) Produces hormones that affect the level of sugar/glucose in the blood.

_____

Recognizing Antonyms.
Complete this exercise by referring back to the original reading to find the appropriate word of opposite meaning.

1) If the verb *secrete* means to "give off" or "emit," what is the opposite verb?

_____

2) If the verb *to conserve* means to protect, to preserve, or to avoid wasting, what is its antonym?

_____

3) If the verb *to eliminate* means to remove or to get rid of something, what is the antonym?

_____

SPEAKING EXERCISE

You have just completed reading another information report. This one was on the gastrointestinal system. The following exercise can help prepare you to speak in English at nursing or medical conferences. The Pronunciation Hints box below will help.

1) Stand in front of a mirror and read the report again, as if you were a teacher telling it to the class. You may glance at your paper from time to time, but do not simply read the report.

2) Now, challenge yourself to look in the mirror and pretend you are speaking to the class. Glance down only momentarily to gather the next sentence or two into your short-term memory, then look up, give eye contact to your reflection in the mirror, and practice speaking aloud to an audience.

PRONUNCIATION HINTS

gastrointestinal – găs"trō-ĭn-**těs'tĭ**n-ăl

cecum – **sē'**kŭm

defecate – **děf**-ě-kā't

saliva – să-**lī'**vă

salivary – **săl'**ĭ-věr-ē

glands – **glănd'**z

jujenostomy – jē"jū-**nŏs'**tō-mē

LISTENING EXERCISE

Go on the Internet. Search for a video clip or newscast of a politician or lecturer giving a speech to an audience. Find an American or Canadian example. Actively listen. The term *active listening* is a professional term that includes listening with your ears and eyes. To do this, be very attentive to the verbal and nonverbal communication occurring. Watch and listen. While you do so, also watch for the cultural norm of glancing at notes but keeping good, direct eye contact with the audience.

WRITING EXERCISE

Use your new vocabulary from this reading selection to describe the purpose and function of the gastrointestinal system. Be careful here with terminology. Differentiate between purpose and function in the context of the question. In this case identify the purpose of the system in general, and then describe how it actually functions. Use logic and describe the functional process in a step-wise progression from the first step to the last.

1) What is the purpose of the gastrointestinal system?

_____

2) What is the function of the gastrointestinal system?

_____

3) What are the steps, from first to last, in the processes of the gastrointestinal system?

_____

_____

_____

_____

_____

_____

_____

_____

_____

_____

Reading Selection 5-2

Read the following aloud or silently to yourself.

NUTRIENTS

Nutrients are the chemicals found within foods that promote the health of the human body. Usually, nutrients are received by the body via the gastrointestinal tract. Once ingested, they must be digested, metabolized, and absorbed to assist the body with maintaining health and repairing the various tissues in the body. Nutrients also assist with the synthesis of enzymes and hormones as well as with other body processes. The field of study that deals with nutrients is called *nutrition*. A health professional who works with people's diets and promotes healthy eating is called a *nutritionist* or *dietician*.

READING EXERCISES

The following exercises will help increase your vocabulary and ability to communicate effectively with coworkers and patients.

Understanding the General Meaning

Read the text again. Think about it. Do you understand it? In your own words, summarize what you have just read here.

_____

_____

Building Vocabulary

Take a moment now to review what you have just read. Circle any words that are new or difficult for you. Jot them down here for future reference. At the end of this section, return to this point and write the definition down beside the words you have chosen.

_____

_____

Determining Meaning from Context.   To build vocabulary, study the following words or terms taken from this text. Discover all you can about them by looking at them in context. Next, choose the correct meaning, and finally, take a look at how these words or terms expand in English.

1. Nutrients *(noun, plural)*

In context:
a) Fast foods and snacks are often lacking in nutrients.
b) Some people believe that all food should be eaten raw so that the body can extract all the nutrients from them.
c) Nutrients provide nourishment for all living things.

Meaning: The best way to explain *nutrients* is
a) savory
b) unsavory
c) edible organic material that is ingested
d) a source of nourishment that promotes growth

Word expansion:
a) The foods we eat provide all the *nutrition* we need on a daily basis. (noun)
b) The *nutrient* value for compounds is based on the amount of heat and energy they produce. (adjective)
c) Fast foods are often lacking in *nutritional* value. (adjective)

2. Synthesis *(noun)*

In context:
a) Cement is the synthesis of sand, gravel, and water.
b) The term synthesis comes from biochemistry.

Meaning: The best way to explain *synthesis* is
a) a chemical reaction
b) the union of two or more elements to create a third substance
c) chain reaction of protons and neutrons
d) a biochemical reaction

Word expansion:
a) In common speech, natural or biological is the opposite of artificial or *synthetic.* (adjective)
b) Nylon is a *synthetic* product. (adjective)

3. enzymes *(noun, plural)*

In context:
a) Enzymes are important for digestion.
b) Synthetic enzymes are manmade compounds that mimic biological enzymes.

Meaning: An enzyme can best be described as
a) an initiator of a chemical reaction
b) a synthesizer
c) molecular biology
d) all of the above

Word expansion:
a) *Enzyme* kinetics is the study of the velocity of enzyme reactions. (adjective, here used with noun *kinetics* to form a term)

Using New Words and Their Derivatives in Sentences. Use a key word from the previous exercise to create a new sentence. The key words to be used are given at the beginning of each numbered line. Change the form of the word given in your new sentence. For example, change *nutrients* to *nutrient* or *nutrition* or *nutritionist.*

1) nutrients _____

2) synthesis _____

3) enzymes _____

SPEAKING EXERCISE

Re-read the short report on Nutrition. Read it aloud and read it quickly. Notice how many times you are required to say nutrition or some other form of the word. Is it easy to pronounce? Take a look at the Pronunciation Hints box below. It will help you with some difficult words.

PRONUNICATION HINTS

enzymes – **ĕn′zīm′z**

synthesis – **sĭn′thĕ-sĭs**

nutrients – **nū′trē-ĕnts**

nutrition – nū-**trĭ′**shŭn

LISTENING EXERCISE

There are a number of resources on the Internet where you can watch and listen to health professionals speak about nutrition. Try that. Go online and search for "nutrition, video clips." Listen carefully to pronunciation. Be sure to look at where the clip is coming from. What dialect of English is being spoken? Is it American, British, Australian, Irish, West Indian, South African, or . . . ? Try to choose a video clip that originates in the English-speaking country with the accent you are interested in hearing.

WRITING EXERCISE—A REFLECTIVE QUESTION

Write your thoughts and reflections here about the video clips you have listened to. Have they been helpful? Have you listened to them more than once? Why or why not?

_____

_____

_____

Reading Selection 5-3

Read the following and be prepared to work with the vocabulary and grammar in the subsequent exercises.

THE PROCESS OF ELIMINATION

All animals (and this includes human beings) must rid themselves of the unhealthy and unnecessary waste products and the nitrogenous byproducts of metabolism. To do so, the gastrointestinal system identifies essential nutrients, metabolizes, and absorbs them into the various body cells, tissues, and systems. Unwanted or used material is then excreted through the processes of defecation and/or urination. The purpose of excretion is to maintain the acid-base (pH) in the body. This promotes homeostasis, or a stable environment, in the organism. Excretion is a biological process that results from metabolism and elimination.

READING EXERCISES

Being able to identify questions, what is being asked and knowing how to answer the questions demonstrate understanding of the meaning of a reading passage or conversation.

Understanding the General Meaning

To show that you understand the meaning of what you have just read, answer the following questions accurately and identify question words.

Answering Questions Accurately. Take a moment now to review what you have just read. Find the sentence in the reading that answers the question and copy it here. The goal of this exercise is to practice answering questions accurately.

1) What is excretion?

_____

2) What does the gastrointestinal system do?

_____

3) What is the purpose of excretion?

_____

Identifying Question Words.   Read the questions that you have just answered again. Identify the question words that helped you arrive at the correct answer.

> **GRAMMAR ALERT: QUESTION WORDS** Question words are those words that when combined cue the responder to reply with the appropriate verb and answer in the plural or singular.
> For example, "Where is the liver located?"
> The key question words *where + verb* in singular form lead to the response: "The liver is located in the abdomen." The answer could also be: "It is located in the abdomen." The singular pronoun "it" is used.
> On the other hand, the question words in the sentence, "Where are the liver and gallbladder?" signal a different response. Here the response depends on the question words of where = verb in plural form. The answer becomes: "The liver and gallbladder are located in the abdomen." The answer might also be: "They are located in the abdomen." The plural pronoun "they" is used.

1) Question 1 question words were: _____

2) Question 2 question words were: _____

3) Question 3 question words were: _____

Building Vocabulary

To build vocabulary effectively you must not only learn to discern the meaning of a word from its context, but also be accurate and comfortable in using the new word in your own communication.

Determining Meaning from Context.   To build vocabulary, study the following words or terms taken from this text. Discover all you can about them by looking at them in context, then choose the correct meaning. Finally, take a look at how these words or terms expand in English.

1. Nitrogenous *(adjective)*

In context:
a) Although the air is comprised of nitrogenous gas and oxygen, the human body only needs oxygen.
b) Nitrogenous gas that is breathed is processed by the body and excreted in the urine.

Meaning: The best way to explain the adjective *nitrogenous* is
a) an inert gas
b) description of a byproduct of metabolism
c) a companion gas to oxygen
d) all of the above

Word expansion:
a) *Nitrogen* comprises 80% of the air we breathe. (noun)

2. Inorganic *(adjective)*

In context:
a) If something is not alive, it is considered inorganic.
b) Most pharmaceutical products are inorganic.

Meaning: The best way to explain the adjective *inorganic* is
a) manmade
b) technical or robotic composition

c) cellular

d) not composed of animal or plant material and/or is inanimate

Word expansion:

a) The heart can now be assisted *inorganically* by the surgical placement of a pacemaker. (adverb)

3. Essential *(adjective)*

In context:

a) Oxygen is essential to life.

b) It is essential that children have adequate nutrition to grow and to stave off some diseases, illnesses, and even allergies.

Meaning: The best way to explain the adjective *essential* is

a) important for life

b) required for a healthy life

c) necessary or indispensable

d) both (b) and (c)

Word expansion:

a) *Essentially,* I have to study hard and long to become a physiotherapist. (adverb)

b) Nitrogen is actually *nonessential* to cellular growth. (adjective)

Using New Words in Sentences. Use a key word from the previous exercise to create a new sentence. The words are chosen for you here.

1) inanimate _____

2) essential _____

3) composition _____

SPEAKING EXERCISE

Go back and read The Process of Elimination aloud. Ask a peer or teacher to help you with pronunciation. Proceed to the following Pronunciation Hints section. This will also help.

PRONUNCIATION HINTS

excretion – ĕks-**krē**'shŭn

inorganic – ĭn″or-**găn**'ĭk

nitrogenous – nī-**trŏj**'ĕn-ŭs

homeostasis – hō″mē-ō-**stā**'sĭs

defecation – dĕf-ĕ-**kā**'shŭn

LISTENING EXERCISE

Listen to the radio or television in English. Listen carefully. You will hear commercials advertising products that help people deal with elimination difficulties. Are you able to discern these? If so, can you understand what the announcer is talking about? This is English in the context of elimination.

WRITING EXERCISE–PARSING VERBS

Work with verbs. Parse or conjugate the following per the instructions.

1) excretion
   a) first person singular, present tense _____
   b) the infinitive form _____
   c) third person singular, present continuous form _____
2) metabolism
   a) the infinitive form _____
   b) second person singular, present tense using "can't"
   _____
3) process
   a) first person, present continuous form _____
   b) third person singular, future continuous form _____
   c) third person plural, simple past tense _____

SECTION TWO | # Common Complaints of the Gastrointestinal/Digestive Systems

This section of Unit 5 explores the language of common complaints of the gastrointestinal system such as constipation, nausea, vomiting, and diarrhea. The linguistic focus is on acquiring language pertaining to signs and symptoms of GI tract disorders and on exploring the efficacy of closed, two-part, and multiple questions in health assessments. A nutritional history interview provides an example of an assessment tool that will enhance communication skills with patients.

Reading Selection 5-4

Read the following discussion of the assessment and pathology of the digestive system.

ASSESSMENT AND PATHOLOGY OF THE GI TRACT

Healthy, adequate nutrition plays an essential role in the health of the GI tract as well as the health of the body as a whole. The digestive system can be negatively impacted by irritants, allergens, toxins, viruses, and bacteria. When this occurs, people are likely to seek home remedies or use over-the-counter, nonprescription medicines to alleviate distressing signs and symptoms of GI upset. At times, it is also necessary to seek out the assistance of a doctor or other health-care professional such as a nurse practitioner. Some of the GI complaints commonly seen in the doctor's office are diarrhea, stomach cramps, nausea, and vomiting. The doctor completes a basic physical assessment, paying close attention to the abdomen and the recent history of food, water, and alcohol consumption by the patient. Elements of the abdominal exam include auscultation and palpation. The doctor uses the stethoscope to auscultate the abdomen, listening across four quadrants. He or she then palpates the abdomen to assess for pain, rigidity, tenderness, or masses. The doctor will also be interested in any pathological evidence available. Pathology is the study of the nature and causes of diseases. Laboratory tests and a stool specimen may be ordered by the doctor for further assessment to, for example, identify any disease-causing bacteria, virus, or toxin. An example of one disease that affects the GI system is *Clostridium difficile,* a highly infectious, virulent bacterial disease that causes diarrhea.

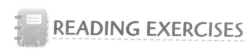

READING EXERCISES

Answering specific questions about the reading selection and being able to recognize common and medical terms for digestive system complaints will help you recognize whether or not you have really understood the reading selection.

Understanding the General Meaning

Read the text again. Think about it. Do you understand it?

1) What is the general purpose or goal of this text?

_____

2) List three key points that were made.

_____

_____

_____

3) What is pathology?

_____

4) According to the text, what do people generally do to treat their own GI complaints?

_____

Building Vocabulary

As you build your English-language vocabulary, you will be able to correctly label and identify the function of different parts of the GI tract and learn how to interpret and understand the meaning of patients' complaints.

Identifying Parts of the Digestive System.   Based on previous exercises in Unit 5, identify which part of the digestive tract is involved in the following symptoms.

1) diarrhea _____

2) stomach cramps _____

3) nausea _____

4) vomiting _____

Defining New Words.   Look at the following words in the context of their sentences. Search for them in the reading on Assessment and Pathology of the GI Tract. Finally, write a definition for the word in your own terms.

1) The patients on Ward 6 seem to have a really virulent strain of the Norwalk Virus. They have been under quarantine for more than 3 weeks now.
   virulent _____

2) When she went whale watching this spring, she couldn't stand the rocking of the boat on the waves. It made her nauseous.
   nauseous _____

3) Sometimes, in the middle of the night, a person wakes up with awful cramps in their stomach and feels an urgent need to defecate. Maybe they ate something that didn't agree with them.
   cramps _____

Mix and Match

See Box 5-1 below.

BOX 5-1 Mix and Match: Patient Complaints and Medical Terms

Draw a line from the common term to the medical term of similar or the same meaning.

COMMON TERM	MEDICAL TERM
cramps	nausea
sore stomach	vomit
"the runs"	passing gas through the anus
throw up	muscle spasms; contractions
burping	bacteria
germs	passing gas through the mouth
feel like barfing	stomach ache
farting	diarrhea

SPEAKING EXERCISE

Practice differentiating the letters "f" and "p." Notice the difference in the slang terms *barfing* and *burping*. These are very commonly used terms. They mean two entirely different things. It is important for the nurse or health-care worker to be able to distinguish clearly what the patient says so that he or she can give the proper treatment, intervention, or assistance.

The sound for the letter "f" is made by pursing the lips very slightly and blowing the air outward between the lips. The jaw is relaxed and the teeth are slightly apart. No vocalization is required.

The sound for the letter "p" is made by bringing the lips together very quickly and making a blowing sound. Air is quickly gathered in the cheeks in front of the teeth and expelled with slight force, in a sudden burst. No vocalization is required.

1) Experiment by speaking these words. Do so in front of a mirror and/or record yourself.

pill	fill
pus	fuss
pew	few
pan	fan

2) Read the following sentences aloud. Repeat them many times to work on pronunciation of the specific consonants. The Pronunciation Hints section that follows will help.

   a) The pharmacists filled my prescription for pills.

   b) The baby is fussing because his wound is infected and oozing pus.

   c) There were very few people sitting in the pews at the chapel for the elderly resident's funeral service yesterday.

   d) Ralph is bedridden. He was absolutely desperate for the bedpan and called the nurse's aide, "Please, please hurry, I need the pan. Hurry." The nurse's aide misunderstood and simply waved at him. Ten minutes later, he brought Ralph an electric fan for his bedside table. Ralph was very angry and embarrassed because in the meantime, he had defecated in his bed.

LISTENING EXERCISE

In the last exercise you needed to watch yourself speak, but did you also hear yourself? Try the exercise again and listen closely to your pronunciation. Are you truly distinguishing between the sounds for "f" and "p"?

In addition, if you would really like to challenge your listening and comprehension skills, watch the video by Loyola University Health System (May 2008) entitled "IPM 1: Physical Exam Series, Abdominal Assessment" with Dr. M. Koller. This video clip is 9 minutes long and uses the language of anatomy and physiology, including words of location and procedure. You can find this at http://www.video.google.com

WRITING EXERCISE

Health professionals, particularly nurses, need to take nutritional health histories as part of their assessment of clients. They must gather holistic baseline data on clients before providing care. In the instance of a gastrointestinal disorder or disease, nutritional data is particularly important.

An example of the questions that might be included in a nutritional history is provided below. However, before going on to that, read the Grammar Alert on types of questions shown on this page.

> **GRAMMAR ALERT: TYPES OF QUESTIONS** There are several types of questions. You are already familiar with closed questions—questions that require a *yes, no, maybe, sometimes,* or *I don't know* type of response. They do not elicit long answers. Closed questions are used by nurses and doctors to gather facts and data. There are also two-part questions and multiple questions:
>
> **Two-Part Questions:** It is very common to ask two questions at the same time. A two-part question is actually two questions joined by a conjunction.
> Two-part questions are not considered a good professional communication strategy. American and Canadian health professionals are aware of the importance of asking clients (patients) one question at a time. In this way, the interviewer can actively and attentively listen to and respond appropriately to each answer before going on to a next question. This activity is referred to as *being fully present.* This strategy is part of professional interpersonal communication and is an example of how it differs from social or conversational communication.
>
> **Multiple Questions:** This type of questioning too is very common. It is not very effective. The problem with multiple questions is that the client may become distracted by their multitude. He or she may only be able to focus on one question. If able to focus at all, it will likely be on the last question asked. The health professional will miss a good deal of important data if he or she continues to use this ineffective communication technique.

Taking a Nutritional Health History. Take the following nutritional health history. Fill in the blanks with your own personal data.

DIETARY HABITS AND PATTERNS

1) Do you eat three meals a day? _____

2) When do you eat? _____

3) Are you a *snacker* and do you like to eat snacks? _____

4) When do you like to eat snacks? _____

5) What kinds of foods do you like? _____

6) What kinds of foods don't you like? _____

7) Are you allergic to any foods? _____

8) How often do you drink fluids and what type of fluids do you drink on a daily basis?
_____

9) Do you drink fluids with meals? _____

10) Do you often eat when you are not hungry? _____

11) If you eat when you are not hungry, do you know why you eat? Is it due to stress, boredom, anger, habit, restlessness, or something else? What is the reason?
_____
_____

12) Do you avoid certain foods because they cause you problems like gas, headache, indigestion, constipation, or diarrhea? _____

13) If you answered "yes" to Question 12, please name those foods.
_____

14) Do you believe you eat a well-balanced, healthy diet? _____

15) Explain your answer to Question 14. _____

Recognizing Types of Questions
Answer the following questions to determine if you can recognize the different types of questions.

1) There are six closed questions in the previous exercise. Have you identified them? Write their numbers down here.
_____

2) There are two two-part questions in this exercise. Identify them by writing their numbers here.
_____

3) There is one example of a multiple question in this exercise. Locate it and identify it by number here.
_____

Congratulations. You have completed the interview. Now, look back and identify your own basic eating pattern over a 24-hour period. Write it here.

_____
_____

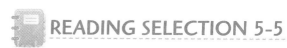

READING SELECTION 5-5

Read the following text discussing the condition of constipation.

CONSTIPATION

Constipation is a commonly experienced condition characterized by infrequent defecation or bowel movements. It may also be diagnosed by the presence of very hard, small, pellet-shaped stools. Sometimes constipation is experienced as difficulty evacuating stools from the bowels. The condition is quite often caused by lack of fluid and fiber in the diet, a sedentary lifestyle, and/or irregular personal bowel habits.

Prior to arriving at a diagnosis of constipation, health professionals need to inquire about the client's medical history. This will include asking about frequency and type of bowel movements (the normal pattern), lifestyle and nutrition, if there is a use of medications that may have a constipating effect, and if the client has any previous or co-occurring disorders that may affect motility in the GI tract. As you know, physical examination of the abdomen using auscultation and palpation will be involved in the assessment processes. Sometimes, a digital rectal exam may also be included.

Motility means movement. In the case of constipation, the bowels, or lower intestines, motility is a term that refers to the ability of waste to proceed down and out through the system as part of the elimination process. In the healthy body, the end process of elimination is referred to as defecation or evacuating the bowels.

READING EXERCISES

An ongoing theme of *Medical English Clear and Simple* is the importance of understanding the general meaning of a reading passage or a conversation as well as the ability to recall specific facts. Remember, health-care professionals must at all times be specific in their questions and in their understanding of responses both from patients and other members of the health-care team; otherwise, serious problems can result.

Understanding the General Meaning

Read the text again and answer the following questions.

1) What is the main topic of the reading selection?

_____

2) What is the general meaning or message of the text?

_____

Learning Specific Facts

1) What causes constipation? _____

2) How common is constipation? _____

3) Is constipation a disease or a condition? _____

Building Vocabulary

Determining Meaning from Context. To build vocabulary, study the following words or terms taken from this text. Discover all you can about them by looking at them in context. Choose the correct meaning. Finally, take a look at how these words or terms expand in English.

1. Evacuation *(noun)*

In context:
a) The police ordered the evacuation of the neighborhood because a flood was imminent.
b) All medical staff and hospital personnel must know the evacuation route for all areas of the hospital in case of a fire.

Meaning: The best way to describe the word *evacuation* is
a) exit outwards
b) entrance inwards
c) escape
d) movement

Word expansion:
a) When the fire alarm rings, you must *evacuate* your patients from the Ward. (verb, present tense)
b) We *evacuated* the building in 15 minutes. (verb, simple past tense)
c) I heard on the news that they are *evacuating* a building downtown because of some strange fumes in the air. (verb, present continuous tense)
d) The building's *evacuees* were housed in the shelter. (noun)

2. Sedentary *(adjective)*

In context:
a) Sarb is unemployed and doesn't look for work. He listens to music and plays videos all day. He leads a very sedentary lifestyle.

Meaning: The best way to describe the word *sedentary* is
a) lifestyle
b) procrastination
c) lethargy
d) sitting a great deal and lacking exercise

3. Digital *(adjective)*

In context:
a) A digital rectal exam requires insertion of a finger into the rectum.
b) Many men are treated for digital amputation due to workplace accidents with machinery.

Meaning: The best way to describe the word *digital* in the context of medicine is
a) luminescent
b) the terminal (end) of a limb
c) numbers
d) analog

Word expansion:
a) Fingers and toes are *digits.* (noun, plural)
b) *Digital creases* are found on the palmar (inside) surface of fingers. (adjective + noun to form a name, plural form)

4. Warranted *(verb, past tense)*

In context:
a) The nurses work so hard. A raise in pay is absolutely warranted.

Meaning: The best way to describe the word *warranted* is
a) proven by evidence, good reason, certainty or authorization
b) reasoning
c) arresting, halting
d) required

Word expansion:

a) I'll *warrant* he won't be back to this clinic, again. We wouldn't give him a prescription for morphine. (verb, with "will" [contraction "I'll"] future tense)

b) When the doctor yelled at the nurse, it *was unwarranted.* She had done nothing wrong. (verb, past tense)

c) The appliance the patient purchased has a 5-year *warranty.* That means if it breaks it will be replaced or repaired free of charge to the patient. (noun)

Mix and Match.   Being able to recognize antonyms is an important language skill for health-care providers since health and its opposite, illness, form the core context of our professional work.

Note: Sometimes words that are actually opposite in meaning sound somewhat alike. It is important that you listen carefully and learn the difference. Some examples are included in the exercise in Box 5-2.

SPEAKING EXERCISE—BREAKING DOWN SYLLABLES

Go back to the last exercise. Locate the words of three syllables or more. In front of a mirror, say each word slowly, syllable by syllable, while watching your mouth. Concentrate on your skills. For example, how are you pronouncing "s" or "a"? How is your diction? Can you see and hear yourself clearly articulate the "t" and "d" in your words? The following Pronunciation Hints box will help.

PRONUNCIATION HINTS

sedentary – **sĕd′**ĕn-tā′rē

immotility – ĭm-mō-**tĭl′**ĭ-tē

evacuation – ē-văk′ū-**ā′**shŭn

LISTENING EXERCISE

Return to your radio or television set. Listen again for commercial ads, but rather than listening for those that treat diarrhea, listen for commercials selling remedies for constipation. Listen to their pronunciation, fluent delivery, and syntax. Compare this to your own.

BOX 5-2 Mix and Match: Antonyms

Draw a line from the word on the left to the word with the opposite meaning on the right.

WORD FROM TEXT	ANTONYM
evacuation	regular
sedentary	inertia
fluid	infrequency
painful	immotility
irregular	conservation
frequency	solid
motility	painless
movement	active

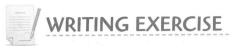

WRITING EXERCISE

Use your new vocabulary. Write a sentence or two by combining new words and medical terms in a meaningful way. Try to stay in the context of the gastrointestinal system.

_____

_____

_____

_____

SECTION THREE Treatments, Interventions, and Assistance: Food Safety and Stomach and Bowel Upset

The content for this section includes a number of case studies designed to use the process of *ruling out* to arrive at a diagnosis. Language skills include common and medical terminology for signs, symptoms, and diagnoses. Vocabulary and concepts related to food safety, health promotion, and disease prevention are introduced. Common remedies for stomach and bowel upset provide insight into cultural contexts for GI upsets. Critical thinking exercises provide an opportunity to use abstract concepts, new language, and medical knowledge to diagnose cases.

Reading Selection 5-6

Read the following four case studies. In each one, the patient presents with gastrointestinal complaints. Read the cases carefully and be prepared to answer the questions that follow.

CASE STUDY A

Patient Mr. Smith complains of a sour taste in his mouth after eating. He particularly notices this after burping. He is also experiencing a burning sensation in the back of his throat. Mr. Smith is a 56-year-old male. He weighs 250 pounds (lbs.), smokes ½ pack of cigarettes per day, is an office worker, and says he "lives for his coffee." You suspect he is suffering from heartburn or gastroesophageal reflux (GERD).

CASE STUDY B

Patient Mrs. Singh arrives at our walk-in clinic. She is a 32-year-old tourist, traveling through your town in the family mini van with her husband and two children. She complains of dizziness, upset stomach, and sudden cold sweats. She often wants to throw up but does not. Mrs. Singh is afraid she is getting the flu. She doesn't want to get sick on her vacation. You diagnose Mrs. Singh with motion sickness or motion-related nausea.

CASE STUDY C

Patient Mueller has an appointment to see you today. He complains of feeling bloated and lethargic. His abdomen is hard, bloated, and painful when you palpate it. He hasn't had a bowel movement for 5 days. Mr. Mueller is a high-powered business man and says he does not have time for regular meals. He "eats on the run" and "grabs a coffee" when he can. He also suffers from what he thinks is carpal tunnel syndrome and has been taking over-the-counter codeine for about a week to control the pain from that. You diagnose the patient with constipation.

CASE STUDY D

Patient Miss Chow has just returned from a 2-week vacation in the tropics. She is in your office now complaining of abdominal pains, watery stool, weakness, and fever. Miss Chow has had these symptoms since midnight. She recalls eating "off and on for about 5 hours at the hotel's farewell buffet and dance" early last evening before her plane ride home. You diagnose Miss Chow with diarrhea that is possibly related to food poisoning.

 # READING EXERCISES

Reading carefully and thoughtfully is essential if a health-care provider is to understand both the general meaning of a passage or report and the specifics contained in it.

Understanding the General Meaning

Read the case studies again. Think about them and answer the following questions. You might want to underline the question words to help you formulate your answers.

1) Why has Miss Chow come to the clinic? _____

2) What brought Mr. Mueller to the clinic? _____

3) What is Mrs. Singh's complaint? _____

4) Where does Mr. Smith experience symptoms of discomfort?_____

_____

5) Who is experiencing abdominal pain? _____

6) Who has poor nutritional habits? _____

7) Who has nausea? _____

8) Has anyone vomited? _____

Building Vocabulary

Patients frequently use slang expressions to describe their physical complaints. It is important that health-care providers be able to interpret these expressions.

Understanding Common Expressions Used by Patients   Here are some terms and expressions taken from the text. Many of them are the subjective reports given by the patients: their own sense of their signs and symptoms. They've come to the clinic for an objective diagnosis. You may not be familiar with some of the expressions, but try to explain them in your own words.

1) He particularly notices . . .
   This means: _____

2) . . . a burning sensation . . .
   This means: _____

3) lives for his coffee
   This means: _____

4) . . . cold sweats . . .
   This means: _____

5) . . . feeling bloated and lethargic . . .
   This means: _____

6) high-powered business man
   This means: _____

7) eats on the run
   This means: _____

8) . . . grabs a coffee . . .
   This means: _____

Determining a Working Diagnosis.   After initial assessment, a doctor or nurse develops a working diagnosis that is used as a framework for pursuing additional subjective and objective data. Read the Vocabulary Alert and then develop a working diagnosis for the patients described in the case studies.

> **VOCABULARY ALERT: WORKING DIAGNOSIS** A working diagnosis is developed after hearing the patient's complaints and doing a preliminary assessment. It is what the doctor or nurse suspects the patient is suffering from or experiencing. It is used as a framework to guide further investigation.
>
> A working diagnosis is not the true or actual diagnosis. Another way to say working diagnosis would be to say provisional diagnosis.
>
> When lab, x-ray, diagnostic imaging, and other tests are completed and compiled with the physician's and nurse's own assessments, only then is a diagnosis reached. To be more precise, the final or confirmed diagnosis comes only after all subjective and objective data has been collected.

Use a key word from the previous exercise to create a new sentence.

_____

Consider each case study. Identify the working diagnosis for each client.

1) Mr. Smith _____

2) Mrs. Singh _____

3) Mr. Mueller _____

4) Miss Chow _____

SPEAKING EXERCISE

Read the Case Studies aloud. Imagine you are giving these short reports to the nurses coming on shift to work for the afternoon. Ask a peer or teacher to help you with pronunciation. Proceed to the following Pronunciation Hints section. This will also help.

PRONUNCIATION HINTS

esophageal - ē-sŏf"ă-jē'ăl

bloated – **blōt'**ĕd

LISTENING EXERCISE

If you have recorded yourself reading the Case Studies aloud, listen to your recording now without looking at the words in this book. Listen only. Do not let the written words be your guide. Evaluate yourself.

- What do you notice about your open pronunciation?

- Are you speaking clearly?

- Are you speaking at a normal rhythm and rate?

If you have not recorded yourself, ask a peer to read any part of this section aloud to you. Do NOT read along with them. Listen only. What do you notice about the way he or she speaks? What lesson do you learn from listening to another?

WRITING EXERCISE

This exercise involves resolving physical complaints and giving professional advice. It requires critical thinking and the use of medical English as well as medical knowledge. Read the explanation of the term critical thinking before proceeding to the exercises.

> CRITICAL THINKING Critical thinking is a composite of attitudes, knowledge, and skills. It includes attitudes of inquiry that involve an ability to recognize the existence of problems and an acceptance of the general need for evidence in support of what is asserted to be true; knowledge of the nature of valid inferences, abstractions, and generalizations in which the weight or accuracy of different kinds of evidence are logically determined; and skills in applying the above attitudes and knowledge (Watson & Glaser, 1980).

1) a) Write Mr. Smith's symptoms here in bulleted form, only.

_____

_____

_____

   b) Review the list you have just written for Mr. Smith. Review the working diagnosis for this patient. Do you agree? Is there some other condition you would still like to rule out?

_____

_____

2) a) List Mrs. Singh's signs and symptoms here.

_____

_____

_____

   b) Review the list you have just written for Mrs. Singh. Review the working diagnosis for this patient. Do you agree? Is there some other condition you would still like to rule out?

_____

_____

3) a) List Mr. Mueller's signs and symptoms here.

_____

_____

_____

b) Review the list you have just written for Mr. Mueller. Review the working diagnosis for this patient. Do you agree? Is there some other condition you would still like to rule out?

_____

_____

4) a) List Miss Chow's signs and symptoms here.

_____

_____

_____

b) Review the list you have just written for Miss Chow. Review the working diagnosis for this patient. Do you agree? Is there some other condition you would still like to rule out?

_____

_____

Reading Selection 5-7

Read the following discussion of common types of pharmacological treatments for GI disorders. Read it aloud or silently to yourself.

PHARMACOLOGY FOR TREATMENT OF DISORDERS OF THE GASTROINTESTINAL SYSTEM

Over a lifetime, everyone can expect to suffer from some type of GI upset at one time or another. When this occurs, our stomachs might produce a sensation of burning or may lead to cramps, noisy sounds that can be heard outside of the body, nausea, and vomiting. Beyond an upset stomach, GI upset can also include painful and embarrassing gas.

Gas is created in the digestive tract in two ways: it is either the result of swallowed air or it is the product of undigested/partially undigested food breaking down in the large intestine. Gas in the lower digestive tract is eventually expelled from the body. En route, however it can cause cramping and pain in the lower abdomen. Passing gas is more properly referred to as "flatulence."

As the products of digestion make their way into the intestines and bowel, stool is formed. Stool is also known as feces. This is solid matter which is eventually evacuated from our bodies through our bowels, rectum, and anus.

When the GI system is functioning normally, stool takes form (it is shaped). Normal consistency and appearance of stool is that it is moderately soft and brownish in color. However, when the body has difficulty metabolizing nutrients or ingested materials, stool can become either very hard or very soft and watery. The result may be cramping, pain, and discomfort. Very loose and watery stool is called diarrhea. Hard and pellet-shaped stool indicates a condition of constipation or impaction.

For all of these conditions, there are home remedies and pharmacological interventions for relief of symptoms. Stool softeners and laxatives help with constipation. Anti-diarrheal medications help stop incidents of diarrhea. Anti-flatulence medication helps with gas, and anti-nausea medications help alleviate the sense of impending emesis (vomiting). Antacids settle upset stomachs and heartburn; some also treat gastroesophageal reflux disease (GERD). While most of the medications are over-the-counter, in severe cases medications may be prescribed by a doctor to help treat the condition.

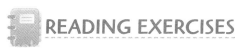

READING EXERCISES

Understanding the General Meaning

Read the text again. Think about it.

1) What is the purpose of this article?

_____

2) What is the focus of the first paragraph?

_____

3) What is the focus of the second paragraph?

_____

4) Identify the introductory sentence for the topic of the article. Copy it here.

_____

5) Identify the concluding statement for the topic here and determine if it ties in with the topic as it was introduced.

_____

6) Do you need a prescription for antacids?

_____

7) Where is stool formed?

_____

Building Vocabulary

Identifying Possible Pharmacological Interventions.   To build vocabulary, study the following words or terms taken from this text. Look at the condition in each question. Identify the pharmacological interventions for each according to the text.

1) nausea _____

2) stomach cramps _____

3) heartburn _____

4) gas _____

5) constipation _____

6) diarrhea _____

Using New Vocabulary to Form Sentences.   Take a moment now to review the vocabulary from this chapter.

Use the words given at the beginning of each question in any form to write a sentence of your own. Remain in the context of the gastrointestinal system. Your own professional background will help you with this exercise.

Note: There are one or two words here you may not be familiar with. Think about the article you have just read and try to draw a conclusion about what the words might mean. You might also consider whether they are nouns, verbs, adjectives, or adverbs.

1) nutrition _____

2) gas _____

3) cold sweat _____

4) intake _____

5) output _____

6) indigestion _____

7) belch _____

8) cramps _____

9) emesis _____

Mix and Match   When patients voice GI system complaints, they may use common speech or slang words and expressions. It is important that all health-care providers be familiar with often-used expressions and understand what is being said. The exercise in Box 5-3 asks you to match common GI complaints with their descriptions.

SPEAKING EXERCISE

Read the Common Complaints in the last exercise. Once again, practice speaking in front of a mirror, watching your mouth as you enunciate each word. How are you doing with your "b" and "p" sounds? Can you see how mispronunciation and misperception of these letters can lead to mistakes in bedside care for the patient? Practice, practice, practice. The Pronunciation Hints box below will help.

PRONUNCIATION HINTS

flatulence – **flăt'**ū-lĕns

impaction – ĭm-**păk'**shŭn

BOX 5-3 Mix and Match: Common GI System Complaints

Draw a line from the common complaint to the description.

COMMON COMPLAINT	DESCRIPTION
I'm going to burp.	I am going to vomit now; throw-up.
I feel sick to my stomach.	I have heartburn.
I have stomach cramps.	I have to have a lot of bowel movements.
I'm going to barf.	My stomach is upset. I have gas.
I'm passing a lot of gas.	I can't have a bowel movement.
I'm plugged up solid.	I have flatulence.
I've got the runs.	I have pains in my gut.
My guts are on fire.	I'm nauseous.

LISTENING EXERCISE

If you would like to hear more native English speakers from the United States and Canada, search the Internet for video clips. Try sites like *You Tube* and search simply using the search word "gastrointestinal" or "digestion." You might like to try the 1 minute clip "Digestive Problems."

WRITING EXERCISE

This exercise addresses multiculturalism and care for a distressed (upset) gastrointestinal system. We all know there are medical treatments for disorders of the digestive system, but we also grew up with a number of home remedies with which our parents and grandparents treated our stomach and bowel aches and pains. Here are a few examples of these. Try to decide what each is for. Write your answer in the space provided.

1) peppermint tea _____

2) licorice tea _____

3) baking soda in water _____

4) fresh apples _____

5) bran cereal _____

6) B.R.A.T. (special diet: eat only bananas, rice, applesauce, and toast)

_____

7) ginger ale to drink and a couple of soda crackers to eat

_____

Now it's your turn. Write some home remedies here from your own background. What did your family do to intervene when you had GI troubles?

_____

_____

_____

Reading Selection 5-8

Read the following dialogue about an incidence of food poisoning. The scene is in the emergency department of a general hospital. A woman and child are seeking medical assistance.

FOOD SAFETY AND FOOD POISONING

Doctor: Hello, I'm Dr. Anderson.

Patient's Mom: Oh, hello. I'm Mary Jenkins and this is my daughter, Kathleen. She's 10.

Doctor: Hello. I see here from your chart that you're feeling sick, Kathleen.

Kathleen: Uh-huh, yeah.

Doctor: What seems to be the matter?

Mom: Well, she woke up at about 3 this morning with diarrhea and she has had it ever since. She's also got pains in her tummy.

Doctor: I see. Any idea what brought this on?

Mom: I'm not sure. Maybe it was something she ate. We barbecued hamburgers yesterday for supper. Maybe it was the meat? But nobody else is sick.

Doctor: Hmmm. Let's have a look, Kathleen. Does your stomach hurt now?

Kathleen: Uh-huh . . . yes.

Doctor: Did you eat today?

Kathleen: No . . . I don't want to.

Doctor: Here. OK, I'm going to use this funny looking thing here to take your temperature. It's not going to hurt at all. I'm just going to hold onto your ear a little bit . . . like this and then . . . wait . . . there. Got it. OK, now I'm just going to take your pulse.

Doctor to Mom: Has Kathleen been able to keep any fluids down?

Mom: Very little. She doesn't want to eat or drink anything today. I'm worried. I don't want her to get dehydrated. Does she have a temperature? She feels hot to me.

Doctor: Yes, she does, but it's not very high . . . just slightly elevated. Have you given her anything to stop the diarrhea?

Mom: Yes, I gave her only 1 teaspoonful of an antidiarrheal medication. The pink, liquid stuff. It doesn't seem to be working.

Doctor: Right. Well, that medication is good, but it's not really the best remedy for this kind of thing once diarrhea starts. Let me suggest a little loperamide. Here is one tablet. I think that's all she'll need. However, and I want you to listen very carefully to me about this first . . . if you give her this loperamide (Imodium), we have to bring that fever down. So, I am going to ask my nurse to give Kathleen a children's acetaminophen first. That should work fairly quickly. Take Kathleen's temperature again when you get home. If it's down, give her the loperamide.

Mom: OK. What do you think she has, Doctor?

Doctor: Well, it's hard to say at the moment. It could be a simple stomach flu or it could be a slight case of *Salmonella.*

Mom: *Salmonella?* You mean food poisoning? Won't we all get it?

Doctor: Not necessarily. Kathleen, your Mom says you had a burger yesterday. Is that right?

Kathleen: Yeah.

Doctor: Do you remember what color that burger was? Did you look at the meat when you were eating it?

Kathleen: Yeah. It was kinda brown and a little black on one side. And, oh yeah, it was a little bit pink and juicy in the middle. And it wasn't really very hot.

Doctor: I see. Mrs. Anderson, I suspect she's got food poisoning. It sounds like that hamburger was not properly cooked. You know, of course, that hamburgers must be well-done on the inside and the outside to kill any bacteria or contaminants like *E. coli,* don't you?

Mom: Well, umm . . . I had heard that. I didn't know hers was underdone. My husband was barbecuing them. Oh, I feel so guilty. I'm sorry, Kathleen. I should have been watching better.

Kathleen: That's OK, Mom. I'll be OK.

Doctor: Right. Here's our nurse and here's your acetaminophen, Kathleen.

Kathleen: OK.

Doctor: And here's that one tab of loperamide I want you to give your daughter when you get home. It works quite quickly once you take it.

Mom: Why can't she just take it now?

Doctor: Well, it's just a pharmacological issue. Some drugs don't mix well and some drugs may mask signs and symptoms of something else going on in the patient. Let's treat Kathleen's fever first and see if that can be remedied.

Mom: I see. OK. I'll do as you say. Thank you.

Kathleen: Mom, Mom . . . I gotta go . . .

Nurse: OK, there's a bathroom just around the corner. Do you want me to take you?

Kathleen: No. Mom, mom . . . mom . . .

Mom: OK, Kathleen, let's go. I know it's urgent. Thank you, doctor, nurse.

Kathleen: Bye!

 READING EXERCISES

As you proceed, remember that being able to understand specific facts as well as the general meaning of a reading selection, conversation, or interview is essential for all health-care workers.

Understanding the General Meaning

Read the text again. Think about it.

1) What is the general story behind the dialogue, the subplot? Summarize it here.

_____

_____

_____

Learning Specific Information

1) What is this dialogue about? _____

2) Who are the characters? _____

3) Where are these people? _____

4) What is the working diagnosis for this girl? _____

5) What is Kathleen's medical complaint? _____

6) The doctor wants the patient to take two types of medication.
   a) What is the acetaminophen for?
   _____

   b) What is the loperamide for? _____

7) According to the dialogue and your own knowledge of pharmacology, why can't Kathleen take both medications together? _____

Building Vocabulary

Understanding and Defining Words from Their Use in Context. To build vocabulary, study the following words or expressions taken from this text. Discover all you can about them by looking at them in context. Then attempt to define or explain them here.

1) teaspoon _____

2) pains in her tummy _____

3) can't keep any fluids down _____

4) kinda brown _____

5) fairly quickly _____

6) juicy _____

Mix and Match. It is important for all health-care professionals to understand that some words may have very similar or the same meaning. These words are called synonyms (which you have studied in earlier chapters) and an exercise is provided for you in Box 5-4.

Using New Words in Sentences. Use words from the dialogue plus the ones given here at the beginning of each line to create a new sentence. Your own medical knowledge will be necessary to write a logical, informed statement.

1) *Salmonella* _____

2) *E. coli* _____

 ## SPEAKING EXERCISE

Read the food safety rules given in the feature on the next page. This is a health promotion activity that includes pamphlets, brochures, lectures, posters, and Internet, television, and radio advertisements. The Pronunciation Hints box following this exercise will help.

BOX 5-4 Mix and Match: Synonyms

Find the synonym for the following expressions or words. Draw a line to link them.

WORD OR EXPRESSION	SYNONYM OR EXPRESSION OF SIMILAR MEANING
It's hard to say . . .	yeah
yes	one tab of . . .
pill	I don't really know
well-done meat	the runs
diarrhea	thoroughly cooked

FOOD SAFETY RULES To prevent gastrointestinal upsets and avoid aggravating existing conditions affecting the gastrointestinal system, safe food handling and storing practices are necessary to prevent unsafe, disease-carrying bacteria or toxins from being ingested. It is important to follow the following rules.

Hygiene

- Wash your hands before preparing all foods. Use both soap and water. If you are interrupted while working, be sure to wash your hands once more before starting to handle food again.

- Wash and dry your hands before eating.

Food Storage

- Do not buy canned food if the can is dented, leaking, or bulging. Such damage can be a sign of bacterial infestation, and the possibility of ptomaine poisoning, among other conditions.

- When purchasing frozen foods, put them in your freezer as soon as possible. Do not allow them to thaw and then attempt to refreeze them since bacteria will have already accessed the food while it thawed.

- Do not eat any leftover foods that have been in the refrigerator for more than 3 days.

- Refrigerate leftover foods within 1 hour. Cover them, as well.

Food Temperatures

- Serve any foods made with dairy products, such as milk, eggs, salad dressings, sandwich spreads, and cheeses, as well as gravies and sauces within 2 hours after refrigeration.

- Do not eat any food items left on a buffet for 2 hours or more when proper food safe temperatures (hot or cold) have not been maintained. This particularly refers to meats, dairy products, and fish.

- Keep hot foods hot at 140°F (60°C) and cold foods cold at 39.2°F (4°C).

- To avoid bacterial contamination, cook frozen foods that have been thawed immediately.

- Never leave poultry (turkey, duck, chicken) sitting at room temperature for more than 1 hour. Refrigerate it immediately.

- Cook all ground meats (burger, sausages, hot dogs) entirely through to the center and only eat when it is well-done in the center.

PRONUNCIATION HINTS

salmonella – săl″mō-**něl**′ă

pharmacological – făr″mă-**kŏl**′ōjĭ-k′l

LISTENING EXERCISE

Go online. Listen to recommendations for Food Safety at the United States Department of Agriculture, Food Safety and Inspection Service website. Click on News and Events, podcasts. There are a wide variety of audio podcasts available that deal with this subject. The site will be very helpful for listening and coming to appreciate the culture and context of health promotion and food safety. http://www.fsis.usda.gov/News_&_Events/Food_Safety_at_Home_Podcasts/index.asp

WRITING EXERCISE

Consider the reading on Food Safety. How does this compare with your country of origin? Does the government in that country make recommendations for health promotion related to food? Discuss this in writing. Compare and contrast.

Anatomy and Physiology

 READING SELECTION 1—THE GASTROINTESTINAL SYSTEM

Understanding the General Meaning

Example: The process of digestion involves the intake of food and fluid into the mouth and down the throat and through other organs where it is broken down and either used by the cells of the body or expelled from the body. Sometimes we say, "In one end and out the other."

Learning Specific Facts

1) Digestion is the process of breaking down or metabolizing foods and materials in the system and filtering nutrients from waste products. Ingestion is the process of taking food or other products/materials into the mouth and then swallowing them to allow them to pass through the rest of the digestive tract.

2) Nutrients are the chemicals found within foods that promote the health of the human body. Waste is undigested products of metabolism that are eliminated (excreted) from the body.

3) The entire process of digestion takes 24 hours from start to finish.

4) A synonym for the gastrointestinal system is the digestive system.

5) Tract refers to a group of organs; a system in which all parts work together to provide a route of passage.

6) The alimentary canal is 28 feet long.

7) excretes, eliminates

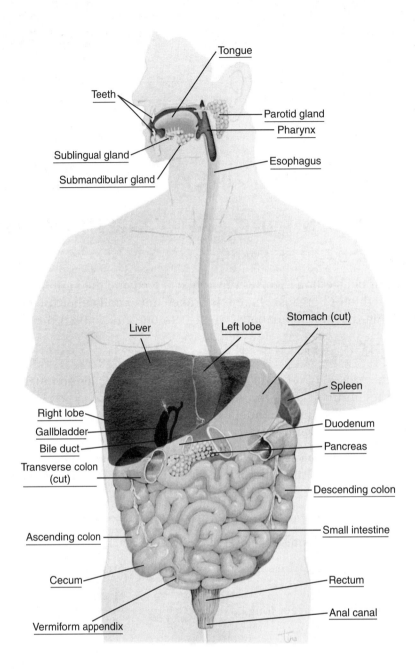

Tongue

Teeth

Parotid gland

Pharynx

Sublingual gland

Esophagus

Submandibular gland

Liver

Left lobe

Stomach (cut)

Spleen

Right lobe

Gallbladder

Duodenum

Bile duct

Pancreas

Transverse colon
(cut)

Descending colon

Ascending colon

Small intestine

Cecum

Rectum

Anal canal

Vermiform appendix

Building Vocabulary

Labeling Anatomical Parts

Determining Meaning from Context

1) c, 2) a, 3) c, 4) c, 5) d

Recognizing Grammatical Structure and Meaning

1) a) "It sits just below the stomach." Rationale: The pancreas cannot actually sit. The word "is" can be substituted for "sits."
   b) The pancreas is located just below the stomach.
   c) Secrete means to generate and separate (a substance) from cells or bodily fluids.
   d) The pancreas is a gland that secretes digestive enzymes and hormones.

2) a) "Salivary glands are found in the mouth and throat."
   b) Saliva keeps the mouth moist.

3) a) "The pancreas lies posterior to the stomach." Rationale: The pancreas cannot actually lie down or lay someplace. The word "is" can be substituted for "lies."

   b) The pancreas is situated behind the stomach. *Or* The pancreas is posterior to the stomach.

4) a) "The liver is a very large organ."

   b) The function of the liver is metabolism.

   c) Detoxify means to remove or counteract the effects of toxins.

   d) These terms are often used interchangeably by health professionals and the public; however, their meaning is not exactly the same. *Excretion* refers to the act or process of eliminating waste matter from the blood, tissues, or organs through discharge or evacuation from the body. Excretion concerns itself with metabolism. *Elimination* means to get rid of, remove, or omit, but it is not strictly tied to metabolism. For example, if a child swallows a coin he will eventually eliminate it from the body, even though before this occurs the body will attempt to metabolize it. Synonyms for elimination are eradication, liquidation, purging, and voiding. The verb *void* is usually used to refer to the elimination of urine, whereas the term *eliminate* is most often used for defecation.

5) a) The gallbladder contains bile which it receives from the liver.

   b) Bile is yellow or green.

   c) It is found behind the liver.

Using New Words to Identify Body Organs

1) large intestine

2) liver and gallbladder

3) stomach

4) rectum

5) pancreas

Recognizing Antonyms

1) to absorb

2) to destroy, neglect, spend, squander, use, waste

3) to retain, keep, accept, include

WRITING EXERCISE

1) The purpose of the gastrointestinal system is to ingest and transport food so that digestion can occur.

2) The function of the digestive system is to provide the body with healthy nutrients and provide a means to expel waste materials and toxins.

3) The steps in the processes of the gastrointestinal system are: Step 1—ingestion of food into mouth; Step 2—salivary glands begin process of digestion; Step 3—food is chewed (masticated) and swallowed to allow passage into the esophagus; Step 4—masticated and partially digested food or fluid enters the stomach; Step 5—accessory organs are stimulated to assist digestion; Step 6—food is digested and metabolized in the stomach; Step 7—digested and metabolized products pass into small intestine; Step 8—nutrients are absorbed in the small intestine and pass throughout the body; Step 9—undigested products pass into large intestine where water is removed; Step 10—rectum is stimulated to feel need to defecate; Step 11—defecation occurs through anal opening.

READING SELECTION 2—NUTRIENTS
Understanding the General Meaning

Sample Answer:
Nutrients are chemicals found in food that our body needs to function well. They usually enter our bodies through the GI tract and are digested, metabolized, and absorbed in the tissues of the body. Nutrition is the study of nutrients, and nutritionists are health-care professionals who specialize in nutrition.

Building Vocabulary

Determining Meaning from Context

1) d, 2) b, 3) a

Using New Words and Their Derivatives in Sentences

Examples:

1) *Nutrients* are extracted from food through the process of metabolism.

2) Pharmaceuticals are actually *synthetic* medicines based on those originating in nature.

3) On television, there is an advertisement that says that *enzymes* in laundry detergent eat dirt and bacteria.

 READING SELECTION 3—THE PROCESS OF ELIMINATION
Understanding the General Meaning

Answering Questions Accurately

1) Excretion is a biological process that results from metabolism and elimination. It refers to the act or process of eliminating waste matter from the blood, tissues, or organs through discharge or evacuation from the body.

2) The gastrointestinal system identifies essential nutrients and metabolizes and absorbs them into the various cells, tissues, and body systems. It then excretes the unwanted or used material through the processes of defecation or urination.

3) The purpose of excretion is to maintain the pH balance of the body.

Identifying Question Words

1) What is . . . ?

2) What does . . . do? (Point of clarification: The question "What does something do?" is asking what job or function it has. For example, if you were asked, "What do you do?" the answer might be "I am a nurse." A short answer to Question 2 would be: "The GI system identifies, processes, and then excretes.")

3) What is . . . ?

Building Vocabulary

Determining Meaning from Context

1) b, 2) d, 3) d

Using New Words in Sentences

Examples:

1) Inorganic material is also inanimate. It doesn't move on its own power.

2) Nitrogen is not essential to human life, but it is helpful to plant growth when it is found as a nutrient in the soil.

3) The composition of air includes oxygen and nitrogenous gases.

WRITING EXERCISE

1) (a) I excrete, (b) to excrete, (c) he (she/it) is excreting

2) (a) to metabolize, (b) you can't metabolize

3) (a) I am processing, (b) He (she/it) will be processing, (c) They processed

Common Complaints of the Gastrointestinal/Digestive Systems

READING SELECTION 4—ASSESSMENT AND PATHOLOGY OF THE GI TRACT

Understanding the General Meaning

1) The general purpose or goal of this reading selection is to explain the process of assessing GI disorders/diseases and to identify the most common GI complaints made by patients.

2) Three key points that were made are (1) that nutrition is essential to the health of the body, (2) that factors/agents (bacteria, viruses, irritants) can affect the health of the GI tract, and (3) that some GI complaints can be treated at home but some need the help of a health-care professional. (Other points could be that the most common GI complaints are diarrhea, stomach cramps, nausea, and vomiting; and that an abdominal exam is part of the GI assessment procedure.)

3) Pathology is the study of the nature and cause of disease.

4) According to the text, people generally try to treat their GI complaints with home remedies or over-the-counter medications.

Building Vocabulary

Identifying Parts of the Digestive System

1) diarrhea—colon, bowels, large intestines

2) stomach cramps—stomach

3) nausea—stomach, also perhaps smell and taste, which can trigger nausea

4) vomiting—stomach, esophagus, mouth

Defining New Words

1) *Virulent* means extremely infectious; hard to treat; potent or fierce.

2) *Nauseous* means affected with nausea, or to feel an uncomfortable feeling in the stomach that leads a person to think he or she is going to vomit. (Note: People who are nauseous do not vomit; they simply feel sick to the stomach.) A synonym for nauseous is nauseated.

3) A *cramp* is a sudden, sharp, and painful muscle contraction that comes and goes.

Mix and Match

BOX 5-1 Mix and Match: Patient Complaints and Medical Terms: Answers	
COMMON TERM	MEDICAL TERM
cramps	muscle spasms; contractions
sore stomach	stomach ache
"the runs"	diarrhea
throw up	vomit
burping	passing gas through the mouth
germs	bacteria
feel like barfing	nausea
farting	passing gas through the anus

WRITING EXERCISE

Recognizing Types of Questions

1) The six closed questions are Questions 1, 7, 9, 10, 12, 14

2) The two two-part questions are Questions 3 and 8.

3) The multiple question in the exercise is Question 11.

READING SELECTION 5—CONSTIPATION

Understanding the General Meaning

1) The main topic of the reading selection is constipation.

2) The general meaning or message of the text is that constipation is common and treatable.

Learning Specific Facts

1) Constipation is quite often caused by lack of fluid and fiber in the diet, a sedentary lifestyle, and irregular personal bowel habits.

2) Constipation is very common.

3) Constipation is a condition that can quite easily be remedied with laxatives or changes in lifestyle and diet.

Building Vocabulary

Determining Meaning from Context

1) a, 2) d, 3) b, 4) a

Mix and Match

BOX 5-2 Mix and Match: Antonyms: Answers	
WORD FROM TEXT	**ANTONYM**
evacuation	conservation
sedentary	active
fluid	solid
painful	painless
irregular	regular
frequency	infrequency
motility	immotility
movement	inertia

Treatments, Interventions, and Assistance: Food Safety and Stomach and Bowel Upset

READING SELECTION 6—CASE STUDIES

Understanding the General Meaning

1) Miss Chow has come to the clinic because she is experiencing abdominal pain, watery stool, weakness, and fever.

2) Mr. Mueller comes to the clinic complaining of feeling bloated and lethargic. (This is a subjective report—Mr. Mueller's personal perspective on how he feels.)

3) Mrs. Singh complains that she feels dizzy and has an upset stomach and sudden cold sweats. She is afraid that she is getting the flu.

4) Mr. Smith experiences discomfort in his throat, esophagus, and mouth.

5) Mr. Mueller and Miss Chow are experiencing abdominal pain.

6) Mr. Smith and Mr. Mueller have poor nutritional habits. There is no evidence that Mrs. Singh and Miss Chow have poor nutritional habits.

7) Mrs. Singh has nausea.

8) No one has yet vomited.

Building Vocabulary

Understanding Common Expressions Used by Patients

1) *Particularly notices* means that one thing stands out as more important and is more salient for him than other things.

2) A *burning sensation* means a sense of hotness or heat.

3) The expression *lives for his coffee* means that coffee is very important to him. He drinks it whenever he can and loves it. He may even have a coffee addiction.

4) *Cold sweats* are a symptom of fever or anxiety in which the person feels cold but actually perspires.

5) *Feeling bloated* is a sensation of feeling larger and perhaps swollen. People often say they feel bloated after a very large meal. Women often complain of feeling bloated around the time of their menstrual period when they have retained excess water in their cells and tissues. When someone is *lethargic*, they are slow moving and perhaps even slow thinking. Lethargy is not the same as lazy.

6) A *high-powered business man* is one who is highly energetic, is extremely busy, is motivated, and who works excessively. Do not be confused by the use of the word "power" in this idiom. Sometimes it refers to the authority the man may have, but not always. The use of the word "power" here can refer to the person's energy level. High energy = high power. Women can be high-powered business people as well.

7) *Eats on the run* means eating and drinking while walking, talking, and driving. In a busy society, we don't always stop to sit down and eat normally. This is very common in the United States and Canada. Many restaurants have drive-through windows for us so that we can drive up in our car, order food or drink to go, purchase it through the car window, and drive off, eating and drinking. You can also eat on the run with food or beverages you prepare for yourself.

8) *Grab a coffee* refers to the habit of buying a coffee for takeout. Because this is done quickly, it is referred to as grabbing a coffee, not getting a coffee.

Determining a Working Diagnosis

1) The working diagnosis for Mr. Smith is heartburn, or gastroesophageal reflux.

2) Mrs. Singh probably has motion sickness or motion-related nausea.

3) Mr. Mueller's working diagnosis is constipation.

4) Miss Chow has diarrhea, possibly related to food poisoning.

WRITING EXERCISE

1) a) • sour taste in his mouth after eating

    • burping

    • burning sensation in the back of his throat

    b) Yes, besides the working diagnosis of GERD, the possibility of a heart attack should be ruled out. Beyond his GI symptoms, Mr. Smith leads a sedentary lifestyle, is significantly overweight, drinks an abundance of coffee, and smokes. He is over 50 years of age. Mr. Smith is a good candidate for heart attack. This needs to be ruled out.

2) b) • dizziness

    • upset stomach

    • sudden cold sweats

    • nausea

   b) Yes, besides the working diagnosis of motion sickness, pregnancy should be ruled out. Mrs. Singh is a 32-year-old married woman and mother of two. It is possible she is pregnant. This needs to be ruled out.

3) a) • feeling bloated and lethargic

    • abdomen hard, bloated, and painful to touch

   b) Yes, in addition to the working diagnosis of constipation, several other conditions should be ruled out. Mr. Mueller has been taking the analgesic codeine for another condition. It may be masking pain in his abdomen. He didn't mention abdominal pain, yet it was evident when the area was palpated. He may have a bowel obstruction and require urgent care. He may have polyps, diverticulosis, or even bowel cancer. All of these potential diagnoses need to be ruled out with more assessments and laboratory tests before he is allowed to leave the office.

4) a) • abdominal pains

    • watery stool

    • weakness

    • fever

   b) No. There is no evidence of unhealthy lifestyle in general or contact with any infectious agents (other than those that may have been contracted through food). The onset and signs and symptoms of the illness fit the criteria for the diagnosis of diarrhea, possibly related to food poisoning.

READING SELECTION 7—PHARMACOLOGY FOR TREATMENT OF DISORDERS OF THE GASTROINTESTINAL SYSTEM

Understanding the General Meaning

1) The purpose of this reading selection is to explain types of GI upsets and what kinds of pharmacological interventions might be available to treat them.

2) The focus of the first paragraph is that whatever we ingest is digested and the results of digestion can sometimes be unpleasant.

3) The focus of the second paragraph is stool is a byproduct of digestion and forms in the lower intestines/bowels. Its consistency depends on what has been digested and/or illness.

4) The introductory sentence for the topic of the reading selection is "At one time or another, each of us will suffer from some type of GI upset."

5) The concluding statement for the topic is, "While most of the medications are over-the-counter, in severe cases medications may be prescribed by a doctor to help treat the condition." Yes, this statement is related to the introductory statement because the latter talks about treatment for GI upset.

6) No, you do not need a prescription for an antacid. Many antacids are available over-the-counter.

7) Stool is formed in the large intestine (colon, bowels).

Building Vocabulary

Identifying Possible Pharmacological Interventions

1) anti-nausea medication

2) stool softeners or antacid

3) antacids

4) anti-flatulence drugs

5) laxatives or stool softeners

6) antidiarrheal medications

Using New Words to Form Sentences

Sample Answers:

1) Proper *nutrition* can help prevent GI upsets, particularly constipation.

2) If you eat a lot of cabbage or beans and you are not used to these in your diet, you may have a very unpleasant bout of *gas*.

3) Some people break out in a *cold sweat* just before they have an incidence of diarrhea or vomiting.

4) Healthy nutritional *intake* requires a balanced diet of fruits, vegetables, and dairy products to obtain proteins, fiber, carbohydrates, and other nutrients.

5) In the hospital, we watch for a healthy balance between the patient's total daily intake and *output* of fluids. We also monitor food intake and output by charting whether or not the patient had a bowel movement each 24-hour period.

6) Eating too much at one time can lead to *indigestion*.

7) Young men seem to like to *belch*. They like the loud noise and the reaction it brings from other people. Belching in public is not socially acceptable in the United States and Canada, but some young men and boys like to test this norm.

8) Stomach *cramps* can come from eating spoiled or rotten food. They are painful and can very often be accompanied by diarrhea.

9) The product of vomiting is called vomit or *emesis*.

Mix and Match

See Box 5-3 Answers on following page.

 ## WRITING EXERCISE

1) peppermint tea—settles indigestion and upset stomach

2) licorice tea—works as a laxative

3) baking soda in water—antacid

4) fresh apples—laxative that provides fiber

The Gastrointestinal System

BOX 5-3 Mix and Match: Common GI System Complaints: Answers

COMMON COMPLAINT	DESCRIPTION
I'm going to burp.	My stomach is upset. I have gas.
I feel sick to my stomach.	I'm nauseous.
I have stomach cramps.	I have pains in my gut.
I'm going to barf.	I am going to vomit now; throw-up.
I'm passing a lot of gas.	I have flatulence.
I'm plugged up solid.	I can't have a bowel movement.
I've got the runs	I have to have a lot of bowel movements.
My guts are on fire.	I have heartburn.

5) bran cereal—laxative that provides fiber

6) B.R.A.T.—special diet given when food allergies are suspected and being investigated and/or postoperatively for some patients when they are allowed solid foods.

7) ginger ale—remedy for diarrhea to hydrate as well as provide basic sustenance until the diarrhea is finished. Ginger ale is often given for nausea and after a bout of vomiting, too.

READING SELECTION 8—FOOD SAFETY AND FOOD POISONING

Understanding the General Meaning

1) The general story, or subplot behind the dialogue is food safety, and specifically, that ground and processed meat must be cooked thoroughly to the center to prevent illness.

Learning Specific Information

1) The dialogue is about the assessment and treatment of a child with diarrhea.

2) The characters are Doctor Anderson, mother, Kathleen (child), and the nurse.

3) The scene of the dialogue is the emergency department of a general hospital.

4) The working diagnosis for the child Kathleen is diarrhea related to food poisoning from the ingestion of undercooked or raw hamburger meat.

5) Kathleen's complaint is diarrhea and pains in her tummy, according to her mother. Kathleen does not voice these complaints. The mother speaks for her.

6) a) The doctor prescribes acetaminophen to reduce Kathleen's fever and to relieve her pain. Acetaminophen works as both an antipyretic to reduce fever and as an analgesic to relieve pain.
   b) The doctor prescribes loperamide as an antidiarrheal.

7) The two medications should not be taken together because one medication may mask the symptoms of another condition.

Building Vocabulary

Understanding and Defining Words from Their Use in Context

1) A *teaspoon* is a measure of a liquid or solid that fits into a kitchen teaspoon.

2) *Tummy* is another word for stomach and most often used with children. It might also refer to the abdomen. *Pains in the tummy* can refer to stomach or abdominal cramps. It is the duty of health professionals to ascertain the exact location of the pain.

3) The expression *can't keep any fluid down* means that any fluids that are ingested are quickly passed through the system and lost through bowel elimination or vomiting. The body quickly becomes dehydrated.

4) The expression *kinda brown* means that the substance was not really brown in color, but rather a combination of pink, gray, and brown.

5) *Fairly quickly* means not instantaneous, but very quickly and not at a normal or regular rate.

6) *Juicy* means moist or consisting of solid and liquid. For example, watermelon is juicy.

Mix and Match

BOX 5-4 Mix and Match: Synonyms: Answers

WORD OR EXPRESSION	SYNONYM OR EXPRESSION OF SIMILAR MEANING
It's hard to say . . .	I don't really know
yes	yeah
pill	one tab of . . .
well-done meat	thoroughly cooked
diarrhea	the runs

Using New Words in Sentences

1) *Salmonella* is a group of bacteria that affect the intestines, causing gastroenteritis or more serious forms of food poisoning.

2) *E. coli* is a bacteria found in food and water contaminated by feces. If ingested in improperly cooked food or in water, it causes food poisoning that can be severe and even fatal. It is sometimes known as the "hamburger disease" because it is often found in improperly cooked ground meat.

Unit 6 familiarizes the health professional who has a non–English speaking background with the vocabulary and grammar necessary to communicate with others regarding the anatomy, physiology, and disorders/diseases of the neurological system. Contextual examples are related to the brain, although reference is made to a variety of neurological diseases and impairments. Terminology related to caring for patients who have suffered injury or impairment is highlighted. Medical prefixes and the language of anatomical location are included, as is reading for gist, or overall meaning. Exercises involving creating and interpreting medical flow charts and writing summaries provide opportunities for familiarizing yourself with form and language.

SECTION ONE Anatomy and Physiology

The ability to discuss the function of the neurological system is important in a wide variety of medical settings as well as in community health care. This section of the unit provides the opportunity for you to acquire the vocabulary used for this system and to improve your grammar through exercises working with verbs, sentence completion, and spelling. These exercises will help facilitate your language and communication skills. A brief introduction to reading for gist and to interpreting or designing flow charts/hierarchical charts is also provided.

Reading Selection 6-1

Read the following in preparation for the exercises that follow. Read it aloud or silently to yourself—the choice is yours.

THE NERVOUS SYSTEM

The neurological system is commonly referred to as the nervous system. It directs all body systems and cells and is responsible for all thought, emotion, sensation, and movement. The nervous system consists of two major subsystems: the central nervous system and the peripheral nervous system. The brain is the center of both.

The central nervous system is most often referred to as the CNS. It consists of the brain, brain stem, and spinal cord. The spinal cord and brain stem function as communication pathways between the brain and the peripheral nervous system. The peripheral nervous system, often referred to by health professionals as the PNS, contains the cranial nerves and spinal nerves that connect the central nervous system to the peripheral organs of the body. The peripheral nervous system can be divided into several subdivisions which will be discussed later.

All the organs of the nervous system are composed of neurons, or nerve cells. Neurons contain a cell nucleus and dendrites and axons. Dendrites receive impulses from the sensory organs, such as the eyes and ears, and from other neurons and transmit them **to** the central nervous system. The central nervous system (either the brain or spinal cord) responds to this sensory input, sending impulses through the axons **out** to the body organs. The gap between sensory, intermediate, and motor nerves is referred to as a synapse.

 READING EXERCISES

The following comprehension and vocabulary-building exercises should help you in improving your English language communication skills. You will also become familiar with identifying and naming in English the parts of the nervous system.

Understanding the General Meaning

In reading reports and in conversation it is important that you both get the gist of the matter (understand its general meaning) and understand the specific details being mentioned.
  Now read about the nervous system again. Think about it.

1) What is the gist of the reading?

_____

2) What is the function of the reading? In other words, what is the purpose or intent of the reading?

_____

3) In general, what is at the center of the entire nervous system?

_____

Comprehending Specific Facts

Once again, review what you have just read. Answer the questions to assess your level of comprehension. You may use short answers.

1) What is the medical term for the nervous system? _____

2) According to the text, what directs all body systems and cells? _____

3) What does PNS stand for? _____

4) What does CNS stand for? _____

5) Based on what you have been learning, is it proper to use the abbreviation NS? You may need to guess. _____

6) How many major subsystems are in the nervous system? _____

7) How are messages relayed from the brain to the body? _____

8) What's another word for neuron? _____

Identifying Parts of the Nervous System

Label the diagram of the nervous system. Refer to the reading for assistance.

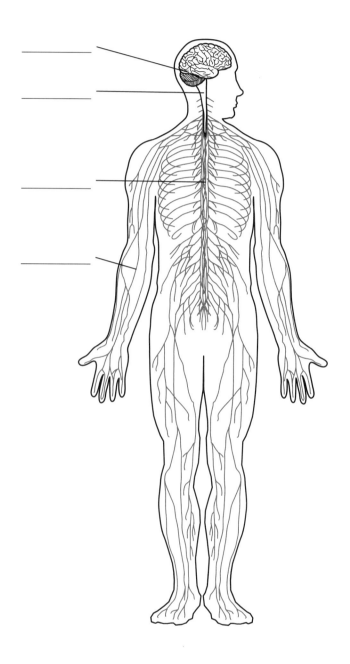

Building Vocabulary

To show that you really are gaining vocabulary, you will be asked to use new vocabulary words in sentences and to identify verbs of similar meaning. Complete the following exercises.

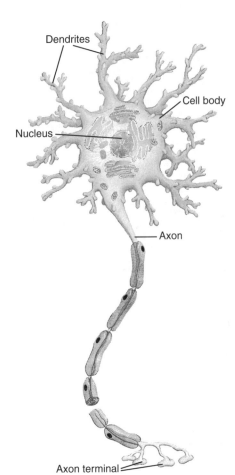

Dendrites

Cell body

Nucleus

Axon

Axon terminal

Sentence Completion. To build vocabulary, use the word from the text in a full complete sentence. Refer to the graphic of a nerve cell shown here for clues in completing the sentences.

1) The _____ between the sensory and motor nerves is known as the _____.

2) _____ and _____ are parts of a _____, or nerve cell.

3) The _____ _____ relays all _____ to and from various levels of the _____ _____.

Identifying Verbs in a Sentence. Identify the verbs in the following sentences.

1) The nervous system directs every body system and cell. _____

2) The central nervous system is most often referred to as the CNS. _____

3) These consist of neurons or nerve cells.
_____

4) The brain stem relays all messages to and from various levels of the nervous system. _____

Recognizing Verbs of Similar Meaning. Replace the following verbs or terms with others of similar meaning. Fill in the gaps. Use the Word Bank to assist you.

WORD BANK

transport

also known as

is comprised

is made up

passes

1) The neurological system is commonly referred to as the nervous system.
The neurological system is _____ as the nervous system.

2) The system consists of the brain, brain stem, and spinal cord.
The system _____ of the brain, brain stem, and spinal cord.

3) Axons carry impulses away from the brain out into the body.
Axons _____ impulses away from the brain out into the body.

4) The brain stem relays all messages to and from.
The brain stem _____ all messages to and from.

Reading for Gist

The general meaning of a text is referred to as its gist. Reading for gist is an important reading skill because it provides an opportunity to predict what the text will be about without having to translate each and every word. The skill is particularly relevant when studying *Medical English*

Clear and Simple. Readings and exercises often call on the reader to use his or her own background knowledge in medicine and health care. The use of this personal knowledge facilitates the reader's ability to comprehend the text about to be read once he or she is prompted by a few key words and phrases. Additionally, when one is able to effectively read for gist, the skill of writing summaries is also enhanced. A good summary based on the gist of the reading can be succinct and informative.

Practicing Reading for Gist. *Read the next few lines in anticipation of a short text.*

WORD ALERT

What is the difference between the words *integral* and *essential?*

Take a look at these examples and try to discover the difference (if there is one).

Example 1   Oxygen is integral to human life.

Example 2   Oxygen is essential to human life.

Example 3   As a stimulus to start the day, many Americans and Canadians see coffee in the morning as essential. However, coffee is not integral to starting the day.

1) Predict what the text will be talking about.

_____

Integral means something is an essential or required part of something larger: a component that cannot be discounted or excluded.

Now read this short text. Essential means important. Sometimes it means basic, like a basic feature or element of something. For example, some doctors and nurses believe it is essential to learn medical English, while others think it is totally unnecessary or unessential. *Medical English Clear and Simple* may be essential to your own career plans, but it is not integral to your ability to practice as a health professional in your country of origin. Command of your native language is integral.

2) Based on your reading of the text, confirm your prediction from Question 1 above. Were you correct?

_____

3) Recall that understanding the gist of a text means the ability to create a short summary of it as well. Do that now. Write a summary of 20 words or less identifying the gist of the text, eliminating any nonessential details.

_____

_____

SPEAKING EXERCISE

Re-read the selection The Nervous System aloud. Ask a peer or teacher to help you with pronunciation. Proceed to the Pronunciation Hints for some help with new words.

PRONUNCIATION HINTS

dendrite – **dĕn′**drīt

axon – **ăk′**sŏn

neurological – nū-rŏl′**ŏjĭk′**l

nerve – **n′ĕrv′**

nervous – **nĕr′**vĕs

synapse – note there are two possible pronunciations for this word:

sĭn′ăps or **sī**-năps

LISTENING EXERCISE

Record yourself saying the words listed in the Pronunciation Hints above. Listen very, very carefully to the words with the letter "v." Are you pronouncing "v" correctly or are you pronouncing it as a "b" sound? In some languages, such as Spanish and Tagalog, "v" and "b" are often used interchangeably. This is not the case in English, and accuracy is impaired when the health professional does not distinguish the correct sound.

1) To pronounce the letter "v" correctly, try this exercise. With your teeth almost closed (partially open) and your lips apart, place a pen or pencil horizontally between your lips. Keep it there. Now make a sound from your throat as you force air out between your lips and the pencil. Can you feel and hear the sound vibrate? You should hear vvvvvvvvvvvvvvv. This is the sound of "v."

2) To pronounce the letter "b" correctly, try this exercise. With your teeth apart, purse your lips, keeping them together in a slight, kiss-like fashion. Push air out of a small opening in your lips rapidly while vocalizing a sound. You should hear "buh." This is the sound of the letter "b."

WRITING EXERCISE

Return to the vocabulary exercise in which you were asked to rewrite various sentences changing the verb or term to something of similar meaning. Use that exercise as a reference to rewrite the entire text of The Nervous System in your own words. Do not simply copy the original text. Replace verbs whenever possible. Be careful not to change the meaning of the text too drastically.

_____

_____

_____

_____

_____

_____

_____

Reading Selection 6-2

Study Figure 6-1 below in preparation for the exercises that follow, then read the text.

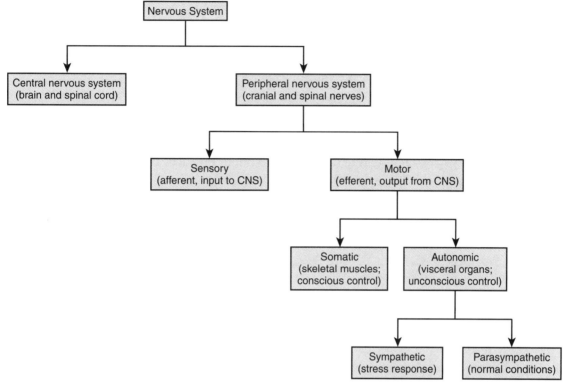

Figure 6-1

DIVISIONS OF THE NEUROLOGICAL SYSTEM

As you know, the neurological system is divided into two major systems—the central nervous system and the peripheral nervous system. Each is vital to human survival and functioning. The central nervous system is divided into the brain and spinal cord. The peripheral nervous system has many subdivisions.

The peripheral nervous system is divided into sensory and motor divisions. The sensory division transmits signals from body organs to the central nervous system, whereas the motor division transmits impulses from the central nervous system to the peripheral body organs. The motor division is further subdivided into a somatic (body) part, in which conscious control of skeletal muscles occurs, and an autonomic part in which unconscious control of smooth muscle and internal organs occurs. The autonomic system is further divided into the sympathetic system, which responds to stress ("the fight-or-flight" response) by releasing the neurotransmitter norepinephrine, and the parasympathetic system, which attempts to maintain normal conditions and a stable internal environment through the release of the neurotransmitter acetylcholine.

 ## READING EXERCISES

As you become more comfortable with reading for gist and general meaning, you will also increase your ability to recall specific details and expand your vocabulary.

Understanding the General Meaning

Understanding the general meaning is very similar to reading for gist—finding the main topic of the reading and identifying what is to be expected in the reading.

Go back. Read the text again. Answer the questions with short-answer responses.

1) What is the general theme of the text?

_____

2) How many divisions are there in the neurological system?

_____

3) Identify the major divisions of the neurological system.

_____

4) Diagram the divisions of the neurological system. To demonstrate your understanding, create a diagram like the one preceding the reading. In your diagram, identify all subsystems of the neurological system and make a brief comment on each. Draw your own boxes.

Reading for Gist. Read the following sentences in anticipation of an upcoming text.

You have now had two opportunities to use charts. These are called flowcharts, meaning they proceed from biggest to smallest elements. They are also sometimes referred to as organizational charts and hierarchical charts.

1) Predict what the text will be talking about

_____

Now read the following Reading Alert.

READING ALERT You have now had two opportunities to use charts. These are called flow charts, meaning they proceed from biggest to smallest elements. They are also sometimes referred to as organizational charts and hierarchical charts. The ability to read and interpret flow charts is essential to health professionals. Many such charts appear on medical and nursing forms and you will be required to complete them frequently.
Look at the chart provided and then the one you have completed. Take a close look at the flow of information: the direction. Draw arrows between the boxes in the direction that each chart flows. Are yours and the textbook's the same? In the United States and Canada,

medical flow charts are usually designed to flow from largest to smallest—<u>from top down to the bottom</u>. This is not so in every country and it is an important feature in North American English to remember. (Note: In some languages, medical flow charts are designed to be read from the bottom up.)

2) Based on your reading of the text, confirm your prediction from Question 1 above. Were you correct?

_____

3) Recall that understanding the gist of a text means the ability to create a short summary of it as well. Do that now. Write a summary of 20 words or less identifying the gist of the text, eliminating any nonessential details.

_____

_____

Building Vocabulary

To be able to write reports—which health-care professionals are often asked to do—they must not only understand new vocabulary but also be able to spell new words and use them properly in sentences. Two words that sound alike or which are spelled similarly may present special difficulties for non-native English speakers. (See Word Alert below.)

> **WORD ALERT: AUTONOMIC VERSUS AUTOMATIC** Autonomic is not a precise or exact synonym for automatic. Take a very careful look at the spelling of the two words. Say them aloud slowly to appreciate the difference. Break them into syllables:
>
> auto - nomic
> auto - matic
>
> The adjective *autonomic* is used to refer to a process of the nervous system that is not controlled by human volition (will). For example, the heart speeds up and slows down in response to neurons and nerve pathways sensing the need to do so. An autonomic response is caused by and initiated by internal stimuli.
> The adjective *automatic* is similar in meaning, but an automatic response can be triggered by an external stimulus. For example, an external stimulus such as a strong light being focused on the eye or someone throwing something at you can cause a defensive automatic blink response, but blinking, in general, is under autonomic nervous system control and occurs continuously throughout the waking day, whether we wish it to do so or not.

Learning the Spelling of New Words. There are a number of medical terms in the text you have just read: Divisions of the Neurological System. Complete the following exercise using these new terms, versions of them, and other relevant vocabulary by unscrambling the words.

1) ninphrneiepero _____

2) nxoa _____

3) dtenedrie _____

4) matpehtciys _____

5) latryvinoun _____

6) smpraahicetatpy _____

7) tttsmnrenruaire _____

8) cimnotuao _____

9) mciuatota _____

Using New Vocabulary in Sentences. Use your knowledge of anatomy and physiology to explain the process or subsystem responsible for the following examples. Write in complete sentences.

1) When the eye opens and shuts automatically

_____

2) When you smell fresh bread baking in the oven

_____

3) When you have the urge to urinate

_____

4) When you stub your toe on the corner of the bed

_____

SPEAKING EXERCISE

Read the Word Alert given above aloud. Repeat this until you can read it without hesitating on pronunciation. You might even want to try to sing it! Singing actually makes reading aloud easier. Try it and see. The Pronunciation Hints box below will help.

PRONUNCIATION HINTS

sympathetic – sĭm″pă-**thĕt′**ĭk

autonomic – aw-tō-**nŏm′**ĭk

automatic – aw-tō-**măt′**ĭk

noradrenergic – nor-ăd-rĕn-**ĕr′**jĭk

adrenalin – ă-**drĕn′**ă-lĭn

hierarchical – hī′**răr**-kĭk′ăl

LISTENING EXERCISE

At this point you again have some homework. Try to find a native English-speaking health professional if you know one or watch an English language television show or film set in an American health-care setting. Listen. The purpose of this exercise is simply to familiarize yourself with how English is spoken in the context of health care.

WRITING EXERCISE

Review the reading Divisions of the Neurological System. Underline key topic words and main ideas. Reflect on these and then write a summary in paragraph form. Refer to Box 6-1 for key features of a summary and hints on how to write one. Be brief. You might want to refer back to the first reading in this chapter to review the concept of reading for gist to help with your summarizing skills.

_____

_____

_____

_____

_____

Reading Selection 6-3

Read the following description of the brain. Concentrate on words that specify anatomical location.

THE BRAIN

The human brain is essential to our ability to function in life. The capacity of the human brain is what sets us apart from other living things. Biological, psychological, emotional, creative, spiritual, and social functioning all arise from the brain. The "mind" is the cognitive capacity of the brain to think, problem solve, reflect, create, imagine, remember, and act in social, moral, and ethical ways.

The brain is divided into two hemispheres and four lobes. The two hemispheres of the brain are most commonly identified simply by their location of left or right. Sometimes they are referred to as "right brain" and "left brain" when describing their function and ability. For example, in very simplistic terms the "left brain" is known for its ability to process mathematical computations and think in strategic ways. The "right brain" concerns itself with more aesthetic functions such as creativity.

The four lobes are the frontal, occipital, temporal, and parietal. The frontal lobe is located in the anterior portion of the cranium (skull). It is responsible for moral judgment, higher order thinking, and short-term memory. Broca's aphasia or difficulty expressing oneself in words can occur when there is damage to the middle of the frontal lobe. The occipital lobe is located at the posterior of the cranium, and it includes the upper end of the spinal cord. This portion of the brain is concerned with homeostasis, coordination of movement, and maintenance and control of the heart rate and breathing, as well as the ability to be alert and fully awake. It plays a significant role in the ability to process visual information. The temporal lobe is actually two lobes—the right temporal lobe and left temporal lobe. They are located anteriorly to the occipital lobe and bilaterally on the right and left sides of the brain. The temporal lobes are responsible for memory, perception, and recognition of auditory stimuli. The ability to receive and understand speech is located within the left temporal lobe. Impairment here is known as Wernicke's aphasia. The right temporal lobe concerns itself with memory for sounds and shapes. The parietal lobe sits superior to the occipital lobe and posterior to the frontal lobe, at the top of the brain. It is situated just under the bony skull cap. It functions in the perception of sensation and spatial relations, as well as in orientation.

READING EXERCISES

Take a moment now to review what you have just read. Use that information to complete the following exercises.

Understanding the General Meaning

Read the text again. Think about it. Do you understand it?

1) What is the core message or thesis of the text?

Learning Specific Facts

Being able to identify and label parts of the brain using medical terminology will demonstrate that you have understood the reading and are knowledgeable about the vocabulary used to describe the anatomy and physiology of the brain.

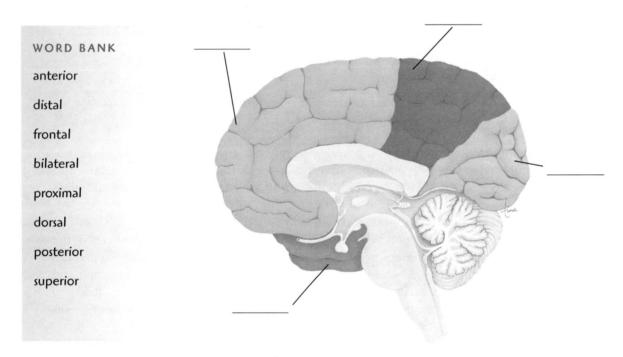

WORD BANK

anterior

distal

frontal

bilateral

proximal

dorsal

posterior

superior

Labeling and Identifying the Lobes of the Brain

Place the words from the following Word Bank next to the appropriate lobe on the same illustration. Label the lobes of the brain based on the reading. Be careful. Some words will not be used.

Using Professional Terminology to Describe the Lobes of the Brain. Now locate the following using professional terminology. Write in full sentences.

1) Where is the parietal lobe located?

2) Locate the temporal lobe.

3) Locate the lobe responsible for heart rates.

Building Vocabulary

Complete the following two exercises to increase your medical vocabulary as well as your ability to describe important centers of the brain. The goal is not to re-learn the anatomy and physiology. Instead, it is to see and use career-specific language in the most appropriate manner in this medical context. While completing the exercises, pay strict attention to the verbs used to describe function and responsibility.

Determining Meaning from Context. To build vocabulary, study the following words or terms taken from this text. Discover all you can about them by looking at them in context, then choose the correct meaning. Finally, take a look at how these words or terms expand in English.

1. Anterior *(adjective)*

In context:
a) The anterior portion of the skull houses the cerebral cortex.
b) The cranium is anterior to the brain.

Meaning: The best way to explain the term *anterior* is to say
a) above
b) opposite
c) external
d) in front of; toward the front of the body

Word expansion:
a) The frontal lobe sits *anteriorly* to the occipital lobe. (adverb)

2. Capacity *(noun)*

In context:
a) The brain does not work at full capacity even though we think it does.
b) Does the human mind have the capacity to heal the body?

Meaning: The best way to explain the term *capacity* is to say
a) ability
b) power
c) ability, adequacy, room, and/or volume
d) agility

Word expansion:
a) Is the human brain *capable* of telepathy? (adjective)
b) We all have the *capability* to be courteous to each other, but some people don't choose to be that way. (noun)

3. Mind *(noun)*

In context:
a) The mind has the capacity to imagine endless possibilities.
b) The study of the mind is called psychology.
c) The medically based field of treatment for disorders and diseases of the mind is called psychiatry.

Meaning: The best way to explain the term *mind* is to say
a) brain
b) brain and cognition
c) cognition and emotion
d) center of thought and emotion, concentration, and imagination

Word expansion:
a) Clients who receive a diagnosis of Alzheimer's disease say they are afraid of losing their *minds*. (noun, plural)
b) *Mindfulness* is a therapeutic technique somewhat like meditation. (noun)
c) A person who is *single-minded* can be rigid in his or her thinking and does not like chaos. (adjective, idiom)

d) Losing your *mind* is an idiom used to express confusion or forgetfulness. (noun used as part of an idiom)

4. Cranium *(noun)*

In context:
a) The brain is housed in the cranium.
b) The cranium is also referred to as the skull or head.

Meaning: The best way to explain the term *cranium* is to say
a) skeletal bones
b) skeletal formation protecting the brain
c) skeletal formation protecting the mind
d) formation of bones protecting the spinal cord

Word expansion:
a) There are 12 *cranial* nerves in the body. They originate in the brain. (adjective)
b) A *craniotomy* is a surgical procedure in which the skull is cut open to expose the brain. (noun)
c) A *cranial* fracture is also known as a skull fracture. (adjective)

Mix and Match.   The exercise in Box 6-2 requires you to use your medical knowledge. The diagram will help if you are not familiar with the English terms.

Using Verbs in Sentences.   The following verbs appeared within the context of anatomy and physiology in the reading. Use them now, in a medical context, in the proper form. Use the words you are given and the verb tense identified to create a new sentence.

1) regulate, heart (past tense) _____

2) maintain, balance, injury (present tense)

_____

3) contain, memory, lost (past tense)

_____

4) pain, relay, fractured tibia (past tense)

_____

BOX 6-2 Mix and Match: Functions of Different Parts of the Central Nervous System

Match the part of the central nervous system to its function.

ANATOMICAL PART	FUNCTION
mid-brain	aids in hearing and vision
cerebellum	waking and maintaining consciousness; alertness
hypothalamus	regulates heart rate and coughing
medulla oblongata	maintains balance and fine and gross motor movements
brain stem	controls the endocrine system
spinal cord	registers mood and pain
thalamus	contains nerve pathways to and from the brain

SPEAKING EXERCISE

Read the exercise Determining Meaning from Context aloud. Ask a peer or teacher to help you with pronunciation. Proceed to the Pronunciation Hints section. This will also help.

PRONUNCIATION HINTS

cranium – **krā**′nē-ŭm

occipital – ŏk-**sĭp**′ĭ-tăl

parietal – pă-**rī**′ĕ-tăl

temporal – **tĕm**′por-ăl

cerebellum – sĕr-ĕ-**bĕl**′ŭm

hypothalamus – hī″pō-**thăl**′ă-mŭs

LISTENING EXERCISE

Go online now. Search for the key words "brain anatomy, audio visual" or research brain anatomy at *YouTube* or any other site that offers free access to video clips. There are a number of online sites that offer good audio examples of the material covered in this section. Listen carefully to pronunciation.

WRITING EXERCISE—CRITICAL THINKING

The author has said that the brain is essential to human functioning. Do you agree? Is the brain essential or integral? Please explain using career-specific vocabulary. State your position and provide your rationale.

| SECTION TWO | # Common Complaints and Disorders of the Neurological System |

This section focuses on building vocabulary that is related to the pathophysiology and dysfunction of the brain and nervous system. The context is that of headaches, migraines, and epilepsy. Descriptors for signs and symptoms are explored in lay and professional language. Concepts of pathways and protocols are introduced. In grammar, medical prefixes, fillers, and interjections are examined. The language for pain and pain scales is also presented.

Reading Selection 6-4

Read the following information regarding pathology of the neurological system.

POTENTIAL CAUSES OF NEUROLOGICAL DYSFUNCTION

Nerve damage, brain damage, and other damage to the neurological system can occur as the result of exposure to a wide variety of toxins. This is an aspect of environmental health. Contributors can include exposure to pesticides and heavy metals such as aluminum, lead, and mercury. Nutritional deficits also fall into the category of environmental health. Deficiencies in vitamins, minerals, and amino acids can lead to diminished capacity to concentrate and to confusion, anxiety, and even depression. Depending on the age of onset, these effects can be permanent and disabling or they can be temporary. Finally, neurological impairment can also result from acute and/or chronic infections. Examples of these can be the results of viral and bacterial meningitis and untreated late stage syphilis. Interestingly, syphilis was almost eradicated in the United States and Canada by the late 20th century, but it has begun to reappear. In the 21st century, the incidence of viral and bacterial meningitis seems to be on the rise in our adolescent population, and public health campaigns now include vaccination against this serious disease.

 # READING EXERCISES

The following exercises test your ability to discern the general meaning of a reading selection and to glean specific facts from it.

Understanding the General Meaning

Read the text again. Think about it. Do you understand it?

1) What is the gist of this text?

_____

2) Critical thinking: Explain how environmental factors are an aspect of environmental health.

_____

Learning Specific Facts

1) Name two potential causes of neurological dysfunction.

_____

2) According to the text, what is on the rise in the United States and Canada among teens?

_____

3) What is meant by the term "heavy metals"?

_____

4) List three heavy metals.

_____

Building Vocabulary

In addition to learning the meaning of a word from its context, you may also be able to determine the meaning of a word by the medical prefixes used.

Determining Meaning from Context.   To build vocabulary, study the following words or terms taken from this text. Discover all you can about them by looking at them in context, then choose the correct meaning. Finally, take a look at how these words or terms expand in English.

1. Toxins *(noun, plural)*

In context:
a) Chemical factories sometimes dump toxins into the public waterways. This is illegal in the United States and Canada.
b) Naturopaths often suggest that bowel cleansing is a good way to clear toxins from the body.

Meaning: The best way to define the term *toxins* is to say they are
a) actualized potential of chemical substances
b) attenuated substances accommodated within
c) accumulated wastes within the body
d) substances that are harmful to the body and can accumulate within it

Word expansion:
a) Excessive ingestion of alcohol is *toxic* to the human body and can cause coma, even death. (adjective)
b) Lithium *toxicity* can be seen when blood levels of the medication lithium carbonate are too high.(noun)
c) *Toxicology* screens are used to assess the level of toxins found in the body. (adjective)
d) *Toxicology* is the study of toxins. (noun)

2. Pesticides *(noun, plural)*

In context:
a) Farmers often use pesticides to protect their crops from insects.
b) Chemical pesticides can be toxic to animals and human beings.

Meaning: The best way to define the term *pesticides* is to say they are
a) abnormal substances used as insecticides
b) chemicals used to kill insects and other pests
c) biological insecticides
d) pest repellent toxicology

Word expansion:
a) Incidents of *pesticidal* toxicity are more common in third-world countries than in the United States. (adjective)

3. Exposure *(noun)*

In context:
a) Exposure to lead paint can cause brain damage in small children.
b) Chemical toxins in the soil in the manufacturing zone of northern Mexico have exposed both the adults and children in the area to increased risk of neurological damage and cancer.

Meaning: The best way to define the term *exposure* in a medical context is to say it means
a) contact
b) frozen
c) life-threatening
d) life-altering

Word expansion:
a) During brain surgery, the brain *is exposed* to the external world. (verb, present continuous)
b) An *exposition* of ancient skulls is on display at the Science Museum. (noun)
c) *Exposing* a person to a severe weather condition such as extreme cold can lead to hypothermia and possibly death. (gerund)
d) *Exposure* to pesticides may cause serious neurological diseases. (noun)

4. Deficiencies *(noun, plural)*

In context:
a) Vitamin deficiencies in children can lead to impaired eyesight and inhibit bone development.
b) Deficiencies in cognitive ability are referred to as learning deficits.

Meaning: The best way to define the term *deficiencies* in the medical context is to say it means
a) lacking in amount or an inadequate supply
b) lacking in time and capacity
c) poorly provided for
d) inadequately supported

Word expansion:
a) A speech *deficit* is one in which a person has difficulty making sound or articulating words. (noun)
b) The patient has numbness and tingling in the extremities because she is *deficient* in vitamin B, not because she has a neurological impairment. (adjective)
c) Neurological *deficits* can occur prenatally and can be screened for via amniocentesis. (noun, plural)

5. Disabling *(adjective)*

In context:
a) The disabling effects of narcotic addiction are more than merely physical.

Meaning: The best way to define the adjective *disabling* is to say it means
a) shortening, diminishing
b) crippling
c) accentuating
d) incapacitating
e) both (b) and (d)

Word expansion:
a) While people with chronic schizophrenia may be *disabled* in psychological and social ways, with proper and adequate treatment they are able to live quite well in the community in group or semi-independent living facilities. They do not require institutional care. (adjective)
b) In the United States and Canada, having a neurological or mental *disability* does not mean life must lack quality. Indeed, many cognitively *disabled* Americans and Canadians have meaningful employment and are able to lead quite normal lives. (noun, adjective)
c) The disease multiple sclerosis is *disabling* over time. It may begin slowly but will eventually *disable* the individual as the disease progresses. (transitive verb, then present tense)
d) *Disabling* the neurotransmitter serotonin is a function of the medications in the serotonin re-uptake inhibitor category. (gerund used as noun)

MEDICAL PREFIXES FOR THE NEUROLOGICAL SYSTEM The prefix *neuro* is frequently found in medicine.[1] It refers to any aspect or condition of the neurological system. Familiarize yourself with some of the more common terms.

Neuronal – an adjective to describe a type of cell as being a nerve cell

Neurological – an adjective relating to the neurological system, as in neurological examination or neurological disease

Neuropathway – a noun that identifies the route of nerve impulse conduction

---

[1] **Neuro** is identified as a prefix in words for concepts or topics that relate to the brain and/or the field of neuroscience. In grammar, it is also referred to as a "combining word" and it functions somewhat as an adjective.

Neurosis – a noun identifying a mental disorder that is mild in nature and very common

Neuropathy – a noun that identifies pathology of/in the nervous system

Neurologist – a noun that names the doctor specializing in disorders and diseases of the neurological system

Neuro-vitals – a descriptive noun that identifies a specific group of vital signs that measure neurological response as well as basic physical signs. It is an abbreviated form of the proper term neuro-vital signs.

Neurosurgery – a noun meaning surgery to any part of the neurological system; it is often used to refer to brain surgery

Neurosurgeon – a proper noun naming a surgeon who specializes in operations on the neurological system.

Neurotransmitter – a noun identifying the chemical that transmits between nerves

Using Medical Prefixes in Sentences. Use each of the terms beginning with the prefix *neuro* to create a logical sentence here. Use the words given.

1) neuronal, cellular

_____

2) neurological, brain stem, damage

_____

3) neuropathway, phantom limb pain

_____

4) neurosis, mind

_____

5) neuropathy, Lou Gehrig's disease

_____

6) neuropathic, autism, mercury

_____

7) neuro-vitals, unconscious

_____

8) neurosurgery, neurologist

_____

9) neurotransmitter, excessive, schizophrenia

_____

SPEAKING EXERCISE

Read the following paragraph aloud. Ask a peer or teacher to help you with pronunciation. The Pronunciation Hints box that follows will help.

Parkinson's disease is a neurological disease that impairs the central nervous system. It is degenerative, which means that it progresses over time and can eventually disable the patient. Its most significant symptom is movement disorder. Muscles become rigid, they may be spastic, and movement is increasingly involuntary and uncoordinated.

> **PRONUNCIATION HINTS**
>
> degenerative – dē-**jĕn′**ĕ-rat′ ĭv
>
> deficiency – dē-**fĭsh′**ĕn-sē
>
> neuropathy – nū-**rŏp′**ă-thē
>
> toxins – **tŏks′**ĭn′z
>
> autism – **aw′tĭ**zm

LISTENING EXERCISE

Watch an English language film about autism. Examples of these include: *Rain Man* (with Dustin Hoffman and Tom Cruise), *Mercury Rising, Bless the Child, House of Cards,* and *Silent Fall.* Listen carefully to the discussion of the illness and its cause. Also listen for the type of care and treatment a person with autism can expect in the United States.

Go online to any medical or health promotion site that offers free audio clips of individuals living with multiple sclerosis and comments from medical professionals. You might want to try Health Talk at http://www2.healthtalk.com or Health Line at http://www.healthlines.com, although there are many sites out there that are helpful. Listen carefully to the discussion of the illness and its cause. Also, listen for the type of care and treatment persons with multiple sclerosis can expect in the United States and how they manage their own signs and symptoms.

WRITING EXERCISE—A REFLECTIVE QUESTION

What type of care and treatment can a person with autism or multiple sclerosis expect in your own country of origin? How does it compare with what you have seen or discovered in the Listening exercise? Write a short paragraph here with your personal reflections on one of the topics.

_____

_____

_____

_____

Reading Selection 6-5

Read the following discussion of pain and headaches in preparation for the subsequent exercises.

PAIN AND HEADACHES

Pain, pain reception, and response are key elements of the neurological system. Pain is perceived by specialized nerve cells called pain receptors. The message is then relayed to the brain where a decision is made regarding the appropriate response. This decision is relayed back to the body via neuropathways. The response may be muscular. For example, in response to burning a finger, we may move our finger instantaneously out and away from the flame. However, not all pain occurs externally. Indeed, headaches are the most commonly known form of internal pain experienced.

Headaches are often the result of stress, but they can also be triggered by external stimuli such as injury to the head, sudden exposure to bright lights, many hours under fluorescent lighting, certain foods and smells, and a myriad of other causes. People describe their headache signs and symptoms with the following descriptors: dizziness, spinning, pounding, hammering, mild, excruciating, and dull. They can usually locate the pain, as well. Headaches are usually of short duration. When suffering from a headache, people often appear cranky, impatient, and irritable. The condition brings with it a decrease in frustration tolerance, or the decreased capacity to tolerate frustration.

One type of headache is a migraine. Migraines are severe and can be quite disabling. They are caused by a constriction of the blood vessels in the occipital area and down into the neck. This decrease in blood flow is experienced as throbbing pain usually felt at first on only one side of the head. Other symptoms include heightened sensitivity and intolerance to light and sound. During a migraine headache, frustration intolerance can be significantly increased. The sufferer may be irritable and unapproachable. It is important for the health-care professional to remember that the migraine sufferer is focused on his or her internal pain. They should not take the client's brusque or unfriendly attitude as personal in any way.

While migraines may need medical and pharmacological intervention, headaches in general do not. Over-the-counter analgesics, changes in one's day or in one's lifestyle to decrease tension, relaxation techniques, balanced nutrition, rest, and exercise can all positively affect resolution of the headache. Pain scales are the method of diagnosing the severity or degree of pain a patient is experiencing. Subjectively, he or she is asked to rate the severity of pain on a scale of 1 to 10, with 1 being the absence of pain and 10 being excruciating pain. While this pain scale may seem simplistic, it is informative and helpful for monitoring the patient's condition.

Understanding the General Meaning

Read the text again. Think about it.

1) What is the gist of this text?

_____

2) What example is used in this reading to illustrate the main concepts?

_____

3) What shouldn't the health professional take personally?

_____

Learning Specific Facts

Take a moment now to review what you have just read.

1) Does all pain occur externally?

_____

2) What is a migraine?

_____

3) As a health professional, you must use language that differentiates. What is the key difference between a headache and a migraine?

_____

4) What is a pain scale?

_____

5) What is frustration intolerance?

_____

Building Vocabulary

Health-care professionals must be aware of the words and expressions people may use to describe their complaints. Sometimes the specific words used can help in diagnosis and intervention.

Identifying Pain Descriptors. There are a number of subjective pain descriptors identified in the text. Complete this exercise by matching the symbol or graphic with the descriptive adjective. Use a word from the Word Bank to fill in the blanks.

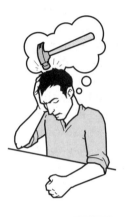

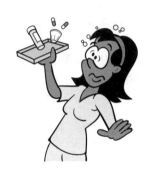

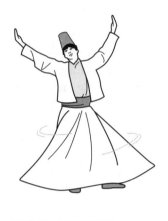

_____

_____

_____

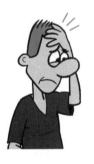

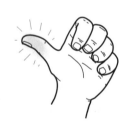

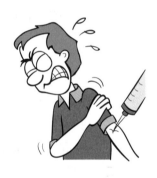

_____

_____

_____

WORD BANK

pounding

light sensitive

throbbing

frustration intolerance

spinning

hammering

excruciating

dizzy

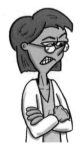

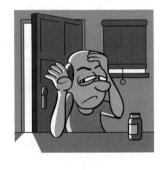

_____

_____

The Neurological System

Explaining Pain Descriptors. In your own words, explain what is meant by the words or expressions used in the last exercise. Consider how these may have originated and how they have come to be used as descriptors for headaches. (Do not simply reiterate what was said in the reading.)

1) pounding

_____

2) light sensitive

_____

3) throbbing

_____

4) frustration intolerance

_____

5) spinning

_____

6) hammering

_____

7) excruciating

_____

SPEAKING EXERCISE

Read the following completed sentences aloud. Ask a peer or teacher to help you with pronunciation. Proceed to the Pronunciation Hints section following. This will also help.

Dizziness is also known as vertigo. When the brain is unable to perceive the body's spatial status, balance is impaired. As a result, the individual experiences a sense of swirling or spinning inside his or her head as well as a lack of balance. Sometimes, if you are watching this person, you will see him or her begin to sway as they lose an internal sense of balance. Vertigo has many causes.

PRONUNCIATION HINTS

neuropathway – nū-**rŏ**-păth-wā

vertigo – **vĕr'**tĭ-gō

LISTENING EXERCISE

Go online. Try to find an audio-video clip made by people who suffer from migraine headaches. Listen to them talk about their signs, symptoms, and health promotion activities. Listen to added commentary by medical practitioners. You might want to try the website Health Talk mentioned in an earlier exercise. Search for the key words, such as migraine videos.

WRITING EXERCISE—A REFLECTIVE QUESTION

Reflect on your own practice as a health-care professional in your country of origin. How do people describe their headaches there? How do these descriptors compare with those of the United States and Canada? Discuss the similarities or differences in a short paragraph.

_____

_____

Reading Selection 6-6

Read the following dialogue to familiarize yourself with the language used to communicate between two friends who encounter a person having an epileptic seizure. Notice that numbers accompany each speaker's words. These numbers relate to a subsequent exercise.

EPILEPSY

Scene: Two men, Art and Brad, are walking in a public park. They see another man collapse to the ground and begin to writhe and twitch. They ask another passerby to call an ambulance and they stay with the stranger to help.

(1) **Art:** Help! Help! Hey you . . . call an ambulance, will you? This guy's passed out. He might be epileptic!

(2) **Brad:** Wow! Look at the way his body is jerking around! Yeah, he must be an epileptic.

(3) **Art:** Yeah. Must be a seizure. What'll we do?

(4) **Brad:** I don't know. Just stay with him I guess, until the ambulance gets here.

(5) **Art:** Wow, I hope they don't take too long. I have NO idea what to do.

(6) **Brad:** Well . . . maybe . . . oh, wow. Look! He's banging his head and rolling his eyes. Hey, Mister, it's all right. We're here with you. An ambulance is coming.

(7) **Art:** Here, here, Mister . . . put this jacket under your head. Gee, Brad, I don't think he can hear us. I think he's unconscious.

(8) **Brad:** Yeah. Hey, he's stopped jerking.

(9) **Art:** Right. Hey, hello. Can you hear me, sir?

(10) **Brad:** Oh, his eyes look clearer now and his breathing's better. I think he's coming around.

(11) **Art:** Hi! Welcome back. I think you had a seizure. We stayed with you. Are you all right now?

(12) **Stranger:** Uh, mmmmm . . . What happened?

(13) **Art:** He's a bit confused, Brad. Listen, an ambulance is coming to help you. Just lay still. Are you an epileptic?

(14) **Stranger:** Epileptic? Yeah. Tired.

(15) **Brad:** OK, well just relax if you want. We'll stay with you until they come.

Understanding the General Meaning

Read the text again. Think about it. Do you understand it?

1) In Art's first speech, exclamation marks are used abundantly. Why?

2) Are Art and Brad health professionals?

3) Do Art and Brad demonstrate a general understanding of how to give aid to a person suffering an epileptic seizure? Explain your answer.

_____

4) In line 6, Brad is distracted from what he starts to say. What distracts him?

_____

5) Art demonstrates one safety measure for caring for a person who is having a seizure. What is that?

_____

6) Use your own medical knowledge. Name two other safety measures necessary for assisting a person having an epileptic seizure.

_____

WORD ALERT Notice the terms used to express the patient's condition.
The man is suffering an epileptic seizure, but it is inappropriate in health care to say he suffers with epilepsy or suffers from epilepsy. The rationale for this is that most of the time the person does not experience negative effects of this neurological condition; therefore, he does not suffer from it. Although we quite often say a person is an epileptic, it is not respectful to do so. We simply say the person has epilepsy.

Recognizing Specifics.   Take a moment now to review the dialogue you have just read. Answer the questions to ensure your level of comprehension.

1) What is the name of the person having the seizure? _____

2) How do Art and/or Brad refer to the person having a seizure? What names or titles do they use? _____

3) In line 1, who does Art ask to call an ambulance? _____

4) In line 5, why is the word "no" capitalized? _____

5) In line 7, does Art actually expect the person seizuring to put the jacket under his head? _____

6) In line 11, to whom is Art speaking? _____

7) In line 13, Art is speaking to more than one person. Name them.

_____

8) In line 15, Brad uses the pronoun "they." To whom is he referring?

_____

VOCABULARY ALERT: SEIZURES In medical jargon, we may turn the word seizure into a verb although it is not grammatically correct to do so. Expect to hear this. It is quite acceptable and career-specific. Here are some examples:

• The patient is seizuring. (medical jargon)
  The grammatically correct way to say this is: The patient is having a seizure.

• He has been seizuring 2 or 3 times a day since being in the hospital. (medical jargon)
  The grammatically correct way to say this is: He has been having seizures 2 or 3 times a day since being admitted to the hospital.

- She seizured during the night but did not incur any injuries. (medical jargon)
  The grammatically correct way to say this is: She had a seizure in the night but did not incur any injuries.

Finally, you may also hear the term "fit" used to describe an epileptic seizure as in, "the patient is having a fit." While this term is very common, it is **extremely improper and unprofessional to use it. Do not use it.**
(Note: you might also have heard the term "fit" in an entirely different context. It is often used to describe a temper tantrum.)

Building Vocabulary

Fillers occur spontaneously in speech when a person is unprepared, hesitant, anxious, or needs a quick pause to think of what to say next. In this instance, they "fill" the silence with words such as "umm" (which isn't really a word at all). Fillers serve no grammatical function. Interjections, on the other hand, are inserted into speech to convey emotions such as surprise. Often, these words stand alone and are followed by an exclamation mark. It is not necessary to use them in sentences, but it is acceptable. On a last note, interjections are rare in professional, technical, or academic writing. They most often appear in dialogues, narratives, and informal writings.

Recognizing Fillers and Interjections. In the dialogue, Art and Brad are nervous. As a result, their speech is full of fillers and interjections. Search for the fillers or interjections and write them here. Label them as one or the other part of speech. You are given a hint by having the dialogue line number identified.

1) Line 2 _____
2) Line 5 _____
3) Line 6 (there are three here) _____ _____ _____
4) Line 7 _____
5) Line 8 _____
6) Line 9 _____
7) Line 10 _____
8) Line 12 (there are two here) _____ _____
9) Line 15 _____

Mix and Match. There are a number of descriptive terms and verbs used in the dialogue that you may or may not be familiar with. Complete the exercise in Box 6-3 by matching descriptors with their meanings.

Understanding Protocols and Pathways. Read the following information about protocols and pathways. It will be relevant to the subsequent exercises.

A medical protocol is standard procedure that is expected to be followed consistently. Protocols are codes of conduct. For example, all staff in the hospital will follow the fire and evacuation protocols. They will adhere to the infection control protocols. They will be aware of and consistently follow protocols for the handling of a patient having an epileptic seizure and for the care of the comatose patient. Medicine is full of protocols. Can you think of a few more?

A clinical pathway is a guideline for the provision of patient care based on the patient's illness or procedures that are being done. While protocols are printed as standard hospital forms, clinical pathways need to be individualized by the attending nurses or doctors. These are flow charts and the pathway flows in a stepwise progression from beginning to end. There are usually two paths on a clinical pathway. One is followed when there are no complications; the other is followed should complications arise. At each step along the path, guidelines are provided for the

BOX 6-3 Mix and Match: The Meaning of Descriptors

Matching the descriptors with their meaning.

DESCRIPTOR	MEANING
writhing	appears conscious, alert, and more able to understand
confused	eyes turn upwards and then return to center
jerking	sudden strong muscle spasms or tics
rolling his eyes	mixed up; not thinking clearly
eyes are clearer	twisting and turning movement

health professional to prepare for and take the next step. If you have not seen a clinical pathway, search the Internet. There are many examples.

1) Describe the protocol that Art initiated when assisting a stranger having an epileptic seizure in a public place.

_____

2) Describe the protocol for assisting a patient having an epileptic seizure in the hospital.

_____
_____
_____
_____
_____

3) Protocol requires that the stranger in this story be transported to the nearest hospital or clinic to be assessed following his seizure. However, he may choose not to do this and he is free to do so. If he goes to the hospital, once there the protocols will continue. A standardized clinical pathway will be initiated to guide his care and to evaluate whether or not the patient is safe and stable for discharge. Based on this information and the Vocabulary Alert, what is a clinical pathway?

_____

SPEAKING EXERCISE

Re-read the information about protocols and pathways aloud. Ask a peer or teacher to help you with pronunciation. Proceed to the Pronunciation Hints section following. This will also help.

PRONUNCIATION HINTS

epilepsy – **ĕp″ĭ**-lĕp′sē

epileptic – ĕp″ ĭ-**lĕp′**tĭk

protocol – **prō′tō**-kŏl

writhing – **rī′**th-ĭng

jerking – **jĕrk**-ĭng

LISTENING EXERCISE

You know about epilepsy and that it is a neurological condition. Record your voice explaining the cause and signs or symptoms of epilepsy, in English. Then, listen. How many speech fillers do you use? Any? Some? Many? None? Use self-reflection to discover why you are doing so. Try to record a second time, this time consciously monitoring your use of fillers. Try very hard to decrease your use of them.

WRITING EXERCISE—CRITICAL THINKING

From the gist of the dialogue and vocabulary work you have just completed, you will have confirmed that Brad and Art were nervous while they were helping the stranger through his seizure. Use critical thinking skills to suggest why this was so. Use full sentences to do so.

_____

_____

_____

| SECTION THREE | Treatments, Interventions, and Assistance |

This section introduces terminology related to brain injury from external or internal causes. Assessing, monitoring, and describing the care and treatment of a patient with a brain injury are presented through language foci of medical prefixes and suffixes, pain scales, and coma and coma scales.

Reading Selection 6-7

Read the following information about head injury, paying close attention to the medical terminology.

HEAD INJURIES

In a general sense, head injuries can be classified as open or closed. They can also be classified by the amount of damage that occurs: the severity of the trauma. In cases of skull fracture, the severity of the injury is determined based on whether or not the protective barriers of the scalp, the skull, and the dura are compromised and the brain is exposed externally. There are three types of skull fractures. A linear fracture is a single, clean break in the skull and is the most common form. A comminuted fracture crushes or splinters the skull into numerous small bony fragments. The third type is the depressed skull fracture. In this instance, trauma (injury) causes the skull bone fragments to be pushed inward onto the brain itself, potentiating severe neurological damage.

Parenchymal injury is the term used when brain tissue is injured. Such conditions include concussion, contusion, and laceration. These may be the result of a blow to the head that causes the brain to move or jostle within the skull, striking the bones of the skull. In degrees of severity a concussion causes temporary dysfunction of the brain. A contusion is caused by a more severe blow and can cause some bruising of the brain and disruption of neural function. A laceration signifies a traumatic tearing of the cerebral cortex and can have very serious neuronal effects.

Closed head injuries can be just as serious as open head injuries due to the potential for alterations in intracranial pressure (ICP). Intracranial pressure occurs when pressure is exerted on brain tissue, cerebrospinal fluid, and brain blood volume. It can be caused by increased cerebrospinal fluid, tumors, or swelling of the brain due to injury or disease. Signs of increasing ICP include headache, altered respirations, deteriorating levels of consciousness, and even visual disturbances. Untreated, intracranial pressure can lead to death. This condition is most often diagnosed with the assistance of a computed axial tomography scan, commonly known as the CT scan or CAT scan.

Coma can occur as the result of disease, severe head injury, or seizure. It can also be caused by metabolic disorders. A coma is an extended period of unconsciousness. Even painful stimulus is insufficient to arouse this patient. Diagnosis involves assessment of the patient's reactivity and perceptivity to external stimuli. Reactivity refers to nervous system response to stimuli such as pain, sound, touch, or movement. Perceptivity refers to responses made to learned stimuli such as responding to language. The comatose patient does not react to either of these types of stimuli. A key evaluative tool for this condition is the coma scale, the most widely known one being the Glasgow Coma Scale. This scale requires frequent monitoring and charting by the attending nurses. It includes neuro-vital signs and measures levels of consciousness (LOC).

READING EXERCISES

As we have stated before, health-care professionals must understand both the general meaning of a reading passage or conversation as well as the specific details included. Remember, health-care workers must ask and answer questions using very specific language. To do this they must build their vocabulary of English words, expressions, and idioms and be able to clearly identify the question words being used.

Understanding the General Meaning

Read the text again. Think about it. Do you understand it?

1) What is the gist of this reading?

_____

2) What key words or prompts led you to believe the answer to Question 1 was correct?

_____

3) In a medical context, what is a synonym that is sometimes used for the word "injury"?

_____

Answering Questions About Specifics

Take a moment now to review what you have just read. Respond with full sentences.

1) When can coma occur?

_____

2) Which type of skull fracture potentiates the risk for severe brain injury?

_____

3) What does the abbreviation ICP stand for?

_____

4) Which type of head injury is most severe?

_____

5) Differentiate between an open and closed head injury.

_____

6) What is a parenchymal injury?

_____

7) According to the text, how does ICP occur?

_____

Review the exercise you have just completed. Circle the question words. Now reconsider your answers. Have you provided answers that are specific to the question word? This is an important language skill to master.

Building Vocabulary

To ensure that you really understand new vocabulary words you have learned, you should be able to use them in sentences.

Determining Meaning from Context.   To build vocabulary, study the following words or terms taken from this text. Discover all you can about them by looking at them in context, then choose the correct meaning. Finally, take a look at how these words or terms expand in English.

1. Bruising *(gerund)*

In context:
a) Bruising around the left eye was evidence of domestic violence and wife assault.
b) Bruising is a constant concern for patients with hemophilia.

Meaning: The best way to explain the word *bruising* is to say it means
a) discoloring of skin
b) bleeding from an organ
c) hemorrhaging under the skin as the result of impact
d) the result of impact or pressure under the skin that damages blood vessels

Word expansion:
a) Spousal assault was the cause of the *bruising.* (noun)
b) Melissa's hip *was bruised* when she bumped into the edge of the desk. (verb with auxiliary verb [was], past)
c) Yvon has a *bruise* on his left arm from fighting. (noun)
d) Some people *bruise* easily. (verb, present)

2. Trauma *(noun)*

In context:
a) The emergency department sees many cases of trauma.
b) Trauma to the brain can result in coma.

Meaning: The word *trauma* means a (an)
a) accidental injury
b) parenchymal injury
c) injury or damage to any part of the body
d) injury or damage to any part of the body or mind

Word expansion:
a) Keesha was emotionally *traumatized* when she saw her pet dog hit by a car. (verb with auxiliary [was], past)
b) *Traumatic* events in childhood can leave emotional scars. (adjective)

c) It *will be traumatizing* for Zena when she discovers she has lost her baby. (verb, future continuous tense)
d) The earthquake *traumatized* the children. (verb, past)

3. Coma *(noun)*

In context:
a) The patient has suffered a severe brain injury and is in a coma.
b) This patient's coma has lasted more than a year and it still continues.

Meaning: The best explanation of the word *coma* is
a) unconscious
b) unresponsive
c) brain death
d) unresponsive and in a state of profound unconsciousness

Word expansion:
a) The patient is *comatose*. (adjective)

4. Potentiating *(transitive verb)*

In context:
a) Global warming may be a potentiating factor for certain diseases.

Meaning: The meaning of the word *potentiating* is
a) to make more effective or active
b) to be impossible
c) to be current
d) to be factual

Word expansion:
a) The *potential* harmful effects of the sun on bare skin cannot be disregarded. (adjective)
b) When two medications are mixed, there is the *potential* for them to interact negatively. (noun)
c) Pain stimulus is a *potent* indicator of the ability of the organism to respond. (adjective)
d) Excessive heat *potentiates* the risk of dehydration for an athlete. (verb, present)

Fill in the Blanks.   Complete the following by filling in the blanks with a word from the Word Bank.

WORD BANK

consciousness

unconsciously

subconscious

profound

1) Brenda often twirls her hair with her fingers when she is thinking. She isn't aware of this habit. She does it _____.

2) Dreams are thought to be the result of the _____ working through personal issues and experiences.

3) After 3 years in a coma, Wilson has finally regained _____.

4) The patient's coma is so _____ that there is absolutely no response to any stimuli.

SPEAKING EXERCISE

Read the following completed sentences aloud. Ask a peer or teacher to help you with pronunciation. Proceed to the Pronunciation Hints section that follows. This will also help.

An acquired brain injury (ABI) is that which occurs after birth. It is not related to disease or a congenital disorder. The most common causes of ABI are motor vehicle accidents, assaults, and workplace accidents. The effects of the injury can be temporary or permanent and can impact the individual's ability to function physically and psychosocially.

PRONUNCIATION HINTS

parenchymal – păr-ĕn′kĭ-măl

concussion – kŏn-**kŭsh**′ŭn

laceration – lăs″ĕ-**rā**′shŭn

contusion – kŏn-**too**′zhŭn

congenital – kŏn-**jĕn**′ĭ-tăl

LISTENING EXERCISE

Record yourself reading the text entitled Head Injuries. It is quite lengthy and full of medical terminology. Next, listen to your recording without looking at the words in this book. Listen only. Do not let the written words be your guide. Evaluate yourself.

- What do you notice about your pronunciation?
- Are you speaking clearly?
- Are you speaking at a normal rhythm and rate?

WRITING EXERCISE

Use some of the symbols shown in Box 6-4 and any medical abbreviations you know to rewrite these sentences. Use short forms, but be sure that what you write is logical and can be read by another health professional.

1) Intracranial pressure is increasing. _____

2) Patient is losing consciousness. _____

3) Patient is increasingly losing consciousness. _____

BOX 6-4 Commonly Used Symbols in Medicine

+	plus or in addition
–	minus
=	equal to
≠	not equal
≤	less than or equal to
≥	greater than or equal to
×	times it occurs (3 x per day = three times per day or tid)
%	percentage of 100
°F	degrees Fahrenheit
°C	degrees Centigrade
↑	increased or increasing
↓	decreased or decreasing

The Neurological System

4) I've checked the patient's eyes. His pupils are equal and reactive._____

5) His temperature is up. It's 101°F. _____

6) Take the patient's vitals three times per shift. _____

7) He rates his pain at more than 10 on the scale. _____

Reading Selection 6-8

Read the following complex and informative text. The goal is not to re-teach you the material, but rather to familiarize you with multiple ways of referring to and communicating about a particular medical incident: a cerebrovascular accident. And while you are reading, take note of how many of the medical terms you are now familiar with. Congratulate yourself.

CEREBROVASCULAR ACCIDENT

The term cerebrovascular refers to the blood supply to the brain. The term is usually used in relation to pathological changes. A cerebrovascular accident (CVA) is a term used to describe an impairment in cerebral circulation. A synonym for CVA is "stroke," and both of these terms are widely used by the medical professional and layperson.

A CVA, or stroke, is an acute clinical event. Its effects can have wide ranging physical, psychological, social, spiritual, and environmental effects. The effects largely depend on where in the brain the decreased circulation occurs. For example, a CVA located in the cerebrum may lead to partial paralysis. In the occipital area, it may disable the autonomic control of breathing and heartbeat, forcing the patient onto life support systems. Should a CVA be located mid-brain, the individual may be unable to think clearly and be unable to integrate information that needs attention and response. A stroke in the frontal and temporal lobe areas may lead to regressed behaviors and responses and impaired memory and communication.

A stroke can last for more than 24 hours and the client needs to be closely monitored during that time. It is imperative that the person experiencing the signs and symptoms of the onset of a stroke seek medical help as soon as possible. With rapid intervention recovery of some, if not all, of lost function is possible. However, an untreated and/or severe stroke can cause devastating brain damage.

Positive patient outcomes after trauma to the brain depend on rapid identification of and response to any signs and symptoms of brain injury whether occurring internally or externally. There are many health promotion campaigns on radio, television, and in the print media in the United States and Canada that teach this important message.

 # READING EXERCISES

As in previous chapters, the following exercises will help you demonstrate your understanding of the reading selection and build vocabulary.

Understanding the General Meaning

Read the text again. Think about it. Do you understand it? Respond to the following in full sentences, using new vocabulary.

1) What is the proper name for a CVA?

_____

2) What is a synonym for a CVA?

_____

3) What causes a stroke?

4) Critical thinking: Why is a CVA discussed in this chapter on the neurological system?

5) What was the declared purpose for reading this text?

Learning Specific Facts

Take a moment now to review what you have just read.

1) List three potentially debilitating effects resulting from cerebrovascular accident.

2) What are the potential effects of a CVA in the occipital lobe and brain stem region?

Building Vocabulary

Determining Meaning from Context.   To build vocabulary, study the following words or terms taken from this text. Discover all you can about them by looking at them in context, then choose the correct meaning. Finally, take a look at how these words or terms expand in English.

1. Ramifications *(noun, plural)*

In context
a) There are serious ramifications to misdiagnosing a CVA.

Meaning: The best explanation for the word *ramifications* is
a) conclusions or consequences
b) complicated results
c) insinuations
d) summations

2. Devastating *(adjective)*

In context:
a) Losing a child in a car accident is devastating to the family.
b) Brain injury can potentially have a devastating effect on a person's personality.

Meaning: The best explanation for the word *devastating* is
a) imploding
b) emotional
c) damaging
d) distressing, overwhelming
e) both (c) and (d)

Word expansion:
a) Hurricane Katrina in the southeastern United States was *devastatingly* severe for many residents. Their homes flooded and were destroyed. Many were left homeless.
b) Paul was *devastated* when he lost full function on his left side after his stroke. (adverb serving as adjective)
c) The degree of *devastation* to the neurological system caused by chronic drug abuse is still not fully known. (noun)

3. Debilitating *(adjective)*

In context:

a) Multiple sclerosis has a debilitating effect on one's ability to walk.

Meaning: The best explanation for the word *debilitating* is

a) dysfunctional
b) dysarthric
c) depleting
d) incapacitating or weakening

Word expansion:

a) Working or walking under the hot sun for a long period of time can *debilitate* a person. (verb)

Differentiating Between Similar Words. Health professionals from non-English speaking backgrounds frequently mispronounce and misuse certain similar words used to describe the effects of a CVA. Read the Word Alert and then complete the exercises below.

> **WORD ALERT: DISORDERS ARISING FROM A CVA** Here are a few words that health professionals of non-English speaking backgrounds often mispronounce and misuse. It is important to understand the differences between these words. Study these and then complete the exercises.

Aphasia is the medical term for total or partial inability to use or comprehend speech.

Dysphasia is the medical term for difficulty understanding <u>language</u>, whether it is written or spoken.

Dysarthria is the medical term for the inability to use the muscles necessary to make speech.

Dysphagia is the medical term for difficulty swallowing.

1) The person with this disorder cannot tell if you are speaking English, Hungarian, Mandarin, or any other language. The disorder is called _____.

2) Alberta needs assistance with eating and protocol requires that a suction machine be near at hand at the same time. Alberta has the disorder known as _____.

3) Since his brain injury, Malcolm's speech is garbled and unclear. It is extremely difficult for him when he tries to make a word, although he understands words clearly. His disorder is called _____.

4) Mrs. Moses is often very frustrated with the nurse. She cannot understand a word the woman says. Mrs. Moses likely has the disorder _____.

Using Similar Words in Sentences. Now alter the form of these nouns. Turn them into adjectives in the following sentences.

1) Ramon used to be able to enjoy a meal of steak and barbecued spareribs. Now he is reduced to eating mashed potatoes and minced meat. He is _____.

2) Since Kim had his industrial accident, he can no longer read the newspaper. This is frustrating and disappointing to him. He is now _____.

3) Belinda believes she is speaking clearly to the family when they visit and she is increasingly frustrated when they don't respond appropriately. This is because she is _____.

4) Tony has learned to keep a writing pad and pen close at hand since he lost his ability to form words. He is _____.

GRAMMAR ALERT: MEDICAL PREFIX, *DYS*– We have been talking about dysfunction, dysarthria, and dysphagia. Have you been able to deduce the meaning of the medical prefix, *dys–* from these exercises?

Dys– at the beginning of a medical term means difficult or disordered. It does NOT mean the absence of something. For example, dysphasia is difficulty, while aphasia is inability.

SPEAKING EXERCISE

Re-read the text regarding cerebrovascular accident aloud. Recall the importance of trying not to hesitate while reading. Also recall that speech fillers are not appropriate for professional speakers. Try to limit these as much as possible. Read the text aloud multiple times until you feel confident and at ease with it. Let the Pronunciation Hints box help you with some of the more difficult words.

PRONUNCIATION HINTS

ramifications – răm″ĭ-fĭ-**kā**′shŭnz

debilitating – **dē**-bĭl-ĭ-tĭng

aphasia – ă-**fā**′zē-ă

dysphasia – dĭs-**fā**′zē-ă

dysphagia – dĭs-**fā**′jē-ă

dysarthria – dĭs-**ăr**′thrē-ă

LISTENING EXERCISE

If you would like to hear more native English speakers from the United States and Canada, search the Internet for audio or video clips of *Stroke Survivors*. These interesting clips are made by individuals who have suffered cerebrovascular accidents of many levels of severity and either recovered fully or came to terms with living with the residual effects of the condition. Listen carefully as they discuss their conditions. Listen even more carefully to discover the holistic impact of a stroke on an individual and his or her family.

WRITING EXERCISE—CRITICAL REFLECTION

Consider all that you have read and learned in this section of Unit 6. In this exercise, you will assess your ability to be able to communicate in English in the hospital setting. Be very honest with yourself. Assess your own developing language skills. Also, reflect on the context and any cultural aspects that may arise from that.

Imagine you are working on a medical unit in an English-speaking workplace. You are assigned to a new patient who suffered a mild, left-sided CVA last evening. She is 55 years old. Her condition is now stable.

---

1) Imagine you have just come on duty and are checking on your patients.
   a) Assess your ability to communicate with your new patient when you first encounter her on rounds.

---

b) Do you have any concerns or worries about your ability to speak to/with this woman in English about her condition and how she is feeling or what she needs at the moment? Describe your thoughts.

_____

2) Imagine you must tell a doctor later this morning about the patient's progress today.
   a) Assess your ability to do so in English.

_____

   b) Describe any concerns you may have about talking to the doctor as another health-care professional, using professional terminology to discuss the patient.

_____

3) Imagine you are ending your shift at work on the medical unit and you must tell the staff coming on duty about your patient's condition.
   a) Assess your ability to do this.

_____

   b) Describe any concerns that you may have about giving a comprehensive, accurate, and appropriate oral report to the oncoming staff.

_____

Reading Selection 6-9

Read the following to discover how pain is assessed in the United States and Canada.

DIAGNOSTIC TOOL: PAIN SCALES

The term _pain scales_ refers to assessment tools used to evaluate the intensity of pain being experienced by a patient. The report is subjective and in no way scientific; however, it allows the nurse and attending doctor to more fully realize the patient's experience. This leads to more effective intervention and treatment that is uniquely designed for that patient. This client-centered approach enhances the quality of care the patient receives and his or her perception of being heard and understood.

Pain scales are assessed and charted by the nurse throughout her or his shift. They are used for all incidents of pain and not restricted to being used for pain associated with any particular disorder or diagnosis. The most common pain scale used in the United States and Canada is a simple Likert scale (a scale with word and number choices) that rates the absence or presence of pain and its degree or severity. The patient is asked to rate his or her pain on a scale from 1 to 10, with 1 being no pain and 10 being excruciating pain. The scale is always rated at 1 out of 10, but sometimes the patient will say a number well beyond 10. This indicates excruciating pain with which they are having difficulty dealing. The nurse records the report as follows:

Jan. 5, 2009 0815 hrs. Pt. is lying in bed, groaning, and holding his stomach near the incision site. He rates his pain at 15 on the scale of 1–10 and is requesting pain medication. —M. Jugaru, RN

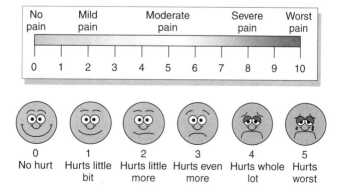

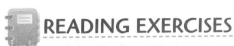

READING EXERCISES

Understanding the General Meaning

You have just read about the assessment tool called a pain scale. Answer the following questions to assess your own level of comprehension.

1) What is the gist of this text?

_____

2) Who uses pain scales?

_____

3) Are pain scales objective?

_____

4) A patient has severe pain following his jaw surgery. He can't say how he rates his pain but he points to a number. Which number is that?

_____

5) What is the benefit of a client-centered approach to care?

_____

6) What is the purpose of a pain scale?

_____

Building Vocabulary

Using New Vocabulary in Sentences.   Use a key word from the previous exercise to create a new sentence. Write in the context of caring for a patient on a neurology unit in the hospital.

1) intensity _____

2) enhances _____

3) tools _____

Fill in the Blanks.   Use the word *pain* in a variety of ways by filling in the blanks with versions of the word.

Jefferson had a _____ in his jaw for many months. It was increasingly _____, particularly of late. He decided to have the doctor look at it. His GP then referred him to a neurologist, suspecting the _____ was the result of cranial nerve impairment. Unfortunately, he had to wait 3 months to get an appointment with the specialist. In the interim, his condition became more and more _____. It got to the point where he couldn't tolerate chewing. There was a dull, _____ ache in his jaw day and night. Finally, the _____ became excruciating and he went to the emergency department. There, the doctor prescribed an injection of morphine. The injection was _____ and within the half hour his jaw was _____, too. Luckily for him, the next day he finally got to see the neurologist who then made a joke that the _____ was "all in his head." Jefferson would have laughed if it had not _____ him to do so. The neurologist smiled and apologized for his attempt at humor. Jefferson smiled and replied that the amount of _____ he had seemed to have taken away his sense of humor and he was a lot more irritable than usual. The doctor examined him, took a history, and then referred him for numerous tests and scans. He also gave him a prescription to treat his condition temporarily until a clear diagnosis could be reached. Jefferson left the office relieved that there was some help on the way for his _____ condition.

VOCABULARY ALERT: LIKERT SCALE The reading mentions a Likert scale. Do you know this English term? Perhaps you will recognize what it is by its description. It is very likely that you have used a version of a Likert scale in your university studies or professional career.

A Likert scale is one in which numbers are used to rate the absence or presence of pain and the intensity of the pain. The numbers are translated into words that describe the pain, from mild to excruciating. Recall that the pain scale has numbers and words.

SPEAKING EXERCISE

Take a moment to read aloud the fill-in-the-blank exercise you've just completed on pain. Using derivatives or versions of the word will facilitate your ability to use it in communication with peers and patients. The Pronunciation Hints box will help also.

> **PRONUNCIATION HINTS**
>
> impairment – ĭm-**pār**′mĕnt
>
> injection – ĭn-**jĕk**′shŭn
>
> diagnosis – dī″ăg-**nō**′sĭs

LISTENING EXERCISE

It's time to go online again. Search for video clips discussing nerve pain. You might try the website *YouTube*. Type in the search words "what causes nerve pain" or "nerve pain." Search **only** for professional video clips. Listen carefully to the terminology. You will be familiar with a good deal of it now.

WRITING EXERCISE

Take a moment now to reflect on how you have enhanced your career-specific English for medical purposes up to this point. Think back to when you first started this book. Congratulate yourself for your progress! Write your reflections here, adding comments on your increasing confidence with the language.

_____

_____

_____

ANSWER KEY

Anatomy and Physiology

 ## READING SELECTION 1—THE NERVOUS SYSTEM

Understanding the General Meaning

1) The gist of the reading is the anatomy and physiology of the nervous (neurological) system.

2) The purpose of the reading is to explain the anatomy and physiology of the system as well as present the reader with new vocabulary

3) The center of the entire nervous system is the brain.

Comprehending Specific Facts

1) The neurological system

2) The neurological system

3) The peripheral nervous system

4) The central nervous system

5) No. This abbreviation does not appear anywhere in the book and is not generally used. The abbreviations for the two parts of the nervous system: CNS (central nervous system) and PNS (peripheral nervous system) are, however, used frequently.

6) Two major subsystems

7) Through neurons via the brain stem

8) Nerve cell

Identifying Parts of the Nervous System

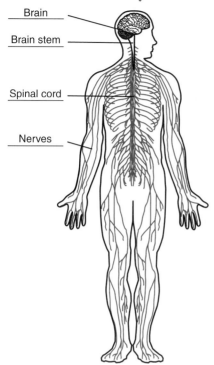

Brain

Brain stem

Spinal cord

Nerves

Building Vocabulary

Sentence Completion

1) The <u>gap</u> between the sensory and motor nerves is known as the <u>synapse</u>.

2) <u>Dendrites</u> and <u>axons</u> are parts of a <u>neuron</u>, or nerve cell.

3) The <u>brain stem</u> relays all <u>messages</u> to and from various levels of the <u>nervous system</u>.

Identifying Verbs in a Sentence

1) directs

2) is referred to

3) consist

4) relays

Recognizing Verbs of Similar Meaning

1) is also known as

2) is comprised, is made up

3) transport

4) passes

Reading for Gist

1) I predict that the text will explain the difference between the two identified words: *integral* and *essential.*

2) Yes, I was correct in my prediction.

3) In summary, the word *integral* means absolutely necessary, while *essential* means important but not absolutely necessary. (16 words)

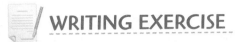

WRITING EXERCISE

A sample of a rewritten reading selection using different/similar verbs and terms.

The Nervous System

The neurological system is <u>also known as the</u> nervous system by health professionals as well as the public. This system <u>coordinates</u> all body systems and cells. It is responsible for all thought, emotion, sensation, and movement. It is <u>comprised of</u> two subsystems, the central nervous system and the peripheral nervous system. The brain is the center of both of these.

The central nervous system is <u>also known as the</u> CNS. It <u>is made up</u> of the brain, brain stem, and spinal cord. The spinal cord and brain stem function as communication pathways between the brain and the peripheral nervous system. The peripheral nervous system is frequently called the PNS by health professionals. It is composed of cranial nerves and spinal nerves that connect the central nervous system to the peripheral organs of the body.

All of the organs of the nervous system contain neurons, or nerve cells. Neurons are composed of a cell nucleus and dendrites and axons. Dendrites <u>accept</u> impulses from sensory organs or other neurons and carry them to the central nervous system. The central nervous system reacts to this input and transmits impulses through axons put to the body organs. The gap between sensory, intermediate, and motor nerves is <u>also known</u> as a synapse.

READING SELECTION 2—
DIVISIONS OF THE NEUROLOGICAL SYSTEM

Understanding the General Meaning

1) divisions of the neurological system

2) two. Rationale: The question is not asking about subsystems or subdivisions.

3) the central nervous system (CNS) and the peripheral nervous system (PNS)

4) create a diagram (Sample)

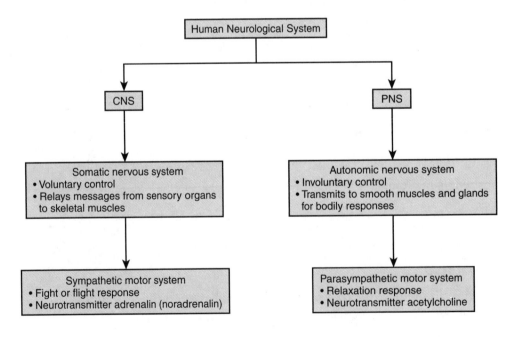

Reading for Gist

1) I predict that the text will be about flow charts and how to develop them.

2) My prediction was correct (or incorrect).

3) It is important to be able to interpret and use flow charts in the health professions. (16 words)

Building Vocabulary

Learning the Spelling of New Words

1) norepinephrine, 2) axon, 3) dendrite, 4) sympathetic, 5) involuntary,

6) parasympathetic, 7) neurotransmitter, 8) autonomic, 9) automatic

Using New Vocabulary in Sentences

1) The eye opens and shuts automatically as a function of the peripheral nervous system.

2) When you smell fresh bread baking in the oven, your olfactory senses are triggered and a hunger message is relayed to your brain.

3) When you have the urge to urinate, you have a great deal of voluntary control over when you choose to do so. Voluntary control of organs originates in the central nervous system.

4) When you stub your toe on the corner of the bed, pain receptors in your toe immediately send a message up through the neuropathways to your brain which, in turn, relays a message back to your toe to retract from the painful stimuli and may even signal you to yell.

READING SELECTION 3—THE BRAIN

Understanding the General Meaning

1) The core message or thesis of this text is the location of the lobes of the brain and some of their functions.

Learning Specific Facts
Labeling and Identifying the Lobes of the Brain

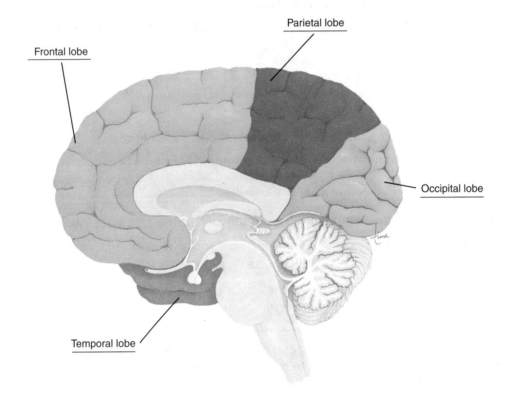

Using Professional Terminology to Describe the Lobes of the Brain

1) The parietal lobe is located superiorly in the cranium, posterior to the frontal lobe and anteriorly and superiorly to the occipital lobe. It is superior to the temporal lobes.

2) The temporal lobes are located anteriorly to the occipital lobe and bilaterally on the right and left sides of the brain.

3) This is the occipital lobe and it is located posteriorly in the cranium.

Building Vocabulary
Determining Meaning from Context

1) d, 2) c, 3) d, 4) b

Mix and Match

BOX 6-2 Mix and Match: Functions of Different Parts of the Central Nervous System: Answers	
ANATOMICAL PART	**FUNCTION**
mid-brain	aids in hearing and vision
cerebellum	maintains balance and fine and gross motor movements
hypothalamus	controls the endocrine system
medulla oblongata	regulates heart rate and coughing
brain stem	waking and maintaining consciousness; alertness
spinal cord	contains nerve pathways to and from the brain
thalamus	registers mood and pain

Using Verbs in Sentences

Sample Answers:

1) A pacemaker regulated Mr. Angelou's heart rate for more than 25 years.

2) I don't know how he maintains his balance after that head injury he got at work yesterday.

3) Recent or short-term memory is contained within the frontal lobe and was lost for Francine when she hit the front of her head in the car accident.

4) Pain receptors immediately relayed the message of excruciating pain to Ralph's brain when he suddenly fractured his tibia.

Common Complaints and Disorders of the Neurological System

 ## READING SELECTION 6-4—POTENTIAL CAUSES OF NEUROLOGICAL DYSFUNCTION

Understanding the General Meaning

1) The gist of the text is the potential causes of neurological dysfunction.

2) Humans are susceptible to all matter and conditions in the environment. It is our external world and affects our ability to survive, to function, and to enjoy a healthy life. Divisions of health-care services concern themselves with assessing the environment for any elements or situations that may threaten our existence. The Public Health Department, Department of Sanitation, and the Food and Drug Administration are examples of such divisions.

Learning Specific Facts

1) Two examples of potential causes of neurological dysfunction are exposure to pesticides and nutritional deficiencies.

2) The incidence of viral and bacterial meningitis is on the rise among teenagers in the United States and Canada.

3) The term "heavy metals" refers to nonorganic compounds that can be toxic to humans.

4) Three examples of heavy metals are lead, mercury, and aluminum.

Building Vocabulary

Determining Meaning from Context

1) d, 2) b, 3) a, 4) a, 5) e

Using Medical Prefixes in Sentences

Examples of possible answers:

1) If we are talking about nerve cells we are discussing matters at the cellular, neuronal level.

2) Neurological impairment occurs when there is damage to the brain stem.

3) Phantom pain receptors trigger the pain message up through the neuropathways to the brain, causing the phantom limb pain phenomena.

4) People who worry a lot or have preoccupations with things "on their mind" may be suffering from mild to moderate neurosis.

5) Lou Gehrig's disease is also known as amyotrophic lateral sclerosis (ALS) and is a debilitating form of neuropathy.

6) Some research points to mercury as the cause of the neuropathic disease of autism.

7) Neuro-vital signs are part of the mandatory protocol for working with unconscious patients.

8) The neurologist has referred Bob for neurosurgery to help decrease his incidence of status epilepticus.

9) There is an excessive amount of the neurotransmitter dopamine being excreted in the brain of a person with schizophrenia.

 ## READING SELECTION 6-5—PAIN AND HEADACHES

Understanding the General Meaning

1) The gist of the text is that pain follows neuropathways and the brain responds by telling the body what to do. Pain comes in many degrees with many symptoms.

2) The example used in this reading selection is *headache*.

3) The health professional should not take it personally when a person suffering from pain is irritable, rude, or intolerant. It is a pain response.

Learning Specific Facts

1) No, all pain does not occur externally.

2) A migraine is a severe form of a headache caused by constriction of blood vessels in the occipital part of the head and down the neck. It usually lasts longer than other types of headaches and is more difficult to treat.

3) The difference between a migraine and another type of headache is the duration and degree of pain.

4) A pain scale is an assessment tool that is informative and helpful for monitoring a patient's level of pain.

5) Frustration intolerance is the inability to tolerate the normal amount of frustration that occurs in everyday life.

Building Vocabulary

Identifying Pain Descriptors

Complete this exercise by matching the symbol or graphic with the descriptive adjective.

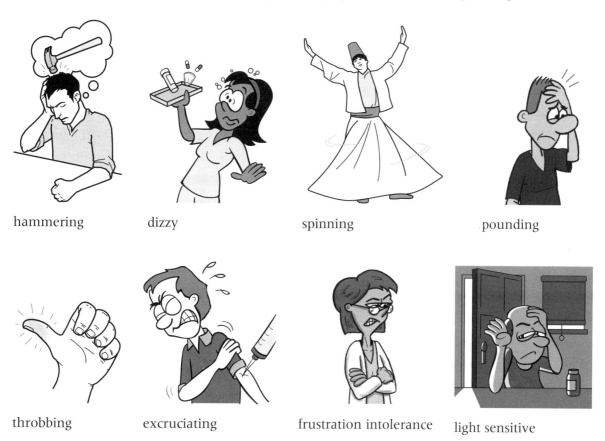

hammering   dizzy   spinning   pounding

throbbing   excruciating   frustration intolerance   light sensitive

Explaining Pain Descriptors

Sample Answers:

1) Pounding is a rhythmic sensation that sometimes sounds like a fist or a hammer being hit on a desk over and over again. It is unrelenting.

2) Light sensitive means that one cannot tolerate normal or average amounts of light that most people can. The sensitivity exacerbates the headache and because of this, people

with migraines will often remove themselves from the light by donning sunglasses and sitting in the dark until the headache passes.

3) Throbbing is a pulsing sensation that people say they can feel and sometimes hear when they have a headache. Throbbing is a descriptor often used to describe the feeling in crush injuries of the musculoskeletal and integumentary systems.

4) Frustration intolerance is the inability to tolerate the expected, normal amount of frustration in one's day or life.

5) Spinning means whirling around or a sense of standing still while the world whirls around you.

6) Hammering means just what it says: a hammering action that is painful. Headache patients will sometimes say they feel like someone is hammering away at the top of their skull.

7) Excruciating is an adjective that describes severe, intolerable pain. Migraine sufferers very often use this term.

READING SELECTION 6—EPILEPSY

Understanding the General Meaning

1) Art is emotional and finds himself in a situation that surprises him. The exclamation marks contribute to the sense of mood he is feeling.

2) No. Rationale: They do not know all of the protocols or procedures for assisting a person having an epileptic seizure.

3) Yes. They do many of the proper procedures, such as calling for help and staying with the person.

4) The stranger having the seizure begins to bang his head and this distracts Brad from what he was about to say.

5) He places something soft under the person's head so that he will not injure himself.

6) Two other safety measures for assisting a person having an epileptic seizure are rolling the person onto his side into the recovery position after the seizure and ensuring that the person's airway remains open and clear. However, do not attempt to reach into the person's mouth. Instead, if the person has difficulty breathing, roll him onto his side.

Recognizing Specifics

1) No name is given.

2) They refer to him as "this guy" and "Mister."

3) He asks someone in the park that we do not know.

4) It is capitalized to emphasize it. It should be read more loudly, with emphasis because he thinks it's important to recognize.

5) No.

6) To the stranger.

7) He is speaking to the stranger and to Brad.

8) The ambulance attendants/paramedics.

Building Vocabulary

Recognizing Fillers and Interjections

1) wow = interjection

2) wow = interjection

3) well = filler, oh = filler, wow = interjection

4) gee = interjection

5) hey = filler

6) hey = filler

7) oh = filler

8) Uh = filler, mmmm = filler

9) well = filler

Mix and Match

BOX 6-3 Mix and Match: The Meaning of Descriptors: Answers

DESCRIPTOR	MEANING
writhing	twisting and turning
confused	mixed up; not thinking clearly
jerking	sudden strong muscle spasms or tics
rolling his eyes	eyes turn upwards and then return to center
eyes are clearer	appears conscious, alert, and more able to understand

Understanding Protocols and Pathways

1) He stayed with him, called for medical assistance (911), and put something soft under his head.

2) Depending upon the protocol at your hospital, the steps in assisting a patient having an epileptic seizure will look something like this:

- Note the time of onset.

- Lower the patient to the bed or ground if he or she has been standing.

- Turn the patient on his or her side.

- Place a small pillow or towel under the head.

- Loosen any tight clothing around the patient's neck.

- Protect the patient from injury by clearing away any furniture or objects nearby that are hazardous.

- Time the seizure.

- Stay with patient until he or she is fully recovered.

- If seizure lasts longer than 5 minutes, call for more assistance and alert the doctor.

3) A clinical pathway is a guideline for the provision of patient care based on his or her illness or procedures that are being done.

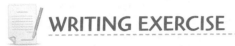

WRITING EXERCISE

Sample Answer:
   Brad and Art were likely nervous because they suddenly found themselves in a situation where they needed to help someone, but they may have felt they lacked the skills and knowledge to be effective. Even so, they did the honorable thing and stayed with the stranger and helped in the best way they could.

Treatments, Interventions, and Assistance

READING SELECTION 7—HEAD INJURIES

Understanding the General Meaning

1) The gist of this reading is that there are many kinds or types of head injuries.

2) The key words that prompted me to know the gist of the reading was the title "Head Injuries." Rationale: Plural use of the word injury and phrase "classified by the amount of damage that occurs," which implies that there are degrees of damage and therefore more than one type of injury.

3) Another word for injury is trauma.

Answering Questions About Specifics

1) Coma can occur when the person has a disease, severe head injury, or seizure.

2) A depressed skull fracture potentiates the risk for severe brain injury.

3) The abbreviation ICP stands for intracranial pressure.

4) A laceration to the brain tissue is the most severe head injury.

5) In an open head injury, the brain may be exposed to the external world; whereas in a closed head injury, this is not so.

6) A parenchymal injury is an injury to brain tissue.

7) Intracranial pressure occurs when pressure is exerted on brain tissue, cerebrospinal fluid, and brain blood volume.

Building Vocabulary

Determining Meaning from Context

   1) d, 2) d, 3) d, 4) a

Fill in the Blanks

   1) unconsciously

   2) subconscious

3) consciousness

4) profound

Writing Exercise

1) ↑ ICP

2) Pt has <LOC

3) Pt is ↓ LOC or Pt is <LOC +

4) Pupils are = and reactive

5) T = 101°F

6) Vitals ×3 per shift

7) 10+ on the pain scale

READING SELECTION 8—CEREBROVASCULAR ACCIDENT

Understanding the General Meaning

1) The proper name for a CVA is cerebrovascular accident.

2) A synonym for a CVA is a stroke.

3) A stroke is caused by impairment in cerebral circulation.

4) A stroke is discussed in this chapter because the accident occurs in the brain, which is part of the neurological system. A stroke can adversely affect neurological functioning.

5) The declared purpose was to familiarize the reader with multiple ways of referring to and communicating about a particular medical incident.

Learning Specific Facts

1) Three potentially debilitating effects of a CVA are partial paralysis, cognitive dysfunction, and regressed behavior. (Can also include impaired memory and communication, need for life support.)

2) A potential effect of a CVA in the occipital lobe and brain stem is death because a CVA in that area of the brain may disable the autonomic control of breathing and heart rate.

Building Vocabulary

Determining Meaning from Context

1) b, 2) e, 3) d

Differentiating Between Similar Words

1) dysphasia

2) dysphagia

3) dysarthria

4) aphasia

Using Similar Words in Sentences

1) dysphagic

2) dysphasic

3) aphasic

4) dysarthric

 # READING SELECTION 9—DIAGNOSTIC TOOL: PAIN SCALES

Understanding the General Meaning

1) The gist of the text is how pain is assessed using a pain scale.

2) Health professionals, especially the attending nurse, use pain scales.

3) No, pain scales are not objective. They are subjective.

4) 10.

5) This client-centered approach enhances the quality of care the patient receives and his or her perception of being heard and understood.

6) The purpose of a pain scale is to assess subjective response to pain and ability to tolerate pain. This will assist the health-care team in intervening when pain is intolerable to promote recovery.

Building Vocabulary

Using New Vocabulary in Sentences

1) Surgeons work with a great deal of intensity when they are performing neurosurgery.

2) The creative use of a variety of communication methods with someone who has left temporal lobe trauma will enhance their ability to communicate.

3) The Glasgow coma scale and a pain scale may very well be used as evaluative tools on this unit.

Fill in the Blanks

Jefferson had a <u>pain</u> in his jaw for many months. It was increasingly <u>painful</u>, particularly of late. He decided to have the doctor look at it. His GP then referred him to a neurologist, suspecting the <u>pain</u> was the result of cranial nerve impairment. Unfortunately, he had to wait 3 months to get an appointment with the specialist. In the interim, his condition became more and more <u>painful</u>. It got to the point where he couldn't tolerate chewing. There was a dull, <u>painful</u> ache in his jaw day and night. Finally, the <u>pain</u> became excruciating and he went to the emergency department. There, the doctor prescribed an injection of morphine. The injection was <u>painless</u> and within the half hour his jaw was <u>painless</u>, too. Luckily for him, the next day he finally got to see the neurologist who then made a joke that the <u>pain</u> was "all in his head." Jefferson would have laughed if it had not <u>pained</u> him to do so. The neurologist smiled and apologized for his attempt at humor. Jefferson smiled and replied that the amount of <u>pain</u> he had seemed to have taken away his sense of humor and he was a lot more irritable than usual. The doctor examined him, took a history, and then referred him for numerous tests and scans. He also gave him a prescription to treat his condition temporarily until a clear diagnosis could be reached. Jefferson left the office relieved that there was some help on the way for his <u>painful</u> condition.

This unit will be somewhat different from the preceding ones. Rather than focusing on the acquisition of language in the context of a body system, Unit 7 looks at three very important topics that affect the daily work of health professionals: wounds, viruses and bacteria, and then viral and bacterial infections. The first section of the unit focuses on the nature and language of wounds and viruses. The second focuses on viral and bacterial diseases however, contextual examples in this section include decubitus ulcers (a type of wound), chickenpox (a viral disease), and tuberculosis (a bacterial disease). The last section focuses on infection, specifically infection control; wound infection. Language skills discussed include the use of participles and conditional forms of verbs, the use of descriptors, charting protocols, interpreting clinical pathways, and interpreting infection control policies. Script writing and fill-in-the-blank exercises focus on communicating with peers and patients.

SECTION ONE   Pathophysiology

This section provides an introduction to the vocabulary of wounds and viruses. Vocabulary building occurs through the naming and use of clear and appropriate descriptive adjectives and adverbs. Opportunities to identify and evaluate types of wounds and viruses are provided.

GRAMMAR ALERT: ADJECTIVES, ADVERBS, AND DESCRIPTORS Adjectives are words that tell us how things sound, look, and feel, as well as their color or quantity. They describe nouns. Adding *er* to an adjective allows us to compare the difference between two nouns. Adding *est* to an adjective lets us compare the greatest differences between them. For example, Sarah is prettier than Jane but Sarah is the prettiest girl in the whole class. Adverbs are used to describe verbs. They identify when, where (time and place), or how things occur. Often they end in *ly*. Health professionals use adverbs to put the patient's injury or situation into context. Context may help explain how or why the patient needs treatments or, perhaps more importantly, what treatment is needed.
For example: As a result of the car accident, the patient is bleeding profusely.
Descriptors are any terms or concepts that describe a phenomenon of concern to the patient's health that requires more than a single word or two to explain. When there is nothing or not much known about the patient's health, emotional status, or socioeconomic conditions, descriptors play an important role in bringing to light salient features of the presenting problems. From this data, nurses and doctors will begin to piece together the puzzle of the patient's health challenge, working toward a diagnosis and treatment.

Reading Selection 7-1

Read the following in anticipation of the vocabulary exercises that will follow.

WOUNDS

Most commonly, a wound is an injury in which the skin is broken. However, a wound can be emotional, too. In this section, we are going to study wounds of the skin and body.

A puncture wound is usually caused by a sharp object and most often occurs to the hands or feet. A common example of this is the wound that results from stepping on a nail. Puncture wounds can easily become infected. It is essential to clean them when they first occur.

A deep puncture wound to a part of the body other than the extremities can cause internal injuries. Organs, veins, and arteries can be compromised. Deep puncture wounds can be life-threatening emergencies. An example of a deep puncture wound is that which results from a stabbing.

A decubitus ulcer, or pressure sore, is also a type of wound. It results when there is lack of circulation to an area and there is pressure on the skin, most often from lying in one position for an extended period of time. That is what *decubitus* means: lying down. These wounds are most often found where a bony prominence is near the surface of the skin. Examples are the coccyx area and the backs of heels. The terms dermal ulcer, bedsores, or pressure sores are commonly used to discuss this type of wound.

READING EXERCISES

Health-care professionals must be able to communicate with one another in a clear, concise manner using the proper vocabulary to describe the status of a patient and his or her disease/disorder or injury. The following will help you to understand, expand, and use vocabulary related to wounds.

Understanding the General Meaning

Take a moment now to review what you have just read. Circle any words that are new to you. Write them down here. Now, work through the following exercises to gain an even better understanding of the reading. In this way, you may find the meaning of those words through the context of a new sentence. If you are still unclear, please check the word in a dictionary or ask an instructor or health professional to help.

_____

_____

Answer the following questions to assess your level of reading comprehension. Short answers are acceptable.

1) This might cause a deep puncture wound. _____

2) These areas are prone to bedsores. _____

3) Wounds are not just physical. What else can they be? _____

4) Is a bruise a wound? _____

5) Is a fracture a wound? _____

6) List three other names for decubitus ulcers. _____

Building Vocabulary

Being able to determine the meaning of a word from the context will help you use the word in sentences. This section emphasizes the identification of types of wounds and their possible causes.

Determining Meaning from Context. To build vocabulary, study the following words and terms taken from the reading. Discover all you can about them by looking at them in these new examples. Next, go on to choose the correct meaning for the word from the choices provided. Finally, take a look at how the words expand in English.

1. Wound *(noun)*

In context:

a) I cut my finger on a piece of glass today. Now I have a wound.

b) Billy has a new wound. He stepped on a nail.

Meaning: The word *wound* can best be described as meaning

a) wrapped

b) uterus

c) tissue trauma

d) none of the above

Word expansion:

a) Ouch! I am *wounded.* (adjective)

b) He accidentally hit the deer with his car, *wounding* it slightly. It ran off into the woods, limping a little. (verb, present participle)

2. Puncture *(noun; verb)*

In context:

a) He has a puncture in his tire. It has gone flat and he can't drive his car.

b) The accident punctured his left lung.

Meaning: The verb *puncture* can best be described as meaning

a) to hit

b) to injure

c) to make a hole

d) to scrape

Word expansion:

a) A mosquito *punctures* the skin when it bites you. (verb, present)

b) You will receive a small *puncture* wound when you get an injection. (adjective)

c) His rib *punctured* his lung. It was an emergency. (verb, past tense)

d) The patient developed an abscess at the *puncture* site where she received an intramuscular injection. (adjective)

> **VOCABULARY ALERT: A MOSQUITO BITE** Please note the English way of expressing the parasitic action of a mosquito. Indeed, the mosquito does not use its teeth to actually *bite* the victim. In truth, the female mosquito punctures the skin with her proboscis or syringe-like mouth and sucks blood into her digestive system from the host. In doing so, she releases an allergen that causes an immune reaction in humans, causing us to itch. Even so, the English term for this is "bite": mosquito bite.

3. Compromised *(verb, past tense; can be used as an adjective)*

In context:

a) Jack's recovery was compromised when his surgical wound became infected.

b) Martin has AIDS. His ability to recover from the wound he received in the car accident may be compromised by his health status.

Meaning: The word *compromised* in a medical context can best be described as meaning

a) having a positive potential

b) jeopardized

    c) having a risk potential

    d) potentially unmet

Word expansion:

    a) Failure to wear gloves when working with patients with open and untreated wounds *can compromise* the health of the nurses and doctors. (verb, future simple tense)

    b) As a health professional, you must avoid the *compromising* position of working with or treating a family member. (adjective)

4. Internal injuries *(term, noun phrase)*

In context:

    a) Intracranial bleeding is one type of internal injury.

    b) In a motor vehicle accident, the steering wheel can cause massive internal injuries when it slams into the chest wall.

Meaning: The term *internal injuries* can best be described as meaning

    a) extreme injuries

    b) intestinal injuries

    c) intracranial injuries

    d) injuries occurring within the body, not always visible on the outside

Word expansion:

    a) Rees was injured *internally* when the hockey puck hit his abdomen. He ruptured his spleen. (adverb)

5. Life threatening *(adjective)*

In context:

    a) Cancer is often a life-threatening illness.

Meaning: The expression *life threatening* can best be described as meaning

    a) dangerous, having the potential to cause loss of life

    b) danger and risk

    c) promoting death

    d) not likely to survive

Word expansion:

    a) The gunman *threatened* the *life* of the employee at the bank. (verb "threatened"; noun "life")

6. Decubitus *(adjective)*

In context:

    a) He assumed a decubitus position in bed.

    b) She assumed the dorsal decubitus position in bed: she reclined on her back.

Meaning: The word *decubitus* can best be described as meaning

    a) stretching out

    b) lying down

    c) sitting up in bed

    d) lying uncovered in bed

Sentence Completion. This exercise is a pre-test. It tests your knowledge and ability to use language about wounds and is a form of self-assessment. Notice that a good deal of the vocabulary required in this exercise comes from this section and previous units in this book. Use the Word Bank, but be careful. There are more words in the Word Bank than are needed to complete the sentences given.

1) A gun shot is considered a _____ type of wound.

2) Stepping on an old rusty nail may lead to _____.

3) After an injury, an infection usually takes _____to appear.

4) If a(n) _____ is punctured, it will spurt blood.

5) Before you put a bandage on a wound, you must _____ it.

6) Numbness and tingling can be a sign of a _____ injury.

7) The body's first line of defense against infection is the _____.

8) A wound you might receive while staying in the hospital is a
_____.

Identifying Types of Wounds.   Continue to expand your vocabulary by looking at the following pictures and labeling them correctly. You will see some of the wounds described in this section, but you will also see some wounds that have not broken the skin. The vocabulary for these was presented in previous units. Recall it here. Identify the type of wound shown in each of the following visual representations (pictures) with a name. Use the Word Bank below and write your choice beside the picture.

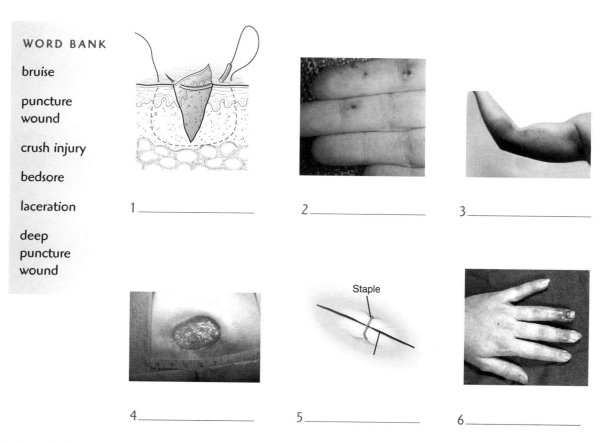

WORD BANK

bruise

puncture
wound

crush injury

bedsore

laceration

deep
puncture
wound

1_____

2_____

3_____

4_____

5_____

6_____

SPEAKING EXERCISE

Read the following complete sentences aloud. Ask a peer or teacher to help you with pronunciation. Proceed to the Pronunciation Hints section following. This will also help.

1) Puncture wounds are not sutured because contamination beneath the surface of the wound is likely.

2) A crush or blow injury to a finger or toe causes blood to collect under the nail bed. This is known as a subungual hematoma. It is an injury and not a wound. Remember that to be called a wound, the surface of the skin must be broken.

PRONUNCIATION HINTS

puncture – **pŭnk′**chūr

wounds – **woond′**z

sutured – **sū′**chūr′d

contamination – kŏn-tăm″ ĭ-**nā′**shūn

subungual/subunguial – note there are two ways to spell and pronounce this word:

sŭb-**ŭng′**gwăl or sŭb-**ŭng**-gwē-ăl

hematoma – hĕm-ă-**tō′**mă

decubitus – dĕ-**kū′**bĭ-tŭs

LISTENING EXERCISE

Take this opportunity to go online. Search for an audiovisual clip pertaining to wounds or wound care and listen to it. You might want to use the words *wound* or *wound care* to search, or try *surgical wound care*. An interesting clip entitled "Post Surgical Wound Care" by Dr. J. Slappy can be seen and heard on the Google video site http://www.videogoogle.com. Listen for technical explanations of the pathophysiology of wounds and for medical terminology for wound care and treatment. Listen without a dictionary close at hand. It is very likely you will be able to understand most, if not all of these clips now.

WRITING EXERCISE

Use your new vocabulary. Write a full sentence or two by combining these words in a meaningful way. You may need to change the form of the word to suit your needs. Stay in the context of the topic of wounds.

1) wound, knife

_____

2) needle, intramuscular, deep

_____

3) decubitus, bony prominence

_____

4) emotional, betrayal

_____

5) spider bite

_____

Reading Selection 7-2

Read the information on viruses. Begin thinking about it, recalling your own health history, medical or nursing knowledge of the topic in preparation for the exercises that follow.

SOME DISEASE-CAUSING MICROORGANISMS: VIRUSES AND BACTERIA

Microorganisms are minute organisms, such as protozoa, bacteria, and viruses. Some microorganisms cause disease. Here we briefly discuss viruses and bacteria. A virus is a disease-causing agent. Viruses are parasitic by nature. Composed of nucleic acids and proteins, they can replicate (reproduce) themselves only in a host organism, eventually interrupting and sometimes even destroying the normal cell function of their host. Virology is the study of viruses.

Viruses often invade the human body via mucous membranes, which are not protected by an outer layer of skin or epidermis. Diagnostic tests to detect and identify viruses include direct detection, serology, and virus isolation (indirect isolation). Common communicable diseases such as measles, mumps, and chickenpox are the result of viral infections, as is HIV. Immunization against viral infection is available for many, but not all, viruses. A great deal of time, effort, and money go into research on viruses each year in the United States and Canada in an attempt to eradicate known viruses and prevent the occurrence of new ones.

Some bacteria are also disease-causing. The major difference between a virus and a bacterium is that a virus cannot multiply without invading a host cell, whereas a bacterium is a one-celled microorganism that is capable of reproducing itself. While some strains of bacteria are harmful, others are actually helpful and necessary to the health of the body. Very often the respiratory disease tuberculosis is referred to as a viral infection but it is not—it is a bacterial disease. Bacterial infections can frequently be treated with antibiotics, while viruses cannot.

 READING EXERCISES

Understanding the General Meaning

Read the text again. Think about it. Answer the questions. You may use short answers.

1) What is the gist of this short reading?

_____

2) What is the purpose of the text?

_____

3) What is virology?

_____

4) Viruses are parasitic by nature. What does this mean?

_____

5) Is there a vaccine or immunization for all types of viruses?

_____

6) Can a virus be life threatening?

_____

7) What is a simple difference between viruses and bacteria?

_____

8) Can viruses be treated with antibiotics?

_____

Building Vocabulary

Determining Meaning from Context. To build vocabulary, study the following words and terms taken from the reading. Discover all you can about them by looking at them in these new examples. Next, go on to choose the correct meaning for the word from the choices provided. Finally, take a look at how the words expand in English.

1. Virus *(noun)*

In context:
a) Bob has a virus. He's been in bed for a week sniffling, coughing, and running a fever. He feels very bad.
b) The effects of a virus are usually temporary, but this is not always so.

Meaning: The best way to explain the word *virus* is to say it is a(n)
a) antibody load
b) infection
c) parasitic microorganism
d) bacterial microorganism

Word expansion:
a) A *virulent* form of the common cold can lead to pneumonia and death in the person who is immunocompromised. (adjective)
b) A *virologist* is a medical professional or scientist who studies viruses. (noun, singular)
c) *Virologists* and epidemiologists may work collaboratively or be the same person. (noun, plural)
d) A *viral* load test is used to monitor and determine the severity of HIV infection in individuals with that diagnosis. (adjective, when used with "load" becomes a term)

2. Serology *(noun)*

In context:
a) Blood serum is examined in serology.
b) Take a sample of the patient's blood and send it to serology for a workup, please.

Meaning: The best way to explain the word *serology* is to say it is
a) the study of blood serum
b) the study of bodily serum
c) the field of blood transfusion
d) all of the above

Word expansion:
a) A *serologist* is the person who examines blood serum. (noun)

3. Immunization *(noun)*

In context:
a) Health professionals need to get keep their immunization up to date to protect themselves.
b) Immunization is important for small children because their immune systems are not fully developed.

Meaning: The best way to explain the word *immunization* is to say it is
a) inoculation
b) invasive

c) injection

d) protection against viral infection

Word expansion:

a) You should get *immunized* against malaria before you go to Africa or other tropical locales. (verb, past participle)

b) *Immunizing* your children is an important obligation you carry. (gerund used as a noun)

c) The public health nurse *immunizes* children against childhood diseases. (verb, present tense)

d) The vaccine injection provided the child with *immunity* from chickenpox. (noun)

4. Bacterium *(noun)*

In context:

a) Bacterium has entered the wound and has caused an infection.

b) The human body needs certain types of bacterium to be healthy.

Meaning: A bacterium is

a) a microorganism that threatens life

b) a microorganism dedicated to the accommodation of disease

c) a multicellular microorganism that can be harmful or helpful

d) a unicellular microorganism that can be harmful or helpful

Word expansion:

a) *Bacterial* endocarditis is a serious disease of the heart. (adjective)

b) *Bacteremia* is a diagnosis given when bacteria is found circulating in the blood. (noun)

c) A *bacteriogenic* illness is one caused by bacteria. (adjective)

d) A *bactericide* is an agent that kills bacteria. (noun)

e) A *bacteriostatic* agent inhibits the growth of bacteria. (adjective)

f) *Bacteriology* is the science of studying bacteria. (noun)

5. Eradicate *(verb)*

In context:

a) Science hopes to discover a means to eradicate the common cold virus.

b) To eradicate human papillomavirus (HPV), a new vaccine has been created that is widely available and highly recommended in the United States and Canada.

Meaning: The meaning of the verb *eradicate* can best be explained as

a) controlling

b) meeting the challenge

c) of great meaning and significance

d) to do away with or destroy; remove permanently

Word expansion:

a) *Eradication* of HIV and AIDS is a goal of scientists, globally. (noun)

b) *Eradicating* the incidence of poliomyelitis is a goal of vaccination programs around the world. (gerund used as noun)

c) For the most part, smallpox has been *eradicated*. (verb, past tense)

Using New Vocabulary in Sentences.   Use the words given to create a sentence related to viruses or virology. You may need to change the form of the word to suit your needs.

1) immunization

_____

2) serology, detection

_____

3) agent of disease

_____

4) parasitic invasion

_____

5) research, eradicate

_____

SPEAKING EXERCISE

Read the following short paragraph aloud. Ask a peer or teacher to help you with pronunciation. Proceed to the Pronunciation Hints section following. This will also help.

HPV is estimated to be one of the most common sexually transmitted infections (STIs) in the United States, Canada, and around the world. Many types of HPV have been identified, with some leading to cancer and others to ano-genital warts. Fortunately, there is now a vaccine available to help prevent infection with some types of HPV and that also offers protection against HPV types responsible for approximately 70% of cervical cancers.

Human Papilloma Virus, Health Canada, 2008

> ## PRONUNCIATION HINTS
>
> varicella – văr"ĭ-**sĕl**'ă
>
> mumps – m**ŭmps**
>
> whooping cough – **hoop**-ing kawf
>
> rubella – roo-**bĕl**'lă
>
> measles – **mē**'zls
>
> polio – **pōl**-ē-ō
>
> eradicate – **ēra**-dĭ-kāt

LISTENING EXERCISE

Go online. Watch the video "When Viruses Become Hijackers" by the Borough of Manhattan Community College/CUNY at http://www.youtube.com or another similar video. This is a discussion of the pathophysiology of HIV. The speaker is a health professional. Listen carefully to the information, but more importantly to her pronunciation. Notice, too, how fluent her speech is and that it lacks fillers and interjections. She is using professional, technical language.

WRITING EXERCISE

Use your new vocabulary to reflect on your own experience with viruses. Use the medium of writing to talk about some of the more prevalent, common viruses in your country of origin. Discuss why this is so: What makes them important for that country? How does their existence affect the health and even the economy of the country?

_____

_____

_____

_____

Common Disorders and Diseases

In this section language learning revolves around some of the more common types of wounds and diseases caused by viruses and bacteria. Medical and lay terminology is presented to enhance the ability of the health professional to communicate with patients and peers. Contextual examples in this section include decubitus ulcers (a type of wound), chickenpox (a viral disease), and tuberculosis (a bacterial disease). Language skills will include use of participles and conditional forms of verbs, use of descriptors, charting guidelines, and protocols.

Reading Selection 7-3

To learn the vocabulary for common wound assessment and description, the example of dermal ulcers is utilized. Read about this common health challenge in preparation for the vocabulary-building exercises that follow.

DECUBITUS ULCERS

Decubitus ulcers can be very painful and difficult to treat. It is important for all health professionals to observe for and protect against them. In North America, you are expected to observe, chart, and treat at all stages of ulceration. The primary focus of care when a pressure sore is discovered is prevention of further skin breakdown. The secondary focus of care is to alleviate the patient's discomfort. When treatment of a decubitus ulcer requires topical medications or highly specific actions to be taken, these orders must be written by either a physician, nurse practitioner, and/or wound care nurse as approved and designated by the health facility.

To assess and diagnose decubitus ulcers correctly, most facilities in the United States and Canada use a scale. This scale is widely recognized and when consistently used provides an excellent means of clear communication between health-care providers. (See Box 7-1, Stages of a Decubitus Ulcer.)

BOX 7-1   Stages of a Decubitus Ulcer—Characteristics and Appropriate Care Interventions

Stage 1
Characteristics

- Warm or hot spot on the body occurs in areas where a bone is close to the surface of the skin: a bony prominence. There is also elevated temperature at the site.
- Affected skin is not broken, but it may be discolored. Pinkness, redness, or even a light purple, bruise color is noticeable and it does not easily go away.
- Patient complains of soreness or discomfort at the site.

Care Interventions (also referred to as Nursing Interventions)

- Reposition the patient at least every 2 hours to take pressure off the affected area.
- Massage to promote circulation at the site may or may not be recommended and will depend on the facility's decubitus ulcer policy.

Stage 2
Characteristics

- Area is warm to the touch and discolored.
- Area begins to show signs of skin breakdown. Skin shows cracks, flakes, or begins to degrade.
- Patient will complain of pain, not simply soreness or discomfort.

Continued

Care Interventions/Nursing Interventions

- More frequent turning/repositioning of patient is needed.
- Appropriate dressing and/or medication (salves or ointments) should be applied according to the treatment policy for this type of wound at Stage 2 and per the doctor's orders.

Stage 3
Characteristics

- Full-thickness skin loss appears. The epidermis has broken down and the wound has become much more visible.
- Discoloration continues but is magnified.
- Wound is more invasive, traveling deeper into the dermis and tissues below. Necrotic damage may occur.

Care Interventions/Nursing Interventions

- Frequent turning or repositioning is required.
- Appropriate, prescribed dressings, powders, ointments, or salves are applied per policy and physician's orders.
- Frequent monitoring of the wound is necessary.
- Vital signs and assessment for signs of infection in this patient are required on an as needed (prn) basis or as per policy dictated by the facility.

Stage 4
Characteristics

- Wound is fully open with full thickness skin loss and extensive destruction of tissue. The wound is said to be *deep*.
- Damage to muscle, bone, and other structures and tissues may occur and will be visible.

Care Interventions/Nursing Interventions

- Wound to be "dressed" following doctor's orders and choice of dressing per Stage 4 protocol. This may include the process of *packing the wound*.
- Topical medication to the wound as well as an oral antibiotic should be administered as ordered by physician.
- Frequent repositioning of the patient will be necessary or the patient may not be allowed to lie on the area at all.
- Necrotic tissue may be removed by the nurse or doctor in a process called *debriding the wound*.

READING EXERCISES

As we have said previously, the non-native English-speaking health-care professional must not only understand the general meaning of a reading selection, conversation, or lecture, but must also learn the specific facts presented. He or she will then learn how to use new vocabulary.

Understanding the General Meaning

Read the text Decubitus Ulcers again. Think about it. Do you understand it? Respond to the questions with short answers.

1) What is the gist of the text you have just read?

_____

2) What key words predicted the gist of this reading for you?

_____

Learning Specific Information

Take a moment now to review what you have just read. Short answers are acceptable when you answer these questions.

1) What is another term for dermal ulcer?

_____

2) Who has the most responsibility for caring for one of these ulcers at any stage of its development?

_____

3) At which stage of development is the wound said to be deep?

_____

4) What is the purpose of debriding a wound?

_____

5) What does necrotic mean?

_____

6) Where are decubitus ulcers most likely to occur?

_____

7) When are decubitus ulcers most likely to occur?

_____

8) As you know from previous studies in biology, medicine, or nursing, the skin consists of a number of layers below which sit muscles, tendons, bones, etc. Knowing this, explain what is meant by the term "deep wound" in the context of a decubitus ulcer.

_____

_____

Building Vocabulary

Reading clinical journals is an excellent way to increase your vocabulary and your ability to use new words in sentences. Many clinical journal articles discuss and provide illustrations of clinical pathways. Clinical pathways are actually procedures developed to treat specific health challenges. Many health-care facilities have designed their own clinical pathways that should be followed by the health-care professionals employed there. Therefore, it is important that you be able to read, understand, and apply the information in a clinical pathway.

Understanding a Clinical Pathway. Study Figure 7-1, which shows a clinical pathway. It has been designed to guide a nurse in the care of the patient with a decubitus ulcer/pressure sore wound. Take note of the language, the direction of flow for this document, and answer the following questions.

1) Once the patient has been deemed by the nurse as being at high risk for developing bedsores, list three of the next clinical steps to be taken along the clinical pathway.

_____

_____

_____

Clinical Pathway for Risk Assessment Related to Impaired Skin Integrity

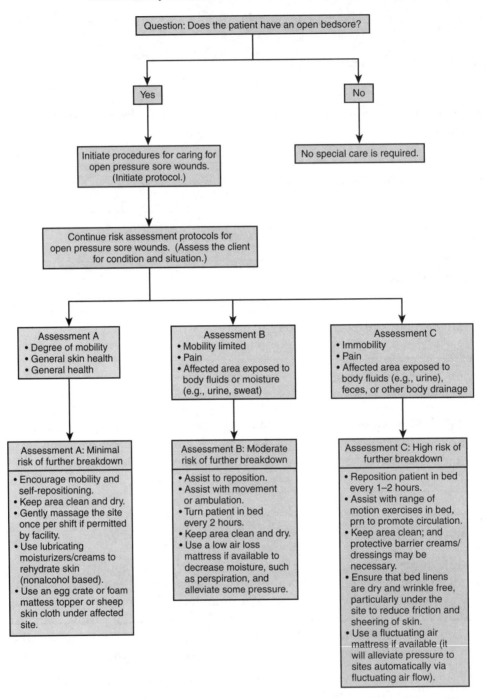

Figure 7-1

2) The patient has limited mobility and spends much time in bed. Based on the clinical pathway shown, what actions should the nurse and care team take to care for this patient and his or her wound?

_____

_____

_____

3) Explain what happens to the patient when he or she is assessed as NOT being at risk to develop a pressure sore.

_____

Wounds, Viral and Bacterial Infections

VOCABULARY ALERT: A SORE

The word *sore* can be an adjective or a noun.

Adjective

In the context of health, people often complain about sore muscles, sore joints, and sore throats. Synonyms include ache, pain, or tenderness at a particular site on the body.

Examples: I have a sore knee today because I fell on it playing basketball yesterday.

My back is sore from lifting heavy boxes.

My muscles are sore and stiff after all the gardening work I did yesterday.

Noun

When someone refers to having a sore, they mean they have an open wound or area of infection. The skin has broken down due to a pathological process, not an injury.

Example: Lying in bed for too long has given me a sore on the back of my heel.

Fill in the Blanks. The language used to describe ulcers is similar to that used to describe other types of wounds. Study the words in the following Word Bank to build your descriptive vocabulary. It includes adjectives, adverbs, and descriptors necessary for explaining or describing wound status to members of the health-care team. Then, in the following exercise, fill in the blanks using those descriptors. Use the words you are given in each individual exercise for your word choices.

WORD BANK

healing

deteriorating

moist

dry

necrotizing

discharging

draining

showing signs of infection

ailing

1) One nurse speaks to another:

Mary, please come take a look at Mr. Howe's toe. He froze it when he got lost snowmobiling. It isn't _____ . It is _____ of _____ . It's actually turning black. I'm sure it's _____ . I think I'd better call the doctor back to look at it, but I'd like your professional opinion first. [necrotic, healing, infection, showing signs]

2) A nurse speaks with the doctor:

Dr. Wilson, Mr. Rubens' abdominal wound is _____ well. The dressing is _____ and there is very little _____ from the Penrose drain. I think we could remove it now. What do you think? [dry, healing, drainage]

3) A doctor speaks with a nurse:

Thanks for calling me, Marge. I've just been in to check Mr. Harcourt in bed 6. His gunshot wound is not _____ . You're right, it has a foul-smelling _____ and is _____ of infection. He looks diaphoretic. What's his latest temperature? [discharge, healing, showing signs]

READING PROFESSIONAL ARTICLES Practice and expand your medical English by reading a nursing or medical journal article on the subject of wounds and wound care. You can go online or to your college library to find the material. This reading will be helpful for you in your career, as well as in language studies, by providing even more exposure to professional writing on this topic.

SPEAKING EXERCISE

Read the following completed sentences aloud. Ask a peer or teacher to help you with pronunciation. Imagine you are telling another nurse, doctor, or health professional what you know about this subject. The Pronunciation Hints box that follows will help.

As you know, decubitus ulcers or pressure sores are a very common type of wound dealt with by health professionals. A great amount of time and effort is spent in care facilities and home care situations in attempts to prevent them. A standard of care expected by professional nurses, allied health care personnel, and by patients is to be free of decubitus ulcers. Some hospitals and care homes pride themselves on their low incidences of bed sores because prevention is challenging, but not impossible. Additionally, there is an abundance of scientific research dedicated to eradicating the development of these wounds. And while we have just read how to assess the staging scale for a decubitus ulcer, it is possible that other scales are applied. This will depend on the facility in which one works. The Braden scale is an excellent predictor of the risk for/potential of a pressure sore occurring. If you are interested in this, search your local college library, nursing or medical textbooks, or the Internet for more information.

PRONUNCIATION HINTS

necrotizing – **nĕ-krŏt′ īz″ĭng**

sore – **sor**

Braden – **brād′n**

LISTENING EXERCISE

Use the Internet again. Search video sites for these words: *debriding a wound*. There are numerous video clips available. Listen carefully to the terminology. You may wish to try to repeat some of them. Play the clips repeatedly so that your ear becomes accustomed to the accent and general pronunciation.

WRITING EXERCISE

Study the information on charting guidelines in Box 7-2 and review the vocabulary in the reading about staging decubitus ulcers given in Box 7-1. Then, write complete but short sentences describing the patients below. You are a nurse caring for them. Use all the information provided in this unit and as many adjectives, adverbs, and descriptors as necessary so that the reader may have a complete picture of what has occurred. Begin with the time and date of your entry (your notation) into the chart. Then, when you have finished noting your observations and clinical activities, sign your name and add your credentials.

1) Paul, age 86, bedridden. Bedsore on coccyx, Stage 2.

_____

_____

2) Kuldeep, 47-year-old woman with cerebral palsy. Wheelchair bound. Decubitus ulcer on spine, Stage 4.

_____

3) Alexi, age 22, just having his leg cast removed. Ulcer to the back of his heel. Stage 3.

_____

4) Sara, 16 years old, recovering from two broken femurs. Stage 1 ulcer to her right elbow.

_____

Wounds, Viral and Bacterial Infections

BOX 7-2 Charting Guidelines

A chart is a document that describes the patient's health status holistically. It follows the patient's care. All members of the professional healthcare team have access to the chart and can make written entries into it. More and more often now, care facilities and clinics are using e-charting programs. These computer programs are designed in much the same way as the standard, handwritten patient chart, but all the patient care records are kept electronically.

All patient charts are legal documents. They identify what care was or wasn't given. As a result, charting guidelines and policies are in place wherever patients or clients are recipients of health care.

While charting guidelines can be different at every health-care facility, basic charting guidelines in the United States and Canada include:

- client name, date of birth, and health number/insurance number clearly identified on each page of the document
- a description of the client's clinical symptoms
- notes on factual, empirical data such as laboratory reports
- notes on subjective data from the client or client's family (which must clearly be identified as being subjective)
- professional opinions with rationale
- date and time for all entries
- the signature and initials of the credentials of the writer for all entries
- consent for treatment forms signed and dated by the client and a witness
- use of abbreviations deemed acceptable by the facility's policies
- no use of common everyday slang or street slang
- nonjudgmental language, including avoidance of the use of personal opinion
- clear and concise documentation that follows the guidelines for charting required by the facility
- all treatments and interventions documented

Reading Selection 7-4

Read the following in anticipation of the exercises to follow.

COMMON VIRAL DISEASES

Most viruses that are found in humans spread through respiratory and intestinal excretions. They can be active or latent. An active virus-caused infection is one in which once the person is infected, he or she will exhibit the signs and symptoms of infection or disease. A latent infection is one in which the person carries the virus but is not physically affected by it. However, this individual may still be able to transmit the disease to others, as a passive carrier.

In either active or latent form, a virus may or may not be contagious. The term contagious refers to whether or not the disease can be passed to another. People with active contagious viral infections may be contagious before, during, and after the presentation of symptoms. Those with latent contagious viral illnesses may pass the disease to another person without having any symptoms himself or herself.

The body reacts to an invasion by a virus by producing antibodies. This occurs through our natural line of defense, the immune system. People with a weakened immune system can have more severe symptoms of the virus and the illness experience may be much more difficult to endure and/or treat. For people with active viral infections, active treatment is initiated. For people with latent infections, there may be treatment if the virus is contagious to help prevent its spread to others, but if it is not contagious, it may be untreated.

Some examples of common viral diseases in North America are:

- The Common Cold. It is contagious and can be contracted by inhaling this airborne virus or touching something contaminated with infected nasal or oral secretions.

- Influenza, also known as "the flu." Influenza comes in many strains, and flu vaccines are developed each year to address the latest strains. The flu is caught through contact with infected droplets in the air from the nose or throat of the individual who has it.

- Human Immunodeficiency Virus (HIV). This virus causes progressive damage to the immune system. Advanced infection is identified as Acquired Immunodeficiency Syndrome (AIDS). HIV is contracted by exposure to infected blood, through sexual contact, through shared needles, and through the birth canal of an HIV-infected woman. Anti-viral medications can help diminish the symptoms of HIV and AIDS, but cannot cure them.

- Hepatitis C, a virus that invades the liver. It may possibly be the most common chronic blood-borne infection in the United States. Often referred to as "Hep C," individuals with this diagnosis can be active or passive carriers of it. Hepatitis C is only transmitted through blood contact. Anti-viral agents may be used to treat symptoms of active hepatitis C. Vaccination can help prevent it.

- Norwalk Virus, a viral infection of the gastrointestinal tract. It is highly contagious and when it occurs in a care facility, the whole hospital floor or entire facility may be quarantined. The Norwalk virus is transmitted via the oral-fecal route. In other words, it is transferred from hands contaminated with fecal matter to the mouth. It can also be passed in the same manner through contact with vomit.

READING EXERCISES

Understanding and using new vocabulary words includes familiarity with basics of grammar, including use of the correct tense of verbs.

Understanding the General Meaning

Read the text again. Think about it. Do you understand it?

1) What is the purpose of this text?

_____

2) Does it serve a social purpose?

_____

3) What is the main theme or thesis of this text?

_____

4) Are all viruses contagious?

_____

5) List the viral diseases named in the reading.

_____

Building Vocabulary

As we have done in previous reading selections, we give you the opportunity to discern the meaning of a word from its context and then to clarify its meaning and use through several exercises.

Determining Meaning from Context. To build vocabulary, study the following words and terms taken from the reading. Discover all you can about them by looking at them in these new examples. Next, go on to choose the correct meaning for the word from the choices provided. Finally, take a look at how the words expand in English.

1. Infectious *(adjective)*

In context:
a) Mononucleosis is an infectious disease sometimes referred to as the kissing disease.
b) If a disease is infectious, it may or may not also be contagious.

Meaning: The word *infectious* in the context of viruses means
a) always communicable
b) leading to contagion
c) caused by invasion of a pathogen
d) spread by airborne droplets

Word expansion:
a) Randy caught a respiratory *infection* when he was on a safari in Africa. (noun)
b) The nurse *was infected* with HIV from a needle stick injury at the hospital. (verb, past participle)

2. Contagious *(adjective)*

In context:
a) Mononucleosis is contagious. You can pass it on through saliva.
b) Vicki is 8 years old. Right now she is contagious. She has the measles.

Meaning: The best way to define the word *contagious* is to say it means
a) capable of being infected
b) an active recipient
c) capable of being transmitted
d) capable of being a donor

Word expansion:
a) The purpose of quarantine is to confine the *contagion* to one locale. (noun)

3. Latent *(adjective)*

In context:
a) Herpes simplex virus is a latent virus. You can carry it for years before a cold sore appears on your lip.
b) For those infected with HIV, its latent tendency makes it difficult to plan a future.

Meaning: The best way to define the word *latent* is to say it means
a) visible, symptomatic
b) noncontagious
c) not visible; present, but asymptomatic
d) noninfectious

Word expansion:
a) A *latency* effect of the *Varicella zoster* virus is that one day it may become active and develop into the condition shingles. (noun)

4. Quarantined *(verb)*

In context:
a) The Seniors' Care Home is quarantined right now because of an outbreak of the Norwalk virus.
b) The ship in the harbor is quarantined. An Ebola-like virus has been reported.

Meaning: The best way to define the word *quarantined* is to say it means

a) isolated due to disease

b) isolated for health promotion

c) categorized as diseased

d) stigmatized and isolated

Word expansion:

a) The Chief Medical Officer at the Public Health Department *quarantined* the home yesterday. No one is to go in or out. (verb, simple past tense)

b) The purpose of *quarantine* is to confine the contagion to one locale. (noun)

5. Contracted *(verb)*

In context:

a) Mrs. Watson contracted genital herpes from her new husband.

b) The staff at the restaurant contracted Hepatitis A from an unspecified contaminant on the premises.

Meaning: The best way to define the word *contracted* in a medical sense is to say

a) gathered

b) acquired

c) received

d) obtained

Word expansion:

a) If you don't want to *contract* malaria when you are on vacation in an area with a high rate of malaria, you should get your inoculations before you go. (verb, infinitive)

b) The village *is contracting* AIDS at a devastating rate. (verb, present participle)

6. Strains *(noun, plural)*

In context:

a) There are multiple strains of hepatitis.

Meaning: The best way to define the word *strains* in the medical context is to say it means

a) microorganisms

b) conditions

c) types or varieties

d) pathogens

Word expansion:

a) Lab tests will determine which *strain* of bacterial pneumonia you have. (noun)

Mix and Match.   Complete the exercise in Box 7-3 to help you clarify the meaning of words and expressions commonly used when discussing a viral respiratory tract infection.

Sentence Completion.   Complete the following sentences by filling in the blanks. Only use the future conditional form for each of the second blanks in the sentences.

1) If a virus _____ (to invade) my respiratory system, I _____ (get) an infection.

2) If a harmful microorganism _____ (to find) a reservoir in the surgical wound bed, it _____ (to contaminate) it.

3) If Jackie can't _____ (to cough), she _____ (to clear, negative form) her lungs of the pathogens.

4) If the postoperative patient _____ (to develop) an infection, he likely _____ (to develop) a fever as well.

5) If the sutures _____ (to break) or don't hold, the patient's wound _____ (open).

SPEAKING EXERCISE

Read the following completed information aloud. Record yourself imagining you are giving a lecture to a group of first-year nursing students.. Use your professional persona to speak clearly, concisely, and with confidence. Repeat the exercise as many times as necessary to achieve this goal. The Pronunciation Hints box following will help.

Chickenpox is a common viral disease of childhood. It is the result of the *Varicella zoster* virus. It is highly contagious and spreads quickly through elementary schools. Signs and symptoms include a red rash on the trunk of the body that soon becomes small, itchy, open sores that erupt. The child may feel irritable and generally unwell. Whenever possible, the child should be prevented from scratching the pox sores as doing so can lead to infection and scarring. Children with chickenpox should not go to school or day care until all of the sores have dried out or disappeared. There is a *Varicella* vaccine available to prevent chickenpox. For more information on this preventative measure, contact your local Public Health Department.

PRONUNCIATION HINTS

quarantined – **kwor'**ăn-tēn'd

pox – **pŏks**

Norwalk – **nŏr'**wawk

immunodeficiency – ĭm" ū-nō-dĕ-**fĭsh'**ĕn-sē

Varicella - văr"ĭ-**sĕl'**ă

LISTENING EXERCISE

Go online to listen to a discussion by a health professional regarding the etiology, signs, symptoms, treatment, and prevention of the childhood disease chickenpox. Search for "How to Diagnose and Treat Chickenpox in Childhood" on the video site *Wonder How to* at http://www.wonderhowto.com. Once there, search for "Diet and Health Medical Diagnosis." Then search for "chickenpox." There are numerous videos available.

Afterwards, listen once more to your own recording about chickenpox. How do your speaking skills compare with those on the video clip? Take a moment or two to reflect on that.

Finally, listen to a discussion of another common virus, influenza, at "The Flu—Maryland Health Today, March 7, 2007" at http://www.video.google.com. Notice the interviewer is a health professional quite capable of using highly academic, technical language; however, in this situation, he is using common English to communicate important information to the public. The goal of the interview appears to be to teach the signs and symptoms and causes of influenza. It is also a health promotion and prevention activity.

 ## WRITING EXERCISE—SCRIPTING A COMMUNICATION

Use your new vocabulary. Read the following scenario and then, in the role of the Public Health Nurse, write a script for the communication you will have with a mother who calls you for advice. Use as many lines as you need to write this script. If this form does not suit your needs, use a separate piece of paper to write your final script. (If you are unsure about the role of a Public Health Nurse in the United States or Canada, research this on the Internet or in your local college library.)

Scenario:

A mother has just phoned for advice. You are speaking with her on the phone now. She informs you that her 8-year-old daughter might have chickenpox. She wants to know if it is true and what she should do about it. She also has to work every day and now is worried she won't be able to care for the child. She is afraid that if the child has chickenpox, the family will be financially affected as well.

Public Health Nurse (PHN): _____

_____

_____

Mother (Mom): _____

_____

PHN: _____

_____

_____

Mom: _____

_____

PHN: _____

_____

_____

Mom: _____

_____

Reading Selection 7-5

Read the following to learn more about infectious diseases. Note the difference between a viral and bacterial infection. In your career be as clear and specific as possible. Always use the correct term.

A COMMON BACTERIAL INFECTION: TUBERCULOSIS

Tuberculosis (TB) is an infectious disease of the respiratory tract. It is caused by the bacteria *Mycobacterium tuberculosis*. This means that TB is a bacterial infection. This is important to remember since the disease is sometimes thought of as a viral disease. While this distinction may not be important to the public, it is important to health professionals and scientists. Clear identification of the cause of an illness leads to a greater understanding of how to treat it. Bacterial infections can usually be treated with antibiotics; viral infections cannot.

Exposure to a person with active TB can be risky. The disease is contagious. It is spread by microscopic droplets and respiratory secretions released into the air by an infected individual. This can occur through coughing, speaking, sneezing, and even laughing. The person with active TB should remain in isolation or quarantine until treatment has eradicated the bacteria. Tuberculosis infection can also be passive or dormant, with no adverse effects of the disease on the person infected. In this form, TB is not contagious and the person can lead a normal life.

Tuberculosis is diagnosed by x-ray and sputum secretion tests. The infection is treated with an antibiotic anti-tuberculosis drug called isoniazid (INH). This is taken on a daily basis for 6 to 9 months. Isoniazid can also be prescribed for persons in direct contact with a tuberculosis patient as a preventive measure. Acute, active cases of tuberculosis can require hospitalization and isolation protocols.

READING EXERCISES

Understanding the General Meaning

Now that you have completed the reading, answer the following questions.

1) What is the main topic of this text?

_____

2) What is one thing that distinguishes bacteria from a virus?

_____

3) People most often refer to tuberculosis by its initials. What are they?

_____

4) What does TB infect?

_____

5) Why is exposure to tuberculosis risky?

_____

6) Can TB lay dormant in the body?

_____

7) Is there a cure for TB?

_____

8) Is there a treatment for TB? If so, what is it?

_____

Building Vocabulary

Determining Meaning from Context. To build vocabulary, study the following words and terms taken from the reading. Discover all you can about them by looking at them in these new examples. Next, go on to choose the correct meaning for the word from the choices provided. Finally, take a look at how the words expand in English.

1. Bacteria *(noun, plural)*

In context:
a) A swab taken from the wound showed that bacteria were present. That is the source of the infection.
b) Gram-negative bacteria can cause respiratory illnesses.

Meaning: The best explanation for the word *bacteria* is that they are
a) unicellular microorganisms that can reproduce themselves
b) unicellular microorganisms that cannot reproduce themselves
c) unicellular pathogens
d) multicellular pathogens

Word expansion:
a) The singular form of the word bacteria is *bacterium.* (noun, singular)
b) A *bacterial* infection is generally treated with an antibiotic. (adjective)
c) *Antibacterial* hand soap actually washes away the good bacteria that lives on our skin and is healthy for us. It's not a good idea. (adjective)

2. Droplets *(noun, plural)*

In context:
a) Water droplets appeared on the window and I knew it was about to start raining.
b) Infected droplets of liquid were expelled when the patient coughed.

Meaning: The best explanation for the word *droplets* in the biological sense is
a) small portions
b) microorganisms
c) small drops of liquid
d) liquids

Word expansion:
a) A drop of water is larger than a droplet. (noun)

3. Dormant *(adjective)*

In context:
a) The *Herpes simplex* virus can remain dormant in the body for years and then suddenly manifest itself as a cold sore on the lip.
b) A dormant virus is still detectable by laboratory tests.

Meaning: The best explanation for the word *dormant* in the medical sense is
a) asleep
b) ineffective
c) incapacitate
d) not currently active; latent

Word expansion:
a) After a long period of *dormancy,* the *Varicella zoster* virus has been activated and the patient is suffering from shingles. (noun)

VOCABULARY ALERT: DIFFERENCE BETWEEN ISOLATION AND QUARANTINE
Clear and proper use of language is essential to providing safe, competent care to clients and patients.

Isolation means separating someone or something from contact with others. It generally occurs in a hospital or nursing home. An isolation room will house one individual or several individuals with the same disease only. It is used when the chances of cross-contamination and infection are extremely high. Isolation protocol is a form of infection control and must be carried out diligently and consistently by the health-care team and any visitors to the patient.

Quarantine means that isolation is enforced or required by some level of authority. That might be the local health department or state, provincial, or federal governmental departments of public health. The goal of quarantine is to contain the people infected with a contagious disease in one location. This does not have to be a hospital or clinic. Quarantines are limited to periods of time until the risk is deemed over by those very same people in authority.

GRAMMAR ALERT: PARTICIPLES Participles are forms of verbs that can modify nouns or act as adjectives or even pronouns.

Participles are used with the auxiliary verbs "be" and "have." They can also appear after (copulative) verbs of perception such as: see, hear, listen, feel, smell, and watch. They also appear after verbs of movement and rest such as: go, walk, skip, come, sit, and stand.

A present participle is formed by adding "ing" to the verb.

Present participles used with auxiliary verbs make progressive, perfect, and passive forms of verbs. Words like attending, bleeding, and changing are all present participles. An example of a present participle used in a medical context is:

The patient was bleeding when he arrived in the ER.

Explanation: past tense of the verb "be" = was + participle form of base word "bleed" = bleeding.

A past participle is formed by adding "d" or "ed" to a regular verb. When a past participle appears in a sentence, the sentence can often be rewritten to make it clearer. Past participles are used with auxiliary verbs to talk about the past or they can have passive meanings when used as adjectives or adverbs. Words like shown, gone, closed, and started are all past participles. An example of a past participle used in a medical context is:

Based on preliminary test results, the patient must remain in isolation.

Explanation: past participle of the verb "base."

To make the meaning and structure of this example more apparent, rewrite the sentence like this:

The decision to remain in the hospital is based on the preliminary test results.

Explanation: past participle of the verb "base" + auxiliary verb "is."

Fill in the Blanks. This exercise is designed to highlight the use of participles in sentences that deal with health care. Complete the following sentences by correctly filling in the blank with either a present or past participle based on the verb identified in brackets.

1) The doctor is —————————— patients. (treat)

2) Look, the nurse is —————————— (cover) her face with a mask while she works with the contagious patient. That is proper procedure.

3) Ann has —————————— (recover) from the virus she caught while on vacation.

4) The x-ray proves he has a —————————— (collapse) lung.

5) I'm pleased to report that the practical nurses are —————————— (remember) to give the patient his medication four times per day.

6) Morris is —————————— (wait) for a lung transplant.

7) The elderly patient felt alone, —————————— (forget) by his family.

8) I believe the family is —————————— (come) into the hospital to see their son.

SPEAKING EXERCISE

Read the following completed sentences aloud. Ask a peer or teacher to help you with pronunciation. Proceed to the Pronunciation Hints section following. This will also help.

> Patients are often reluctant to comply with the treatment for tuberculosis because it is a lengthy process of recovery over 6 to 12 months. In the United States, it can also be a costly process if the patient does not have adequate medical insurance. In the acute phase, hospitalization of 14 days or longer may be required. A daily regime of medication will be prescribed with frequent monitoring through laboratory testing for the remainder of the year after that. This can put economic pressure on the patient and lead him or her to discontinue treatment. The repercussions of this to society can be problematic. Tuberculosis is contagious and this patient has the potential to spread it to all those with whom he or she comes into contact. The person also risks his or her own life because if left untreated, death is possible.

PRONUNCIATION HINTS

tuberculosis – tū-bĕr″ kū-**lō′**sĭs

repercussions – rĕ-pĕr-**kŭsh′**ŭns

laboratory – **lăb′**ră-tor″ ē

LISTENING EXERCISE

Go online to listen to experts talk about infections. Try *MD Kiosk (2007)* at http://www.mdkiosk.com. Listen to the introduction on the home page. It's instructional and interesting. Then, choose the menu button for videos. Once there, type in the title, "Acute Otitis Media." You will be taken to a short audio-visual clip discussing ear infections in children.

WRITING EXERCISE

Write a teaching and learning script. You are a nurse practitioner, community health nurse, or family doctor. Imagine a male patient has been diagnosed with TB and you have made arrangements for him to be admitted to the hospital today. Explain the course of the disease and the treatment plan. Teach the patient the importance of adherence to the care plan, including compliance with the treatment and the medication regime. Write in script form. You are the nurse. You must write for the patient, too. Remember that in English-speaking North America the patient is an informed consumer and will very likely ask you many questions about his or her condition.

   a) Begin with a draft of the points you wish to make. Recall the genre of *explanation* to guide you in this task.
   b) Answer the questions posed following completion of your draft.
   c) Critique your draft by reviewing it in light of the questions you've just answered. This is a form of critical reflection.
   d) Write the final teaching and learning script.

1) Draft

_____

_____

_____

_____

_____

_____

_____

_____

_____

2) Reflective questions:
   a) Is your interaction client-centered? How often are you focused on what the client wants to know rather than on what you want to teach?
   b) Have you demonstrated to the client that you have heard and understood what he or she has asked or said? How so?
   c) Did you use a majority of open-ended or closed-ended questions? Which one was more facilitative to communication?
   d) How did you determine how much information you would include in your teaching?
   e) Did you use language that the client would understand?
   f) How did you assess that the client learned what you taught?
   g) Have you followed the format for writing an explanation?

3) Amend or edit your draft based on your reflections to the questions asked above.

4) Write the completed teaching and learning script here. Use as many lines as you need. If this form does not suit your needs, use a separate piece of paper to write your final script. Be as creative as you like. There is no right or wrong answer if you have followed directions and applied the answers to your reflective questions.

Health Provider (HP): _____

_____

Patient: _____

_____

_____

HP: _____

_____

_____

Patient: _____

_____

HP: _____

_____

Patient: _____

_____

_____

HP: _____

_____

_____

Patient: _____

_____

HP: _____

_____

Patient: _____

_____

_____

HP: _____

_____

_____

Patient: _____

_____

| SECTION THREE | # Treatments, Interventions, and Assistance |

The reading selections and exercises in this section focus on vocabulary and concept building related to infection control and wound healing. The language and concepts of Standard Precautions and asepsis are introduced. There are also opportunities to practice charting. Exercises in grammar include working with gerunds and spelling. Critical thinking exercises and case studies facilitate the skills of using language in meaningful ways.

Reading Selection 7-6

Read the following information about infection in preparation for vocabulary building exercises. Some of the information will be a review. Remember, we are not focusing on content, but on the acquisition and improvement of your English language skills.

CHAIN OF INFECTION AND INFECTION CONTROL

As stated earlier, microorganisms are minute organisms, such as protozoa, bacteria, and viruses. Those that cause disease are called pathogens. Viral and bacterial infections, some of which you have just read about, are both spread in basically the same ways—through what is known as a chain of infection.

Health professionals will be very familiar with the chain of infection. This is a cyclical process that explains the life and transmission of a pathogen. To begin the process, an agent that has the capacity to cause disease (a pathogen) is required. The first link in the chain occurs when the agent finds a reservoir (a home) where it can multiply. The next link in the chain occurs when that pathogen finds a mode of transportation to expand throughout the organism it has infected and to multiply. If it cannot find this, it looks for a portal of entry into another reservoir where it can continue its life cycle, starting another chain of infection. An object that is free of microorganisms is said to be sterile. The elimination of microorganisms from a site (e.g., the site of a wound) is called surgical asepsis.

Infection control is a set of policies and procedures adhered to in health care to prevent the spread of harmful microorganisms. It is achieved by following the principles of asepsis or clean technique. This includes using protection such as gloves, gowns, and masks whenever the risk of contact with a pathogen is likely.

Standard or Universal Precautions are medical asepsis protocols used with all patients whether or not they have or are known to carry pathogens. Medical asepsis is a standard of practice followed by all members of the health-care team. Standard Precautions are preventative actions applied to everyone equally to promote health, prevent the spread of infection, and avoid the problems of stigmatization for patients with infections and/or those who harbor organisms that are contagious.

The treatment for viral infection is anti-viral medications, interferon, vaccines, and immuno-globulins, if available. The treatment for bacterial infection is antibiotic medication. Wound infections are most often due to bacterial infection. The interventions for wound infection include clean and sterile dressing changes, aseptic and sterile techniques, and strict attention to infection control protocols for wound care. Assistance strategies include keeping the environment clean, placing bio-hazardous materials in the appropriate waste bins (rather than the common garbage or trash), and limiting contact with other potentially infectious agents.

For more information on infection and disease control, visit your local Center for Disease Control or search for them online. The Center for Disease Control and Prevention is an excellent resource of information and provides a multitude of opportunities to enhance your career-specific English language vocabulary.

VOCABULARY ALERT: THE WORD "MINUTE" The word "minute" appears in the first sentence of this reading. In this context, *minute* does not refer to a measure of time and it is not a noun. It means very small or tiny and is commonly used as an adjective to describe an organism. It also is not pronounced the same way as the word meaning a measure of time. It is pronounced: meye-**noot.**

The word is also commonly used to describe very fine details of a subject, as in: Being a lawyer, she read all the minute details of the criminal report.

 # READING EXERCISES

Understanding the General Meaning

1) Explain what you have just read in a short summary of 20–40 words.

_____

_____

_____

2) List the terms that deal with sterile technique in the reading.

_____

3) Based on the reading, draw the chain of infection.

Building Vocabulary

Determining Meaning from Context. To build vocabulary, study the following words or terms taken from this text. Discover all you can about them by looking at them in context. Choose the correct meaning. Finally, take a look at how these words or terms expand in English.

1. Agent *(noun)*

In context:

a) Medical research can be an agent of change in health and health care delivery.

b) A pathogen is an agent of disease.

Meaning: In the context of the reading selection, the word *agent* means

a) an accomplisher
b) the means by which something occurs
c) the means of obstruction
d) the conspirator

Word expansion:

a) The rate of recovery can often be altered by the *agency* of medication. (noun)

2. Causative *(adjective)*

In context:

a) A causative factor in the spread of infection is lack of hand washing.

b) The causative agent in the disease typhoid is *Salmonella typhi.*

Meaning: The best way to define the word *causative* is to say it means

a) responsible
b) neglectful
c) ordinary
d) assistive

Word expansion:

a) The principle *cause* of the spread of disease is poor hand-washing hygiene. (noun)

b) The bacteria *Mycobacterium tuberculosis causes* tuberculosis. (verb, present tense)

3. Asepsis *(noun)*

In context:

a) Understanding the need for healing to occur in a clean, sterile environment, hospitals promote asepsis.

b) Wound asepsis requires that specific protocols be followed by the nurse and doctor when examining the wound or changing the dressing. This will avoid contaminating the wound.

Meaning: The word *asepsis* means

a) accumulative
b) causality
c) influential
d) sterility

Word expansion:

a) The operating room is aseptic. Pathogenic organisms are absent. (adjective)

Practicing Spelling. Unscramble these words from the text.

1) orasscirmmniog _____

2) lcialycc _____

3) deom _____

4) hegpoant _____

5) crtiaabel _____

6) sismniotnras _____

7) eelrtsi _____

8) uscavetia _____

9) souteifnic _____

10) rresverio _____

GRAMMAR ALERT: GERUNDS Gerunds are verbs that function as nouns. They end in *ing*. Here is an example of a gerund used as a noun in the medical context:
Bleeding from a laceration to the face can be profuse.

Fill in the Blank Complete the following grammar exercise by filling in the blanks. The word preceding every blank is a preposition. You may want to circle these as a grammar reminder to yourself. You are given the first letter of the gerund as a hint.

1) Frieda is afraid of **l** _____ her leg from gangrene.

2) The patient is insisting on **h** _____ more pain medication.

3) The elderly man doesn't believe in **s**_____ in the hospital.

4) I wish I could call in sick today. I don't feel like **w**_____.

5) Beth is afraid of **c**_____. It hurts her lungs too much.

6) It is important to focus on **r**_____, not staying in the hospital.

READ MORE Expand your vocabulary by reading more about antibiotic-resistant infections. An excellent resource can be found at the New York State Department of Health website at http://www.health.state.ny.us. On the home page, select "Infection Control." Scroll through the choices and click on "Multi-Drug Resistant Organisms."

SPEAKING EXERCISE

Read the following completed sentences aloud. Ask a peer or teacher to help you with pronunciation. Proceed to the Pronunciation Hints section following. This will also help.

Fever is the most obvious sign of infection and disease. It is the body's reaction to illness and attack by pathogens. In the immune system, chemicals called pyrogens are released into the blood stream in response to a threat to health. These affect the hypothalamus in the brain where temperature is regulated. Temperature will rise and fall as necessary to fight the battle.

PRONUNCIATION HINTS

reservoir – **rĕz'**ĕr-vwor

infectious – ĭn-**fĕk'**shŭs

pathogens – **păth'**ō-jĕnz

microorganisms – mī-krō-**or'**găn-ĭzmz

causative – **kawz**-atĭv

LISTENING EXERCISES

Here are three good sites on the Internet on which to listen to examples of the terminology and grammar included in this section. Whichever resource you use, listen carefully to the style of language. Who is the intended target audience? What style of language has the speaker chosen to use to engage this audience in particular? Remember, your choice of language will facilitate or inhibit your ability to communicate with your audience—be it a patient, a peer, or a community group. You should match your style to the intended receiver or target audience.

1) Go online to the website: http://www.ResearchChannel.com. Search for the video in the Howard Hughes Medical Institute Holiday Lecture Series, "2000 and Beyond." Search for the video title, "Emerging Infections: How Epidemics Arise." You can also find this video at http://www.video.google.com.

2) Search the Internet video sites. Look for any clip entitled "MRSA." There are more than one of these, but the author recommends the NBC news presentation *Ask the Doctor, October 2007*, by Dr. John Hong at http://www.video.google.com. That clip is called "MRSA: The 'SuperBug.'"

3) Search for yeast infections on the website *Medical News Today, Healthology* at http://www.medicalnewstoday.com. Click on the menu selection that includes videos.

 ## WRITING EXERCISE

Read the following short stories and answer the questions that follow each. Remember to remain within the context of this chapter; namely, wounds, viruses, and viral and bacterial infections. Use full sentences and provide the rationale or explanation for your answer.

1) Janice cut herself on a piece of wire fencing the other day. You attend night school with her and have noticed that she was wearing a small bandage across the top of her right hand. It's now been 3 days since she injured herself. Today she tells you that the cut is red and "oozing some yellow stuff." It's beginning to throb too, she says.

a) What are your first thoughts about this situation?

_____

b) What is the gist of the story?

_____

c) Who is the main character in the story?

_____

d) As a health professional, what is your working diagnosis?

_____

e) What treatment, intervention, or assistance would you recommend for the person who is ill?

_____

f) What is night school?

_____

2) You are on vacation on a trip to the tropics. Steven is a 55-year-old gentleman sitting on the airplane, sniffling. As the flight continues, you hear him occasionally cough and sneeze. You discover you are staying in the same hotel and observe he is getting sicker when you see him the next day. His color isn't good and he seems irritable. By the third day, you hear this man is sick in bed with the flu and that the doctor had to be called. He has a high temperature and is weak and congested.

a) What are your first thoughts about this situation?

_____

b) What is the gist of the story?

_____

c) Who is the main character in the story?

_____

d) As a health professional, what is your working diagnosis?

_____

e) What treatment, intervention, or assistance would you recommend for the person who is ill?

_____

f) What is your prognosis for yourself and the others who were on the airplane with this man?

_____

3) Zarah is a 32-year-old patient newly admitted to your ward for assessment and monitoring of her epilepsy. You notice she has been coughing a lot over her first 36 hours in the hospital. Sometimes the cough is productive; at other times, her cough seems to be "stuck in her throat." You notice that she occasionally sounds short of breath or her breathing is a bit raspy. You check her records and find she is newly arrived here in the United States from Nigeria. She has no other signs of a cold or flu.

a) What are your first thoughts about this situation?

_____

b) What is the gist of the story?

_____

c) Who is the main character in the story?

_____

d) As a health professional, what is your working diagnosis?

_____

e) What treatment, intervention, or assistance would you recommend for the person who is ill?

_____

Reading Selection 7-7

To differentiate between signs and symptoms of an infected wound and a healthy one, it is important to study the language of both. Describing, planning, and guiding the treatment of wounds are the purview of the nurse, or, in other words, within the nurse's realm of responsibility. The following readings and exercises deal with healthy and infected wounds and the treatments, interventions, and assistance required to promote healing.

WOUND HEALING

The term used to describe how open wounds heal is "intention." Intention begins when the edges of the wound are brought together through the process of approximation. There are three stages of intention. Although wound healing is a natural process, closure of the wound can also be mechanically induced. These procedures will now be discussed. The clinical decision made regarding which type of intention will promote optimal recovery is based on the amount of tissue loss, risk for infection, and expected amount of scarring.

Primary intention occurs when the edges of a wound or surgical incision are close together: in close proximity to one another. To promote closure and healing, an adhesive

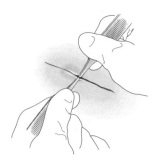

approximation

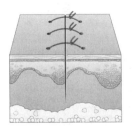

sutures

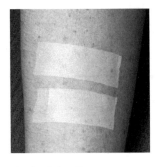

steri-strips/tapes

may be used to seal the edges together. Primary intention healing is facilitated by the use of sutures, staples, tapes, or steri-strips. This can only occur if the edges of the wound approximate.

Secondary intention healing occurs when the wound site has extensive damage and tissue loss. In this case, healing must occur in the wound bed first before the wound closes, but the edges of this type of wound will never approximate. Through the natural processes of granulation (formation of new connective tissue) and contraction (wound bed closes), scar tissue eventually fills the wound bed. Depending on the time it takes for tissue and skin to re-cover the area, the wound remains at risk for infection. Dressings or some form of sterile covering are required. Secondary intention healing is the goal of wound care when treating skin ulcers.

Tertiary intention healing occurs when trauma or contamination to the site is extensive and the tissue is no longer viable (alive) or useful to the healing process. In this situation, the wound edges will be surgically closed and secured with sutures, staples, or tapes. A temporary drain may be placed *in situ* to facilitate the healing by providing a route of evacuation for purulent or sero-sanguinous drainage. The wound may also require debridement of dead or contaminated tissue for an extended period of time. Sometimes this type of wound healing is referred to as "delayed primary intention healing."

 READING EXERCISES

Understanding the General Meaning

Complete the following exercises using short answer responses.

1) What is the topic of the first paragraph?

_____

2) What is the topic of the second paragraph?

_____

3) What kind of wound or incision would require this type of healing?

_____

4) What is the topic of the third paragraph?

_____

5) What kind of wound or incision would require this type of healing?

_____

6) What is the topic of the fourth paragraph?

_____

7) What kind of wound or incision would require this type of healing?

_____

Understanding Specific Information

Complete the following exercises based on your readings.

1) Sometimes, a wound must be closed by suturing. This is known as _____ intention healing.

2) When the skin or tissue surrounding a wound is no longer able to heal, and granulation and contraction are not likely to occur, _____ intention healing must be considered.

3) Sometimes referred to as an open wound, _____ intention healing does not necessitate sutures or tapes.

4) Drains can be surgically placed in wounds. They are placed *in situ*. Based on the context of the reading and your own medical knowledge, define the medical term *in situ*.

VOCABULARY ALERT: PURVIEW The word *purview* means domain of responsibility.

Building Vocabulary

Determining Meaning from Context. To build vocabulary, study the following words taken from the reading. Discover all you can about them by looking at them in these new examples. Next, go on to choose the correct meaning for the word from the choices provided. Finally, take a look at how the words expand in English.

1. Incision *(noun)*

In context:
a) A surgical incision is required in a cesarean section to facilitate successful delivery of the baby.
b) A small incision was made to the crush injury site to release pressure on the tissues.

Meaning: The word *incision* can best be explained as
a) a precise cut by a sharp instrument
b) a surgical opening
c) a medical laceration
d) an imperfect cut made by an instrument

Word expansion:
a) The man arrived in the emergency department with an *incised* wound to his finger. He is a butcher. He accidentally sliced himself with a very sharp knife. (adjective)
b) To ascertain whether or not the mole on her face is cancerous, an *incision* biopsy will be performed. (adjective; medical term)

2. Intention *(noun)*

In context:
a) Whenever possible, small facial wound edges are approximated with steri-strips and left to heal by primary intention. This minimizes scarring.

Meaning: The word *intention* used in the context of wound healing or surgery can best be explained as saying it is
a) a process of combining
b) a process or operation
c) skin grafting
d) integumentary repair

Word expansion:
a) An *intention* tremor is caused by neurological disorder and occurs when a person is doing a precise, voluntary movement. (adjective)

3. Granulation *(noun)*

In context:
a) The wound bed shows signs of granulation. It has begun to heal.
b) Granulation does not occur in a simple wound that can heal by primary intention.
c) Granulation tissue formation occurs in second stage healing.

Meaning: The word *granulation* in a medical context can best be explained as
a) tissue exudate
b) small abscesses that occur in the process of wound healing
c) formation of purulent material that must be drained from the wound
d) formation of small grains that form connective tissue in the process of wound healing

4. Approximate *(verb)*

In context:
a) The plastic surgeon believes she can approximate the wound edges with little or no residual scarring.
b) The nurse was able to approximate the edges of the open wound while the nurse practitioner prepared to suture.

Meaning: The word *approximate* used in a surgical context can best be explained as
a) to be nearby the wound site in preparation for healing
b) to bring together into a desired position for healing or suturing
c) inclusion of each edge of the wound
d) linking tissues and cells

Word expansion:
a) The edges of the wound were jagged and torn. They could not be approximated. (verb, past participle)

5. Coagulate *(verb)*

In context:
a) A wound spontaneously stops bleeding when blood begins to coagulate.

Meaning: The meaning of the word *coagulate* is
a) to transform from murky liquid to clear liquid
b) to join or combine
c) to change from a liquid to a gel or solid
d) to cover and connect

Word expansion:
a) An important blood test taken prior to surgery is *coagulation* time. (adjective; medical term)
b) A *coagulant* is an agent that promotes or stimulates the thickening or coagulation of blood. (noun)
c) An *anticoagulant* is a pharmaceutical agent (a medication) used to decrease the clotting time in blood. (noun)

6. Tissue (noun)

In context:
a) Connective tissue is only one of four types of tissue in the body.
b) When tissue has died it is identified as necrotic.

Meaning: The word *tissue* used in a medical context can best be explained as
a) an aggregate of proliferous microorganisms
b) a collection of similar cells that together form skin, muscles, and other organs
c) integument
d) a collection of organic material

7. Purulent *(adjective)*

In context:
a) Purulent discharge from a wound is commonly referred to as pus.
b) The wound is discharging a malodorous (foul smelling), green-colored substance.

Meaning: The word *purulent* can best be explained as
a) consisting of or containing pus
b) heated or elevated temperature
c) rotting or decomposing
d) all of the above

Word expansion:
a) A nurse or doctor is qualified to assess a wound for *purulence.* (noun)

VOCABULARY ALERT: THE WORD "PUS" Pus is a fluid-like substance that results from decaying or decayed cells, dead tissues, and inflammation. A pustule is a small, raised spot on the skin that contains pus. A common example of a pustule is a pimple. Pus does not have to be encapsulated in a pustule and can be found in wound beds.

Answering Specific Questions. Take a moment to review the reading. Answer the following questions in your own words.

1) Explain the term "coagulate" in a medical context.

_____

2) What are sutures?

_____

3) What are steri-strips?

_____

4) Define tissue loss.

_____

5) Why would someone prefer steri-strips to sutures?

_____

Mix and Match. Using your previous knowledge from nursing and medicine, and that which you have learned through *Medical English Clear and Simple,* connect the word or term in Box 7-4 with the proper explanation.

BOX 7-4 Mix and Match: Wound Healing

Connect the word or term with the proper explanation. Draw a line to connect the answers.

WORD OR TERM	EXPLANATION
tissue	pebbly tissue that forms in and over a wound
approximation	epithelial and connective tissue that re-covers a wound
granulation	most visible layer of a wound
contraction	movement inward of the wound's edges
wound bed	two straight edges come together

Communicating Descriptions to Peers. When the nurse removes the dressing from a patient's wound, she or he must observe any drainage or discharge for color and smell. She or he must also note the overall status of the wound by describing it as healing, deteriorating, necrotizing, or showing signs of infection. Wounds also drain and discharge in the healing process. It is the responsibility of a health professional to recognize and report abnormalities.

For each exercise below, write a full sentence. Imagine that you are a nurse and this is the sentence you want to say to another nurse. You want to communicate your message clearly and simply. To succeed, you will need to recall vocabulary from all chapters in *Medical English Clear and Simple,* particularly this one.

1) Your patient is a soldier. He was wounded overseas, treated at the hospital there, and has now been sent home to your hospital. He had a piece of shrapnel (fragment of a bomb) in his left calf. The wound is not healing.

   a) Use the noun *necrosis* in a full, complete sentence. Tell another nurse about your findings.

   _____

   b) You notice that the wound also has a foul smell. In a full sentence, describe what you will say to the same nurse.

   _____

2) A wound is described as purulent when it is discharging yellow- or green-colored pus. A badly infected wound will remain purulent until treated.

   a) Use the adjective *purulent* in a full, complete sentence to describe a man who has an infected wound. This is the sentence you will use to communicate your findings to a colleague.

   _____

   _____

   b) Include two other symptoms this man may be experiencing as a result of an infected wound. Tell your colleague this, too.

   _____

3) You were a student assisting Nurse Robby today. In your company, he removed the dressing from Mr. Stanfield's abdomen (who is 2 days post-surgery). In a team conference later that morning, he reported that the patient's dressing was minimally wet with serosanguineous drainage and had no odor. The wound itself appeared moist and healing. Subjectively, the patient said he was comfortable.

   a) Write sentences that will help you describe to another student nurse what Nurse Robby reported.

   _____

4) When a nurse lifts the dressing off a wound, she inspects the dressing for signs of drainage or discharge. Today, as the student nurse, you note your patient's dressing has a light pink, watery looking color to it. You know this means it contains both blood and serum and is called serosanguineous drainage.

   a) In a full, complete sentence tell a medical intern what you found in this mutual patient.

   _____

5) Your patient is 6 hours postoperative. You find him moaning in bed. He is diaphoretic and not fully conscious. You check the surgical site. The dressing is wet and very red.

   a) Tell a colleague immediately what you have found.

   _____

b) Tell the doctor what you have discovered and what you want.

6) To discharge something is to excrete, secrete, or evacuate it. In the case of a wound, natural healing includes all of these processes.

   a) In a full, complete sentence name one process in which the body excretes materials into the wound bed to protect it from infection and identify what it excretes. Use one of these choices: antibiotics, immunity, granulation.

7) Wounds can smell, particularly when they are infected or necrotic. The term for this is "foul smelling."

   a) Manuel has a deep decubitus ulcer on his coccyx from lying in bed for 1 month after his accident. You are the home care nurse. As you begin to cleanse his wound, you notice a smell. Tell a colleague about your findings.

SPEAKING EXERCISE

Read the following short paragraph aloud. Ask a peer or teacher to help you with pronunciation. The Pronunciation Hints box that follows will help.

Inflammation is a natural response to infection. It is a process generated by the immune system. It stimulates and sends an increased blood supply to the site to promote healing. This gives the area a reddish color. We can say the site looks "angry." Leukocytes and other fluids accumulate and the site of infection swells. A localized area of warmth is part of the inflammatory process and a generalized fever indicates that the immune system is at work to battle infection.

PRONUNCIATION HINTS

sanguineous – **săng**-gwĭn′ĕ-ŭs

foul – **fow′l**

tissue – **tĭsh′ū**

sutures – **sū′chūrz**

purulent – **pūr′ū-lĕnt**

LISTENING EXERCISE

Go back online. Listen to professionals discuss wound care.

1) Try Google or a similarly popular search engine. At the top of the Google screen is a menu. Click on VIDEO. You will be sent to Google's video search engine. Search for these key words: wound care, wound care nurse, wound treatment. You will find a wide variety of video clips. Choose one or two to listen to and study the way language is both used and pronounced.

2) You might also like to listen to some simple discussions of wounds and wound care on "Expert Village" at http://www.expertvillage.com.

3) For a more professional, technical discussion of wounds look up the Penn Wound Care Center videos by Dr. Kirksey. Find these on *YouTube* at http://www.youtube.com or simply type in the search words: Penn Wound Care Center videos.

WRITING EXERCISE

We have come to the end of Unit 7. It has been quite comprehensive and, at times, technical. Take some time now to write down your thought about this chapter. Reflect on how your ability to talk about wounds, viruses, and infections has improved through the readings and exercises herein.

_____

_____

_____

_____

Pathophysiology

READING SELECTION 1—WOUNDS

Understanding the General Meaning

1) stabbing with a knife

2) bony prominences (could also say coccyx and back of heel)

3) emotional

4) No, it's another type of injury

5) No, not unless the skin is broken, as in a compound fracture

6) dermal ulcer, pressure sore, bedsore

Building Vocabulary

Determining Meaning from Context

1) c, 2) c, 3) b, 4) d, 5) a, 6) b

Sentence Completion

1) puncture

2) tetanus

3) 12–24 hours

4) artery

5) cleanse

6) crush

7) integumentary system

8) bedsore

Identifying Types of Wounds

1) deep puncture

2) puncture wound

3) bruise

4) bedsore

5) laceration

6) crush injury

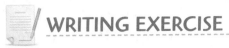

WRITING EXERCISE

Examples of possible answers:

1) A knife can cause a stab wound.

2) An intramuscular injection uses a long needle which causes a small but deep puncture wound.

3) Areas around bony prominences are candidates for skin breakdown and the formation of decubitus ulcers.

4) The act of betrayal can cause a deep emotional wound to the psyche.

5) A spider bite is a type of puncture wound.

READING SELECTION 2—SOME DISEASE-CAUSING MICROORGANISMS: VIRUSES AND BACTERIA

Understanding the General Meaning

1) The gist of the reading is that viruses can invade cells of a host where they can then reproduce and cause disease. Viruses can be studied and detected and the diseases they cause treated and immunized against. In contrast, bacteria do not need to invade a host cell in order to reproduce.

2) The purpose of the text is to provide information about viruses in a brief overview of the subject. It is an information report.

3) Virology is the study of viruses.

4) They live off, feed off, or exist off and can destroy or take over a host organism.

5) No. Rationale: There are vaccines for some, but not all, viruses

6) Yes. Rationale: Some virus-caused diseases may be untreatable and lead to death. This may occur slowly or rapidly, depending on the disease and the health of the infected individual.

7) A simple difference between viruses and bacteria is that viruses need to invade a host cell in order to reproduce; bacteria do not.

8) Viral infections cannot be treated with antibiotics. They are treated with different types of medications. Bacteria-caused infections are often treated with antibiotics.

Building Vocabulary

Determining Meaning from Context

1) c, 2) a, 3) d, 4) d, 5) d

Using New Vocabulary in Sentences

Examples of sentences:

1) Immunization programs are occurring around the world in an attempt to combat child-hood diseases.

2) To detect whether or not a virus is present in the blood, serology tests are ordered by the physician.

3) A pathogen is an agent of disease.

4) In the tropics, intestinal worms are examples of parasitic invasion of the intestinal tract.

5) Worldwide, a great deal of money goes into research in an attempt to discover how to eradicate and prevent viral infection and disease.

Common Disorders and Diseases

READING SELECTION 3—DECUBITUS ULCERS

Understanding the General Meaning

1) Decubitus ulcer wounds progress in stages, can be assessed using a scale, and can be very hard to treat once they occur.

2) Key words: "can be very painful and difficult to treat," "prevention of further skin deterioration," and "use a scale."

Learning Specific Information

1) decubitus ulcer or skin ulcer

2) the nurse

3) stage 4

4) to remove necrotic tissue

5) dead

6) near a bony prominence such as coccyx and back of the heel

7) when the patient spends a long time in one position, particularly lying down

8) A deep wound is one in which there is full thickness skin loss and extensive destruction of tissue. There may also be damage to muscle and other underlying tissues.

Building Vocabulary

Understanding a Clinical Pathway

1) Any three of these are correct:

- Reposition in bed every 1–2 hours.

- Assist with range of motion exercises in bed prn to promote circulation.

- Keep area clean and protective barrier creams/dressings may be necessary.

- Ensure bed linens are dry and wrinkle free, particularly under the site to reduce friction and sheering of skin.

- Use a fluctuating air mattress if available (it will alleviate pressure to sites automatically via fluctuating air flow).

2) Any of these actions are correct:

- Assist to reposition.

- Assist with movement or ambulation.

- When in bed, turn every 2 hours.

- Keep area clean and dry.

- Use a low air loss mattress if available to decrease moisture such as perspiration and alleviate some pressure.

3) No special care is required.

Fill in the Blanks.

1) Mary, please come take a look at Mr. Howe's toe. He froze it when he got lost snowmobiling. It isn't <u>healing</u>. It is <u>showing signs of infection</u>. It's actually turning black. I'm sure it's <u>necrotic</u>. I think I'd better call the doctor back to look at it, but I'd like your professional opinion first.

2) Dr. Wilson, Mr. Rubens' abdominal wound is <u>healing</u> well. The dressing is <u>dry</u> and there is very little <u>discharge</u> from the Penrose drain. I think we could remove it now. What do you think?

3) Thanks for calling me, Marge. I've just been in to check Mr. Harcourt in bed 6. His gunshot wound is not <u>healing</u>. You're right, it has a foul-smelling <u>discharge</u> and is <u>showing signs</u> of infection. He looks diaphoretic. What's his latest temperature?

 # WRITING EXERCISE

Charting examples:

1) 3 July 2008 at 10:25 <u>am</u>. Pt. is bedridden and complains of pain in area of coccyx. Site is reddened, skin is breaking down, and the area is the size of a penny. Possible Stage 2 bedsore: doctor notified and orders are pending. Will turn every 2 hours. M. Johnson, RN.
<u>Rationale:</u> Components of this charting include date and time of assessment, subjective data from patient, objective data obtained through observation and knowledge of patient's situation, evidence of a clinical judgment (in this case, to call the doctor) based on sound nursing knowledge that the wound may need a dressing. Identifies a nursing plan to intervene to protect the site. Nurse signs her name to end the entry. The patient's age and name are not written into the notes. They will appear at the top of each and every page in his chart. Pt. is an acceptable abbreviation for patient in many facilities.

2) 18 October 2008 at 2:44 pm. Pt. is currently lying on her side in bed, resting. No complaints of pain or discomfort. Decubitus ulcer to spine examined. No change from yesterday. Size and color remain constant. Cleansed. Clean dressing applied per doctor's orders. Pt. will remain in bed today to avoid aggravation to the wound site from sitting in her wheelchair. —M. Johnson, RN.
<u>Rationale:</u> Many of the core features of this charting entry are similar to those in the last example.

3) 15 February 2008 at 16:00 hrs. Seen in cast clinic for removal of cast to left leg. Skin dry, cracked, and flaking, but not open. Color and shape are good. Wound posteriorly to heel where it has rubbed against the cast. Stage 3 ulcer. Pt. complains of soreness at site. Doctor notified to assess. Pt. teaching done. Wound cleansed. Awaiting doctor's visit. —M. Johnson, RN.
<u>Rationale:</u> The nurse includes objective and subjective data and makes an assessment of the patient's condition based on that. Information is included regarding notifying the doctor to legally demonstrate the nurse has taken all action required to assist the patient. Patient teaching is an essential element of all care and is expected to be given by both nurses and doctors in the United States and Canada. Here, the nurse charts that she has done so. She includes it because it is part of the expectation of care and she has provided it. The word *posteriorly* is used to describe the location of this wound. While this is not grammatically correct (nor is the word recognized in most dictionaries), it is acceptable medical jargon in many places.

4) 12 September 2009 at 0800 hrs. Given morning care and bed bath. Assessed for skin breakdown. Reddened area to right elbow, only. No complaints of discomfort re: same. High risk for bedsores: bedridden for 2 weeks. Suspect Stage 1 ulcer developing. Area gently massaged to promote circulation. Right and left arms both repositioned to alleviate pressure to the

areas. Pt. teaching done regarding same. Monitor every shift.   —M. Johnson, RN.
<u>Rationale:</u> Many of the core features of this charting entry are explained in the previous examples. **Please note: Some facilities have very strong policies that massage is NOT recommended and NOT to be done in these circumstances. Please clarify same with your employer or clinical site.**

READING SELECTION 4—COMMON VIRAL DISEASES

Understanding the General Meaning

1) The purpose of this text is to explain viruses and how they are spread and to identify some common types of viral diseases.

2) Yes, it provides basic information about viruses and how they are transmitted.

3) The main thesis of this text is that viral diseases are common and they can be contagious.

4) No, all viruses are not contagious.

5) Common cold, influenza, HIV/AIDS, hepatitis C, Norwalk virus.

Building Vocabulary

Determining Meaning from Context

1) c, 2) c, 3) c, 4) a, 5) b, 6) c

Mix and Match

BOX 7-3 Mix and Match: Reporting a Viral Respiratory Infection: Answers

raspy voice	a scratchy, rough sound
productive cough	expels or dislodges mucous
congested	blocked sinuses; hard to breathe
feverish	showing signs of having a fever; diaphoretic
sniffling	nose is runny; doesn't blow it
SOB	shortness of breath
ashen	pale, grey color to skin

Sentence Completion

1) If a virus <u>invades</u> my respiratory system, I <u>get</u> an infection.

2) If a harmful microorganism <u>finds</u> a reservoir in the surgical wound bed, it will <u>contaminate it</u>.

3) If Jackie can't <u>cough</u>, she <u>won't clear</u> her lungs of the pathogens.

4) If the postoperative patient <u>develops</u> an infection, he likely <u>will develop</u> a fever as well.

5) If the sutures <u>break</u> or don't hold, the patient's wound <u>will open</u>.

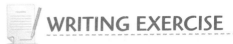

WRITING EXERCISE

Script writing example:

Public Health Nurse (PHN): Good morning, Public Health Clinic, Marjorie speaking.

Mother (Mom): Yes, hello. I wonder if you can help me? I think my little girl might have chickenpox. She's got a rash on her belly and its itchy and . . .

PHN: All right. Let's see if I can help you. How old is your little girl?

Mom: She's 8 years old.

PHN: Has she had any immunization: any vaccine for chickenpox in the last few years?

Mom: No, we didn't get her that. You know, she started feeling kind of fussy—you know, irritable and cranky yesterday. She didn't want to get up in the morning and she really didn't want to go to school, but I made her. She didn't really look sick at the time.

PHN: And how does she look today?

Mom: Well, she's warm to the touch. I took her temperature and it's up a little. It's 100°F (37.7°C). That's not too high, is it?

PHN: No, that's not too high. Any other symptoms? You said she has a rash.

Mom: Yes, she has red spots on her belly. Well, not like measles, though. I know what they look like: small red spots and lots of them all over. This is different. Bigger spots and not so many of them. She says they itch.

PHN: Uh-huh. And how does she say she feels?

Mom: Sick, she says she's sick and she wants to go back to bed and its only 3:00 in the afternoon! She must be sick to say that!

PHN: Yes, that's a bit unusual for a child, all right. You said you think your daughter has chickenpox. What leads you to believe that? Has she been in contact with anyone else with that disease?

Mom: Oh, well, unfortunately, yes. Four or five of the kids in her grade 2 classroom have come down with it. They're away from school this week, but they got it last week.

PHN: Well, that sounds like your culprit, but I can't say for sure over the phone. I am assuming the child has never had chickenpox before?

Mom: No.

PHN: All right, then here's what I suggest. Chickenpox in young children is pretty un-complicated, but that doesn't mean you shouldn't watch her. Keep her home from school. Those red bumps she has will turn into little blister-like sores that will break open, dry, and crust over. That's normal in this illness. You must keep her away from other people until all of the sores have crusted over to prevent spreading the disease, OK?

Mom: OK. You want me to keep her at home and also away from contact with other people. Gee, I don't think I can get that much time off work without being docked pay. Gee . . .

PHN: That sounds like a problem for you. Is there anyone else in the family that can help?

Mom: Well, her dad could stay home a few days. He's out of town on business, but he'll be back tomorrow. Yes, OK ... maybe he and I can split our days off from work and it won't be so financially difficult.

PHN: That sounds like a good plan. And try not to let your daughter scratch. She could cause an infection in one of those sores. Use a soothing lotion to stop the itch. The pharmacist at your local drugstore can suggest one. Most importantly, give your daughter's physician's office a call just to notify them. The doctor may or may not want to see her. I'll contact the school and follow-up on how many cases of chickenpox are being reported there right now.

Mom: OK. How long will this last? About a week or so?

PHN: Yes, about a week.

Mom: OK, thanks. Bye.

READING SELECTION 5—A COMMON BACTERIAL INFECTION: TUBERCULOSIS

Understanding the General Meaning

1) The main topic of this text is tuberculosis.

2) Bacteria can reproduce themselves; viruses cannot: they must invade a host cell in order to replicate. Another difference is that bacterial diseases can be treated with antibiotics, whereas viral diseases cannot.

3) TB

4) TB infects the respiratory tract primarily.

5) Exposure to TB is risky because the disease is contagious and you could catch it.

6) Yes, TB can lay dormant in the body.

7) Yes, there is a cure for TB.

8) Yes. The treatment for TB is take medications (often isoniazid) for an extended period of time until all of the TB bacteria have been eradicated from the body. (Note: Only after this treatment can a person say they are cured.)

Building Vocabulary

Determining Meaning from Context

1) a, 2) c, 3) d

Fill in the Blanks

1) treating – present participle of the verb, treat + auxiliary verb (is)

2) covering – present participle + auxiliary verb (is)

3) recovered – past participle of the verb, recover + auxiliary verb (has)

4) collapsed – past participle of the verb, collapse + auxiliary verb (has)

5) remembering – present participle of the verb, remember + auxiliary verb (are)

6) waiting – present participle of the verb, wait + auxiliary verb (is)

7) forgotten – past participle of the verb, forget. Can be revised as: He felt forgotten by his family. "Felt" is a verb of perception.

8) coming – present participle of the verb, come + auxiliary verb, be (is) + base form of verb, come (coming)

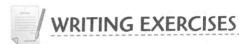

WRITING EXERCISES

Examples of possible answers:

1) Draft:

- TB is contagious.

- TB is passed by droplets in the air through coughing, sneezing, even laughing or shouting.

- TB sometimes just seems like it is the symptoms of a chest cold.

- TB is treatable but it takes a long time. You must comply with treatment or you won't be cured.

- Untreated, you may get very, very sick and could possibly die and that is why I am sending him to hospital to be admitted today. (I've got to teach him this so he will comply with treatment right through to the end.) Here's how I think I'll start . . .

Health Provider (HP): Hi, Mr. Webster. Nice to see you again.

Mr. Webster: Hi. Did my lab results come back yet? I assume that's why you called me and wanted me to come in today.

HP: Yes, that's correct. Please, have a seat. Mr. Webster, your tests have come back positive to TB. You have tuberculosis.

Mr. Webster: Damn! What does that mean? Expensive treatments and hospital bills?

HP: Well, Mr. Webster, well, actually it does mean you have to go to the hospital. Is that OK?

Mr. Webster: No!

HP: I mean, Mr. Webster, let's talk about the illness first . . .

2a) Yes, I am trying to be more client-centered. I can see that I have knowledge about tuberculosis that I want to share with my client so that he will get better. I can see that I have to ask him first about his own level of knowledge about the illness. That is the respectful thing to do. I can't assume he has no knowledge whatsoever. Once I find out what he knows about the disease I will be able to supplement what he knows. I want to be respectful and not treat him like he isn't smart or knowledgeable. I also want to think about how I engage him in conversation. I must treat him as an equal, with respect and sincerity.

2b) If I let him know I honestly care about him and his health, then I think he will be more open to sitting with me to discuss his illness and the need for treatment in the hospital. I will use good eye contact, sit with him to talk (not behind my desk). I think it's a very good idea if I ask him about his life in general. Maybe there are circumstances such as work, family, and finances that will make him reluctant to being admitted to the hospital. I'll want to explore this with him. If we work together on this, I hope he will see that it is OK to be admitted. I will also use communication skills of paraphrasing, summarizing

Wounds, Viral and Bacterial Infections

or reflecting back to the client what he has said to me to be sure I am understanding him correctly. This will let him know I am understanding him and hearing him.

2c) I have a tendency to use closed-ended questions and am trying to break this habit. I will use open-ended questions whenever possible in my script because they are more facilitative.

2d) I will determine how much information to include in the teaching by asking the client what he knows, first.

2e) What kind of word choices will I need to make so that he can clearly understand me? In my final script I will use words that are clear and appropriate for the type of communication style my client has. I will not use words he does not understand, but I won't speak in very simple terms to him if he is capable of much more. I must be careful about this not to talk above or below my client.

2f) I asked him what he has learned today and if he had any questions.

2g) Yes, sort of. I followed the format for writing an explanation, but I changed it to fit the format of a script; a dialogue.

Completed Script: A Dialogue

HP: Hi, Mr. Webster. Nice to see you again.

Mr. Webster: Hi. Did my lab results come back yet? I assume that's why you called me and wanted me to come in today.

HP: Yes, that's correct. Please, have a seat. Mr. Webster, your tests have come back positive for TB. You have tuberculosis.

Mr. Webster: Damn! What does that mean? Expensive treatments and hospital bills?

HP: Well, Mr. Webster, let's start from the beginning. What do you know about TB?

Mr. Webster: Well, I know something about it. It's a disease of the lungs. It makes you cough and sometimes you cough up dark, ugly stuff from your lungs. That's what I've been doing.

HP: Yes, that's correct. And it was that sputum from your lungs that we sent in for testing.
What else do you know, Mr. Webster?

Mr. Webster: Well, I know from commercials on TV that TB is contagious and I have to take pills for it. How much do they cost? How long do I have to take them? Damn! My medical coverage is not very good. How am I going to pay for that?

HP: I can see you have some serious concerns about your finances, Mr. Webster.

Mr. Webster: Yeah, that's for sure.

HP: Perhaps we can talk a bit about that in a minute. First, though, we need to talk about your treatment. I'm afraid that your TB is serious enough to require admission to the hospital.

Mr. Webster: What? You must be kidding! No way! Impossible! I've got a wife and three kids to feed. No chance! I can't afford that!

HP: I can hear your anxiety, Mr. Webster. Let's try to work this out together so we can find a healthy solution for both you and your family, all right?

Mr. Webster: Like what?

HP: Well, as you know, TB is contagious. That means your family is also at risk for acquiring it. We'll need to test them.

Mr. Webster: You mean I could make my family sick?

HP: Well, not you per se. . . the disease. It's best then that you don't remain in the home. I have made arrangements for you to be admitted to County General Hospital today.

Mr. Webster: Oh my God!

HP: Yes, I know it's a lot to think about, Mr. Webster. I can see your concern. How can I help you with that?

Mr. Webster: Just give me the pills to take. I promise I'll take them. I can't leave my job and go to the hospital.

HP: I'm afraid it's not as simple as that. Patients with acute TB need to be hospitalized for their own protection and that of others. You wouldn't want to spread it at home, work, and even in your neighborhood.

Mr. Webster: You're right, but what choice do I have? I have to work!

HP: OK, let's talk about that for a bit. I know you have medical insurance because you've come to see me. Treatment for TB takes quite awhile, but you will be able to go back to work before your treatment is completed. It is just for now, the next month or so, that you will need to be in hospital. If this is going to be a very big hardship financially, I can refer you to someone in our office that is very helpful for finding additional resources for you. If you need a note for your employer, I'd like you to know we can say you are off on medical leave, but your diagnosis will be completely confidential from your employer.

Mr. Webster: Oh . . . I'll have to think about all of this. What a mess! I really am going to need some help.

HP: All right, Mr. Webster. Let's get planning. After we talk a bit more, you'll need to head to the hospital where they are expecting you, OK?

Mr. Webster: Well, it's not really OK, but I know I need to get better. I need to get better for my wife and kids.

HP: Yes, Mr. Webster. Let's begin . . .

Treatments, Interventions, and Assistance

READING SELECTION 6—CHAIN OF INFECTION AND INFECTION CONTROL

Understanding the General Meaning

1) Minute organisms (microorganisms) that cause disease are known as pathogens, and their life cycle follows the chain of infection. When there is no infection present, an organism is said to be aseptic or sterile. (33 words)

Wounds, Viral and Bacterial Infections

2) surgical asepsis, asepsis, clean technique, medical asepsis, Standard Precautions, Universal Precautions.

3)

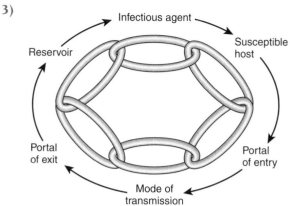

Building Vocabulary

Determining Meaning from Context

1) b, 2) a, 3) d

Practicing Spelling

1) microorganisms

2) cyclical

3) mode

4) pathogen

5) bacterial

6) transmission

7) sterile

8) causative

9) infectious

10) reservoir

Fill in the Blank

1) losing

2) having

3) staying

4) working

5) coughing

6) recovering

Writing Exercise

1a) My first thought about this story is that the woman's wound is infected.

1b) The gist of this story is that a woman cut herself and now the wound is infected.

1c) Janice is the main character of the story.

1d) My working diagnosis is wound infection.

1e) I am not her nurse or doctor, so I would suggest she have the wound looked at by a medical professional as soon as possible. I might then suggest that she cleanse it again and apply a new, clean bandage in the meantime.

1f) Night school is a term used to describe classes that are only taken at night (i.e., between 6:00 and 10:00 p.m.). Night school can be held at any school, college, or university. Usually, only adults attend night school.

2a) My first thought about this situation is that Steven has contracted a virus that is making him sick. I base this on his signs and symptoms.

2b) The gist of this story is that a man with a virus was traveling on a plane with other people and he may have infected other people on the plane.

2c) Steven is the main character in this story.

2d) My working diagnosis is a viral respiratory infection. I base this on his respiratory symptoms.

2e) I would suggest he isolate himself from others until the acute phase of this illness is over. I would also suggest he contact a doctor or nurse practitioner for assessment and treatment. My rationale for this is to stop the spread of the virus if indeed it is contagious. (I don't actually know if it is or not.)

2f) My prognosis is that all passengers on the plane have been in some degree exposed to the virus and may fall ill.

3a) I wonder if she has tuberculosis. I base this on my knowledge of TB and that it has not been eradicated or well controlled in many Third World countries such as Nigeria.

3b) The gist of this story is that an immigrant woman has an undiagnosed cough secondary to her epilepsy, but because the cough is more acute and obvious it is the focus of the story.

3c) Zarah is the main character of this story.

3d) My working diagnosis is tuberculosis, but I would want to rule out the common cold, influenza, and allergies before arriving at a final diagnosis. My rationale for this: I have no proof this woman has been in contact with someone with tuberculosis who may have exposed her to it. I understand I may have assumed too much because of where she has came from. As a professional, I must remain nonjudgmental and open-minded and search for the truth. I will do so by completing a comprehensive health assessment.

3e) My initial response to the situation (suspecting TB) is to put this patient into an isolation room. However, this is not standard protocol based on suspicion. I will leave her in a regular bed on the unit while completing the assessment. I will minimize her contact with others in the interim. I will provide tissues, hand sanitizers, a basin or container into which she can cough, and encourage her to cover her mouth when coughing. I will explain to the patient why she should and must (at least temporarily) limit her contact with/exposure to others.

READING SELECTION 7—WOUND HEALING

Understanding the General Meaning

1) how wounds heal

2) primary intention healing

3) superficial (not deep) wounds where the edges are easily placed back together alongside each other

4) secondary intention healing

5) a wound that is a little or moderately deep and the edges can't be easily moved back together again. There is tissue loss between the two edges. This wound might be wide.

6) tertiary intention healing

7) a very deep wound where there is loss to epithelial, muscle, and maybe even bone tissue

Understanding Specific Information

1) primary

2) tertiary

3) secondary

4) *in situ* means in place or situated in a place; dwelling or residing in a specific place

Building Vocabulary

Determining Meaning from Context

1) a, 2) b, 3) d, 4) b, 5) c, 6) b, 7) a

Answering Specific Questions

1) To coagulate is to thicken, to gel, or to clot.

2) Sutures are the links in a surgically made process to bring two edges of surfaces (i.e., tissue) together and hold them there until healing can occur. Note: A suture is a specific material (such as catgut) that is used to re-join surfaces in a process similar to sewing. The synonym for sutures comes from the language of sewing. It is stitches. Each suture is a stitch.

3) Steri-strips are a type of adhesive dressing that comes in small strips. They are used instead of surgical stitches to approximate the edges of superficial lacerations or wounds, particularly on the face.

4) When tissue is lost, it has either been removed from the site (via trauma, disease, infection, or surgery) or it has died and it is therefore unable to replace or regenerate itself.

5) They are often the treatment of choice by patients, doctors, and nurses to avoid scarring of the skin.

Mix and Match

BOX 7-4 Mix and Match: Wound Healing: Answers

WORD OR TERM	EXPLANATION
tissue	epithelial and connective cells that re-cover a wound
approximation	two straight edges come together
granulation	pebbly tissue that forms in and over a wound
contraction	movement inward of the wound's edges
wound bed	most visible layer of a wound

Communicating Descriptions to Peers

Sample answers:

1a) This morning, I noticed the patient's wound has begun to blacken around the edges and show signs of necrosis.

1b) The first thing I noticed besides the poor wound color was the slight smell of decay: a foul smell.

2a) I treated a man in the clinic today whose wound was purulent and discharging pus.

2b) That same man was diaphoretic, had a fever, and was complaining about pain at and around the wound.

3a) Nurse Robby reported to the team that his patient's wound was healing well, that there was minimal serosanguineous drainage, and the wound bed was still moist.

4a) When I changed the patient's dressing, it was wet with slight serosanguineous discharge, which I think can be expected post-surgery.

5a) My patient is deteriorating. He's showing signs of bleeding at the surgical site and he's in pain. I'll stay with him. Please alert the doctor.

5b) Doctor, the patient is bleeding at the surgical site, he's diaphoretic, moaning, and no longer oriented to time or place. Please come.

6a) Through the process of granulation tiny grains of connective tissue are excreted by the body into a wound.

7a) Manuel's wound isn't healing well. It is increasingly foul-smelling and the tissue around it is now very red and angry.

UNIT 8

This unit contains an introduction to the language of pharmacology, the actions of medications, and related concepts. It contains a great deal of terminology that may be new to you. The focus is on the written word. The ability to read, write, or transpose medication orders both correctly and safely is paramount to the health professional's career. The ability to discuss medications and the underlying principles of pharmacology are also essential to good patient care. In this regard, Unit 8 will be extremely helpful to those who wish to communicate with English-speaking health professionals and patients about this important subject.

Pharmacology, Pharmacodynamics, and Pharmacokinetics

An understanding of the language of pharmacology, pharmacodynamics, and pharmacokinetics is crucial to safe and effective health-care delivery. These subjects provide the foundational knowledge required for prescribing and administering medications. Language competencies in these fields can positively or negatively affect patient outcomes.

Reading Selection 8-1

Read the following text aloud or silently to yourself. Observe the use of the roots pharma *and* pharmac *in preparation for exercises that follow. This will help build a vocabulary repertoire (a collection; a resource) for the root. You might want to circle each word that contains the root word as you read.*

ALL THINGS PHARMACOLOGICAL

Pharmacology is the study of the science of drugs, the mechanisms of drug actions and interactions, and the conditions under which drugs can be used. Pharmaceutics is a branch of pharmacology wherein drugs are manufactured and identified as medicinal by pharmaceutical companies. They make up the pharmaceutical industry.

Pharmacodynamics, on the other hand, is the study of how drugs manipulate cells in the body: how they affect cells. In this field, drugs are studied for their positive or negative effects on organisms. A positive effect may make it medicinal in nature. This is known as a therapeutic response. A negative or fatal effect of the drug on cells will inform scientists of the dangers of the drugs and/or certain drug combinations. Sometimes a drug targeted to affect one type of cell will be found to inadvertently affect others, leading to the discovery of a secondary effect. The medication acetylsalicylic acid (aspirin) is a good example of this. Identified primarily for its analgesic and antipyretic effect, it has more recently been recognized as an effective anticoagulant.

Knowledge of pharmacokinetics is essential for health professionals when administering, monitoring, or teaching about medications. Pharmacokinetics is the study of the biological processes or movement that occurs once a medication enters the body. These processes include:

- absorption – how the drug enters the body and enters into the bloodstream. How is it absorbed?

- distribution – how the drug is distributed and where it goes in the body after absorption.

- metabolism – how the drug is changed or broken down into metabolites by the body and how long this takes.

- elimination – how the drug or its metabolites leave the body.

Finally, pharmacotherapeutics is the study and use of drugs that promote health and healing. Pharmacotherapeutics are commonly referred to as "drug therapies" by professionals and lay persons alike. Medicines are used for their therapeutic effects on the body and mind. In the United States and Canada there is an increasing demand by consumers for alternative medicines of more natural origins rather than synthetic medications created by the pharmaceutical industry. Health professionals must be alert to this fact, knowledgeable about alternative medicines, and prepared to discuss the implications of their use or concurrent use with manufactured, synthetic medications. The best resource for expert advice on the medicinal use of drugs is a compendium of pharmaceuticals or a hospital formulary. The expert to consult is the pharmacist.

VOCABULARY ALERT: MEDICINE OR DRUG? The terms *medicine* and *drug* are often used interchangeably. The plural forms are medicines and drugs.
The term *meds* is commonly used by health professionals and is quite career-specific. Clients who have long-term, chronic illnesses are familiar with this term and they too may refer to their *meds* when speaking to others.

 READING EXERCISES

The sometimes confusing vocabulary associated with pharmacology and medication administration can be learned through a variety of exercises including those about the use of prefixes, suffixes, and roots in forming words; about how similar sounding words have different meanings; and by building vocabulary through determining the meaning of a word from its context.

Understanding the General Meaning

Read the text All Things Pharmacological again. Think about it, then answer the following questions.

1) There are two main themes in the text you have just read. Identify them.

_____

2) What example was used to support the claim that an unexpected therapeutic effect of a drug can be accidentally or inadvertently discovered?

_____

GRAMMAR REVIEW: ROOT WORDS, PREFIXES, AND SUFFIXES IN MEDICAL TERMINOLOGY A *root word* is the basic element of a word upon which all meaning is built. Sometimes two root words may appear together in one word.
   A *prefix* is an element of a word that is added to the beginning of a root word to make it more specific.
   A *suffix* is an element of a word that is added to the end of the root word to make it more specific.

Linking or combining vowels placed in between word parts helps with pronunciation. Take a look at the following example of the root words *pharma* and *pharmac*. The roots *pharma* and *pharmac* originate in Greek as the word *pharmakon*, meaning drug. Hence, all words containing these root words in English will refer to drugs. The root word *pharma* requires other word elements to have meaning. It cannot stand alone as a word. Notice how new words and meanings are created from the root words:

pharmac + ology = pharmacology (root + suffix)

pharmac + eutical = pharmaceutical (root + suffix)

pharmac + o + dynamics = pharmacodynamics (root + linking vowel + root)

pharmac + o + kinetics = pharmacokinetics (root + linking vowel + root)

Mix and Match. The many terms used to describe the subdivisions of pharmacology can be confusing. Use the exercise in Box 8-1 to help you learn the distinctions between somewhat similar terms.

Fill in the Blanks. Fill in the blanks with the appropriate term.

1) A ———————— dispenses meds from the ————————.

2) A ———————— company manufactures and may do research into drugs.

3) The desired ———————— effect of a medication taken only at bedtime is sleep.

4) Chemotherapy is a type of ———————— that kills dividing cancer cells.

5) Identifying when and how all traces of a drug have been eliminated from the body is the realm of ————————.

6) Each and every hospital unit, clinic, and licensed care home will have this book or one like it, easily at hand for reference. It is called a compendium of ————————.

7) The study and research foundational to chemotherapy for cancer is part of the scientific field called ————————.

> **VOCABULARY ALERT: PHARMACOLOGICAL VERSUS PHARMALOGICAL** The term *pharmalogical* is heard from time to time in common speech. It is not a proper word and should not be used by health professionals. The proper and correct term is *pharmacological.*

Building Vocabulary

Determining Meaning from Context. To build vocabulary, study the following words and terms taken from the reading. Discover all you can about them by looking at them in these

---

BOX 8-1 Mix and Match: Words Derived from *Pharma*

Complete the following exercise, linking a term beginning with/deriving from the root pharma to its definition.

WORD	DEFINITION
pharmacokinetics	science of drugs, their actions, and interactions
pharmacotherapeutics	movement of drugs through the body
pharmaceuticals	helping or healing effects of drugs
pharmacodynamics	understands and dispenses medications
pharmacology	synthetic or manufactured drugs
pharmacist	how drugs affect cells

new examples. Next, go on to choose the correct meaning for the word from the choices provided. Finally, take a look at how the words expand in English.

1. Mechanisms *(noun, plural)*

In context:
a) The mechanisms of transport for antipsychotic medications are the neurotransmitters.
b) The mechanisms of action for antibiotics explain how these medications work.

Meaning: The best way to explain the term *mechanisms* in the context of pharmacology is to say it means
a) the way in which an effect is obtained
b) the workers affecting a process
c) the means by which an effect is obtained
d) the means by which a process occurs
e) all except (b)
f) all of the above

Word expansion:
a) When a patient's heart stops, *mechanical* intervention must be started. This could be chest compressions or defibrillation. (adjective)
b) The patient with an acute brain injury was just put on *mechanical* ventilation. He cannot breathe on his own. (adjective)
c) Cardiac pumping *mechanics* are interrupted during a myocardial infarction. (noun)

2. Medicinal *(adjective)*

In context:
a) When a client says he is taking a medicinal cure, he means he is taking medications that he hopes or expects will cure his condition.
b) Herbal teas are often said to have medicinal properties.

Meaning: The best way to explain the term *medicinal* is to say it means
a) inguinal
b) healing
c) positively effecting
d) potentially healing
e) both (b) and (d)
f) doctor's orders

Word expansion:
a) *Medicine* is the field of study taken by doctors. (noun)
b) *Medicine* is another name for medication. We commonly say, "I need to take my medicine." (noun)
c) Belinda takes *medication* for her springtime allergies. (noun)
d) If you suffer from headaches from time to time, you probably *self-medicate* with over-the-counter analgesics. (verb)
e) Rochelle is away at *medical* school. She wants to be a doctor. (adjective)
f) The doctor wants to *medicate* the child to help him calm down before beginning to suture his wound. (verb, infinitive form)
g) *Medical* terminology is difficult to learn if you do not have an opportunity to use it in a communicative fashion. (adjective)
h) Mr. and Mrs. Dhaliwal have large *medical* bills. This worries them. (adjective)
i) *Medically* speaking, we should wait another 24 hours before operating. (adverb)

3. Analgesic *(noun)*

In context:

a) The patient was given an analgesic to help him cope with his pain.

b) In simple terms, an analgesic is a painkiller even though it does not completely destroy the sense of pain.

Meaning: The best way to explain the term *analgesic* in a pharmacological sense is to say it is

a) a chemical compound

b) any compound that reduces or alleviates pain

c) a medicinal compound that metabolizes in the intestine

d) an anti-inflammatory medication

Word expansion:

a) The goal for this patient is *analgesia*. We don't want him to experience any more pain than absolutely necessary. Use prn (as needed) liberally. (noun)

b) The *analgesic* effect of morphine is significant, but the adverse effect of addiction is always a risk. (adjective)

4. Antipyretic *(adjective or noun)*

In context:

a) The child's high temperature required administration of an antipyretic medication.

b) The fever subsided in direct response to the use of an antipyretic medication.

Meaning: The best way to explain the adjective *antipyretic* is to say it means

a) heat moderating

b) fever reducing

c) heat stimulating

d) temperature immunosuppressive

Word expansion:

a) An *antipyretic* is indicated when a small child has a very high fever. (noun)

b) The *antipyretic* effect of this particular drug is extremely valuable to health professionals and patients. (adjective)

c) Febrile is the medical term for feverish. A synonym for the term *antipyretic* is antifebrile. (adjective)

5. Compendium *(noun)*

In context:

a) Nursing standards are listed in a compendium produced by a nursing regulatory body. Check your local state or provincial nursing organization to see an example.

b) Students in the health sciences often purchase a compendium of medications to help them with their studies.

Meaning: The best way to explain the noun *compendium* is to say it is

a) a collection of pharmaceuticals

b) a comprehensive list and collection of knowledge and information

c) a formulary

d) formulations of responses and actions

Word expansion:

a) The Health Sciences section of the university library has a number of pharmaceutical *compendia* on hand. (noun, plural)

6. Formulary *(noun)*

In context:

a) Dr. Watson was considering changing the patient to a new drug, but he was not sure if it would adversely interact with the patient's other current meds. He referred to the hospital formulary for more information.

b) Health insurance programs often produce their own formularies of medications. Within it they identify which medications they will or will not approve for payment under their medical plans.

Meaning: The best way to explain the term *formulary* is to say it is

a) a list of drugs approved for prescription and their formulas

b) the pharmacist

c) a restricted guide for usage of medications

d) a scientific database of formulas and drug trials

Word expansion:

a) The chemical formula for many new drugs is kept highly secret by the pharmaceutical research company that discovered them. (noun)

7. Therapeutic *(adjective)*

In context:

a) The therapeutic effect of sleep cannot be underestimated in the healing process.

b) It was very therapeutic for Police Officer Delarose to take 3 or 4 weeks off from work after his partner was fatally injured in the line of duty. He needed time to reflect and grieve.

Meaning: The best way to explain the term *therapeutic* is to say it means

a) nonsynthetic intervention and assistance

b) chemical intervention

c) able to treat, ameliorate, or cure

d) psychological intervention

Word expansion:

a) Mr. Hull's diabetes can be *therapeutically* managed at home with the help of his family. (adverb)

b) Walter has been referred to *physical therapy* for his hand injuries, but also for some *psychotherapy* for his mind. He is recovering from an attack by a pit bull dog. He has a severe hand wound and post-traumatic stress disorder. (adjective, noun)

c) Exercise time spent in a swimming pool is a well-recognized *therapy* for patients with limb or joint injuries and diseases. (noun)

> **GRAMMAR ALERT: ROOT WORDS: *MEDIC, MEDICO*** From the Latin, *medicus* and *medicalis* mean physician. Recall the Grammar Review featured at the beginning of Unit 8 as you continue to learn more about the structure and form of medical terminology. All words containing these root words in English will reference something to do with a physician or the work of physicians. (Note that the origin of the term is ancient. Today, nurse practitioners, paramedics, pharmacists, and other qualified health professionals may also be considered along with the physician as part of the reference when the root word *medic* appears.)

Mix and Match.   Complete the Mix and Match exercise in Box 8-2 to help you determine the meaning of a word from its root.

Fill in the Blanks.   Use the appropriate term from Box 8-2 to fill in the blanks and make complete sentences.

BOX 8-2 Mix and Match: Words Derived from *Medic*

Draw a line linking a term beginning with/deriving from the root word medic *to an appropriate explanation. Treat this exercise as a word puzzle.*

WORD	APPROPRIATE EXPLANATION
medicate	most often found working in an ambulance
medicinal	a way to speak
medical	something you take to get better
medically	health promoting
medicine	type of school for doctors
medication	something the nurse or doctor administers
medic	performs medical duties in the armed forces
paramedic	administer

1) Emergency Medical Services (EMS) employ _____ to work in ambulance and rescue services.

2) If you think you are having a heart attack or stroke, you should consider this a _____ emergency and seek _____ help immediately.

3) Cough remedies often taste bad. People complain that they taste "like _____."

4) A patient prescribed antibiotic _____ must be taught the importance of completing the regime: taking all of the pills or capsules he or she is given.

5) Bob was a _____ in the Army and he loved it. When he came home, he entered _____ school to become a doctor.

6) _____ speaking, the patient's prognosis for recovery is very poor.

7) The psychotic patient needed to be _____ in the emergency room so that his admission to the hospital could be complete. He was too anxious and disturbed to be managed, otherwise.

8) The doctor decided to _____ the cardiac patient with an antihypertensive.

9) Janis complains of grogginess in the morning. It is difficult for her to wake up and feel alert. She believes it is a result of her sleeping _____ and she wonders if she is over-_____. She wants to lower the dose.

10) A wide range of _____ and recommendations for their use can be found in a compendium of pharmaceuticals.

GRAMMAR ALERT: MEDICAL PREFIX: *ANTI* Use of the prefix *anti* is very common in health care and medicine. Words beginning with it are sometimes written with hyphens and sometimes not.
Anti can mean opposite. If it occurs in front of a word naming a symptom or disease, it means healing, relieving, or curing. For example, an antidepressant medication relieves the symptoms of depression.
Anti can also mean opposed to or against. For example, the term anticoagulant is opposite to the term coagulant. An anticoagulant medication is given to decrease the clotting ability of blood. In other words, it is opposed to clotting. However, a coagulant is given to enhance or improve the ability of the blood to clot. Can you see how the misunderstanding of these terms could lead to the patient's death?

Using Common Medical Prefixes. Use the prefix *anti* in a meaningful way. In this exercise you will see words you have become familiar with through *Medical English Clear and Simple.* Use the prefix *anti* with each one in a complete, full sentence that explains the term. Each new word you create is the term used to refer to a type of medication. For example, when the prefix *anti* is added to the word *tussive,* a type of medication is named—specifically an antitussive, which is a drug that alleviates or eases a cough.

1) epileptic

_____

2) hypertensive

_____

3) cancer

_____

4) toxin

_____

5) anginal

_____

6) viral

_____

7) bacterial

_____

8) diarrheal

_____

9) inflammatory

_____

10) pyretic

_____

Fill in the Blanks. Use a key word from each of the previous two exercises to create a new sentence. Fill in the blanks to achieve this.

1) Rachel has springtime allergies. Her doctor has prescribed some _____ _____ to alleviate the symptoms.

2) Frances is a nurse and she is pregnant. She has morning sickness and wants the vomiting to stop. She would like to ask her doctor for an _____, but she knows very well that this is not safe for her unborn baby.

3) After the hurricane, a _____ from the Army Reserves helped my grandmother with the serious laceration she incurred to her right arm.

4) Chevonne has high blood pressure. The doctor put her on an _____ yesterday.

5) _____ speaking, prescribing an _____ to treat a virus is not the appropriate method of treatment.

6) The patient diagnosed with hypomania needs a mood stabilizer. The psychiatrist on duty has commenced her on an _____ for that purpose.

7) Glenn and Marge never go on holidays without taking some _____ _____ with them. They are afraid of stomach upsets and diarrhea.

SPEAKING EXERCISE

Go back and read all of the fill-in-the-blank exercises in this section. Read them once silently to refamiliarize yourself with the material. Then, read them out loud at a normal, fluent pace. The more you speak these words aloud in full sentences, the more comfortable you will be when speaking to others about these topics.

PRONUNCIATION ALERT: PREFIXES ENDING IN THE LETTER "I"

The prefix *anti* is commonly pronounced with a long "i" sound in the United States. However, in Canada that is not so. *Anti* is pronounced with a short "i" or "e" sound. It is wise to be prepared to hear and understand it with both pronunciations. Here is an example:

antibiotic = ăn″**tī**-bī-ŏ t′ĭk (American pronunciation)
antibiotic = ăn″**tī**-bī-ŏt′ĭk (Canadian pronunciation)
semiconscious = sĕm″**ī**-kŏn′shŭs (American pronunciation)
semiconscious = sĕm″**ē**-kŏn′shŭs (Canadian pronunciation)

LISTENING EXERCISE

If you would like to hear more native English speakers from the United States and Canada, search the Internet. A good resource for the North American English accent you are looking for can be heard on the clips produced by:

- The MedicCast Podcast Extra video series. Search for their home website. On the left side of their webpage, type in the following search words: EMS Medication, Pharmacokinetics. You can also access their videos on sites such as *YouTube*.

- The Online Community of Clinical Excellence. These clips include "Introduction to Pharmacology," "Cardiac Pharmacology," and "CNS Pharmacology: Introduction." Go to their website, http://www.o2demand.com. On the right side of the webpage where it says "search," type in the title of one of these videos. Click and listen. (Please note that the language on this site is advanced, technical English and best suited for medical students or internationally educated doctors seeking to improve their English language skills. The main site is dedicated to anesthesiology, the study and use of anesthetics.)

WRITING EXERCISE—SELF-REFLECTION

Use your new vocabulary. Write some comments here about your sense of personal competency administering medications using the English language. Is this a concern for you? Why or why not?

_____

_____

_____

_____

Reading Selection 8-2

Read the following reading selection in preparation for learning new vocabulary words, how to use them in sentences, and some important grammar points.

SIDE EFFECTS OR ADVERSE EFFECTS?

Medications have the potential to adversely or negatively affect the body and in some instances, lead to death. While these adverse effects are often referred to as side effects, the terms are not synonymous. Side effects are the action of the drug on cells other than the ones the medication was targeting. These side reactions may be weak and may cause some minimal discomfort or disruption to a person's general level of functioning. An example of this might be the sleepiness or the dry mouth that occurs as a side effect of the allergy medications antihistamines.

An adverse effect has undesirable and/or severe effects on a person's ability to function physically or mentally. Examples of adverse effects can range from severe diarrhea to gross tremors (shaking) of the hands. Each of these can affect the client's ability to think, work, and function as he or she normally would. Side effects and adverse effects are the result of the body's reaction to the drug (pharmacodynamics).

Toxicity is not a side effect. It is not an adverse effect of a medication either, although it might seem to be so. Toxicity is directly related to the amount of a medication that has been taken into the body. The word "toxin" means poison. The toxic effect of a medication means literally that the cells or systems it reaches are poisoned by it. Sometimes a very small amount of a medication will prove toxic. Toxicity can be fatal. Immediate laboratory screening tests of blood and urine are required to identify the level of toxicity so a treatment may be initiated. These tests are called toxicology screens.

READING EXERCISES

As in other units, these exercises will allow you to test your ability to understand the general meaning of a reading selection, learn how to use new vocabulary, and pick up some important grammar and word usage details.

Understanding the General Meaning

Read the text Side Effects or Adverse Effects? again and answer the following questions about its general meaning. Respond with short answers.

1) What is the general meaning of the text? Its focus?

_____

2) What is the purpose of this text?

_____

3) Explain the term *adverse.*

_____

4) Provide a synonym for *toxin.*

_____

5) Are adverse effects of drugs mild, moderate, or severe?

_____

6) Of the three effects described in the reading, which one is most deadly?

_____

Building Vocabulary

Determining Meaning from Context.   To build vocabulary, study the following words and terms taken from the reading. Discover all you can about them by looking at them in these new examples. Next, go on to choose the correct meaning for the words from the choices provided. Finally, take a look at how the words expand in English.

1. Potential *(noun)*

In context:

a) Science and research have the potential to cure cancer.

b) The true, long-term potential of the new vaccine against the human papillomavirus is still unknown.

Meaning: The best way to explain the term *potential* in a chemical sense is to say it

a) has guaranteed results

b) is capable of action but not yet doing so

c) has lasting effects

d) has adverse effects

Word expansion:

a) Crack cocaine is a *potent* drug with the power to cause almost immediate addiction. (adjective)

b) The *potency* of an intramuscular injection of epinephrine for a severe allergy reaction is extreme. Relief can be instantaneous. (noun)

c) The *potentially* debilitating side effects of chemotherapy must be seriously considered prior to commencing this treatment regime. (adverb)

d) To discover if *potentiation* is going to be a factor when combining two or more medications, the compendium of pharmaceuticals can be an excellent resource. (noun)

e) Estrogen *potentiates* the metabolism of vitamin D. (verb)

f) Morphine is *potentiated* by alcohol. Taken alone, neither drug is likely to cause severe harm. Taken together and at high levels, they increase the risk of death. (verb, present participle)

2. Gross *(adjective)*

In context:

a) As Petra's Parkinson's disease worsens, she notices that she can no longer hold a coffee cup safely in her hands. Her fine hand tremors have now become gross tremors.

b) Gross motor skills are those skills which use the large muscles of the body.

Meaning: The best way to explain the term *gross* in a medical context is to say that it means

a) obese, obtuse, and ocular

b) disgusting and discomforting

c) large or coarse and visible to the eye

d) handicapping and debilitating

Word expansion:

a) Cirrhosis of the liver from years of alcoholism has *grossly* affected the ability of the patient's liver to metabolize and detoxify. (adverb)

b) Sudden and extreme changes in dietary intake can potentially cause *gross* damage to organs such as the heart and eyes. (adjective)

c) *Gross anatomy* is a synonym for the general anatomy only at the level of what is large enough to be seen and examined by the eye. (adjective forming a term)

3. Poison *(noun)*

In context:

a) The detection of poison in the body is not always a simple task. A toxicology screen is necessary.

b) The poison arsenic causes hair to fall out and fingertips to turn blue.

Meaning: The best way to explain the term *poison* in a medical context is to say it is

a) a substance excreted by reptiles to injure or kill

b) a substance that enters the body that is injurious to health or potentially fatal

c) a marine animal that if ingested is injurious to health or potentially fatal

d) an illegal chemical substance or household cleaner

Word expansion:

a) The man was bitten by a *poisonous* snake in the desert. (adjective)

b) *Poisoning* can cause brain damage in children. (noun; gerund)

c) The traveler was *poisoned* by a venomous snake. (verb, past participle)

d) The Centers for Disease Control has an extensive data bank identifying *poisons* and their antidotes. (noun, plural)

e) *Poisoning* is a rare crime in 21st-century North America. (gerund)

f) We had a case of accidental *poisoning* in the ER last night. (noun)

4. Tremors *(noun, plural)*

In context:

a) Petra's gross hand tremors cause the coffee in her cup to splash and spill out all over her.

b) The client's tremors began last month and have gotten increasingly unbearable. That's why he came to the clinic today.

Meaning: The best way to explain the term *tremors* in a medical sense is to say it means

a) shakes and spasms

b) rapid, involuntary movements

c) lack of flexion and contraction

d) abnormal, repetitive, involuntary shaking movements

Word expansion:

a) Because her hands are *tremulous,* Auntie Eva no longer enjoys knitting. (adjective)

b) Bonnie was so frightened from the assault that she *was* still *trembling* when she was speaking to the nurse. (verb, past continuous tense)

c) Many people are afflicted with an essential *tremor*. Their hands and head shake uncontrollably. (noun))

d) Walking alone on a dark street in the center of a big city makes some women *tremble*. (verb, present tense)

> **VOCABULARY ALERT: TREMOR VERSUS TREMBLE** You may have noticed in this last exercise that when you have a tremor, you tremble. In health care, we refer to this type of involuntary movement as a *tremor* or *tremors*. The word *tremble* is a verb and cannot and should not be used as a noun. Here are a few more examples to clarify:
> "I have a tremor and right now I am trembling. Can you see? My hands are tremulous. My tremor is greater and I tremble more when I am anxious or afraid. Even my voice is beginning to tremble. Can you hear? It's more tremulous now. I must admit I am anxious about hearing my diagnosis today."

Using New Vocabulary in Sentences. Use a key word from the reading and previous exercise to create a new, complete sentence.

1) poison

_____

2) adverse

_____

3) anxious

_____

4) reaction

_____

5) fatal

_____

6) sleepiness

_____

SPEAKING EXERCISE

Work on pronunciation of letters "p," "v," and "b" by reading the following aloud. The Pronunciation Hints box that follows will also help.

I went to the pharmacy to see the pharmacist. I needed pharmaceutical advice. I had purchased two over-the-counter antipyretics but didn't understand how they were different. The pharmacist told me that medications vary by their pharmaceutical formulas. She said that I should always read the product label on the box before I buy. The label identifies the compounds and the amounts of various medications that together comprise the formula. The pharmacist also pointed out that pharmaceuticals also vary by their side effects and risks. She pulled out a folder paper from each of my two boxes. She explained that each piece of paper was a product description. This paper is officially known as the product monogram. I saw that the purpose of the drug was identified as well as the various effects, side effects, adverse effects, toxic effects, and cautions for use of the medication. Because of this, I found the differences between the two bottles of pills. I appreciated the time and patience the pharmacist took to improve my level of understanding about pharmaceuticals.

PRONUNCIATION HINTS:
A REVIEW OF THE LETTERS "P," "B," AND "V"
Recall the following information from previous units in this book.

Letter "p"
The sound for the letter "p" is made by bringing the lips together, quickly gathering air in the cheeks in front of the teeth, and expelling the air with slight force, in a sudden burst. Smile.
Continue to smile and put your two lips together very quickly. In a short burst, blow out through your lips, making a blowing sound "p." It should make a sound like "puh." At no time should your smile disappear. Do not move your jaw. No vocalization is required: do not use your vocal cords. The sound is made by air escaping.

Letter "b"

Next, continue to smile with your lips together. Repeat the exercise, but this time you will say the letter "b." Push the air out through your mouth, but this time make an audible sound and say "buh." This is how to pronounce the letter "b." Do not move your jaw. Notice that "p" has almost no sound: it is air, but "b" is a definite sound and you must forcibly and consciously make it.

Letter "v"

Now, continue to smile, but this time place a pen or pencil horizontally between your lips. Hold it there. Blow the air out of your mouth again, but this time say the letter "v." Do not move your lips or your jaw! Notice that as "v" escapes the mouth it makes an audible vibration sound. This absolutely distinguishes it from the letters "b" and "p."

LISTENING EXERCISE

If you would like to hear more native English speakers from the United States speak on the topic of medication safety, search the Internet for a video clip for pharmacy students or listen to and watch the following video clips:

- "New Studies on Antidepressants in Pregnancy" (March 5, 2007) by the U.S. Food and Drug Administration. You can find this video at their website, http://www.fda.gov/psn or at http://www.video.google.com

- "FDA Studying Potential Safety Issues with Several Drugs" (June 27, 2008). This news release can be found on the U.S. Food and Drug Administration's website at http://www.accessdata.fda.gov/scripts or video.aol.com

WRITING EXERCISE—REFLECTION

Take some time now to think about all that you have read, heard, and learned in this section. All of the information is set in the context of American and Canadian perspectives on pharmacology and pharmaceuticals. Reflect on your own days at college or university. You very likely studied pharmacology. In a short paragraph, write down your thoughts about the value of that component of your education. Comment on whether or not you think your current level of pharmacological knowledge is sufficient to begin working in an English-speaking country. Is this a result of your pharmacological knowledge and skills base or of your English language knowledge and skills base?

_____

_____

_____

_____

_____

_____

Reading Selection 8-3

In Unit 8, you have learned that an excellent resource for information about medications is a compendium of pharmaceuticals. In your professional practice, however, there may be times when you are called upon to find evidence that informs your medication administration safe practices. In other words, you will desire or require more information and evidence about safe practices, new methods of medication administration, and issues and concerns related to the implications of and use of medications than is provided in a compendium. To do this, you will want to search the peer-reviewed journals written by and for the health professions. You will access the articles through specific search engines on the Internet via computers in the hospital, university, or your professional associations' libraries. You will search by key words in your topic and then begin to sort through abstracts of the journal articles for their relevance to your needs. The following exercises will assist you in that linguistic process.

> **VOCABULARY ALERT: ABSTRACT** An abstract is a brief descriptive summary of the essential information in an article or report. It provides the first impression of the document with just enough information to alert the reader to the contents of the text. By doing so, the abstract allows the reader the opportunity to anticipate the text and whether or not to read it in its entirety. Abstracts are short and can range from 25 to 250 words maximum. As such, they must be concise. The information contained in each sentence must be meaningful and relevant to the thesis (main theme) of the article it is describing.

Read the following abstract of a research study. As you do so, circle any words that you think are key words or cues that allow you to anticipate what the full article is about. Then proceed to the exercises to confirm your prediction.

ABSTRACT

Survey of Nursing Perceptions of Medication Administration Practices, Perceived Sources of Errors and Reporting Behaviours

Armutlu, M., Foley, M., Surette, J., Belzile, E., and McCusker, J. (2008).
Healthcare Quarterly, Vol 11, Special issue, 2008, p 58–65.
Longwood Publishing, Toronto, Canada

Abstract: In January 2003, St. Mary's Hospital Center in Montreal, Quebec, established an interdisciplinary Committee on the Systematic Approach to Medication Error Control to review the whole process of medication administration within the hospital and to develop a systematic approach to medication error control. A cross-sectional survey on medication administration practices, perceived sources of errors, and medication error reporting of nurses, adapted from a nursing practice survey and medication variance report (Sim and Joyner, 2002), was conducted over a two-week period in February 2004.

The results were analyzed by years of experience (greater or less than five years) and patient care unit of practice. The perceived source of error most often cited was transcription (processing), and the second most frequently cited source was the legibility of handwritten medication orders (prescribing). The results demonstrate no significant difference in medication safety practices or in perceptions of errors by years of experience. Nurses appear to adapt to the safety culture of the unit rather quickly, certainly within their first five years on the unit. Good medication error reporting behavior was noted, with no differences between all comparative groups within both years of experience and unit of practice. Quality improvement initiatives to improve the safety of medication administration practices have included the development of a nursing medication administration handbook, the revision of policies and procedures related to medication administration safety, the standardization of solutions and limited variety of high-risk medication dosages, and the reduction of handwritten reorders. The need for ongoing education and information sessions on policies and procedures specific to safe medication practices for all nurses, regardless of years of experience, was identified.

Review the abstract again and determine if it contains the main structural features of an abstract, which are given in the Grammar Alert on this page.

GRAMMAR ALERT: STRUCTURE OF AN ABSTRACT An abstract contains five basic structural features:

- Title
  ↓
- Introduction
  ↓
- Methods
  ↓
- Results
  ↓
- Conclusion

READING EXERCISES

This abstract is written in the genre of an informational or declarative report. It provides information about purpose or intent, scope, and method(s) of research. Complete the following exercises to illustrate your understanding of the general purpose of the article and of specific details included.

Understanding the General Meaning

Respond to the following questions with short answers. You may copy the answers directly out of the abstract where appropriate.

1) What is the title of this journal article project?

_____

2) What is the general intent of the research it describes?

_____

3) What are the results of this review?

_____

_____

4) Who is or are the intended reader(s) of this text: the target audience?

_____

5) What type of research is this?

_____

6) Are the authors health professionals?

_____

7) Under what circumstances would a nurse, doctor, pharmacist, or administrator look for an article like this?

_____

8) Generally, a short list of key words appears at the end of an abstract to help the reader clarify once again what the text of the article will be about. No key words are provided here. Suggest the key terms you would use for this abstract. Use the words you circled while reading.

_____

Understanding Specifics in the Abstract

Answer the following questions using short-answer responses. Base your answer directly on the abstract you've just read.

1) At St. Mary's Hospital Center in Montreal, how do years of nursing experience factor into the amount of medication administration errors that occur there?

_____

2) What factors led to errors at this facility?

_____

_____

3) What is the conclusion of this research?

_____

Building Vocabulary

GRAMMAR ALERT: LINGUISTIC CHOICES Linguistic choices are the word and style choices an author makes based on his or her intentions, the genre type, and the communicative situation (i.e., for whom it is written). In preparation for writing, the author goes through a selection process, considering which language or linguistic possibilities are available; selects appropriate words, structure, and style; and then composes the text.

Linguistic choices for research papers require formal, academic, scientific, and technical language without the use of jargon or abbreviations. This same rule applies to the abstract.

Sentence Completion. The abstract you have just read uses words and concepts that are expected to be understood by the targeted reader. In this exercise, interpret some of these language choices. Match the meaning of a term or concept used in the abstract with the actual word or words. Use the Word Bank.

WORD BANK

standardization

cross-sectional survey

systematic approach

medication variance

1) The _____ is also known as the analytical approach—breaking down a problem to see various aspects of it and how they interrelate.

2) In this case, this term refers to the study of a specific group of people at one instance in time to discern certain aspects or elements of their characteristics or activities. The term is _____
_____.

3) When a discrepancy occurs between the medication order and the administration of that med, a _____
is said to occur.

4) _____ refers to a process of developing, implementing, and following set guidelines and practices.

Reading and Interpreting an Abstract

Review the abstract by Armutlu, Surette, Belzile, and McCusker. Have they included all five of the basic structural features of an abstract?

_____

Peruse the same abstract now, looking for the main purpose of each sentence.

_____

1) Copy a sentence here that identifies the objective of the research survey conducted by the authors.

_____

2) Copy a sentence here that describes the methodology used in the research.

_____

3) Copy a sentence here that identifies the main findings or conclusion of the research.

_____

SPEAKING EXERCISE

Go back and read the abstract aloud now, just as you did in the previous Speaking Exercise. This time, work on your fluency, once again trying to eliminate moments of hesitancy and stumbling. The Pronunciation Hints box below will also help.

PRONUNCIATION HINTS

variance – **văr′ē**-ăns

cross-sectional – cros-**sek′**shun-al

systematic – sĭs′tĕ-**măt′ĭk**

LISTENING EXERCISE

If you would like to hear more native English speakers from the United States and Canada discuss their research into medication administration and safe practices, search the Internet for a conference near you. Try to attend. If this is not possible, seek out a pharmacist and ask him or her to talk to you about these issues, in English. Listen carefully for the terminology and concepts.

WRITING EXERCISE

Read the following conclusion section of a research article written by four medical professionals. Then, use your new vocabulary and linguistic knowledge to write your own abstract for it. Begin with a draft, and then write the complete abstract.

Opportunities for performance improvement in relation to medication administration during pediatric stabilization

Morgan, N., Luo, X, Fortner, C., Frush, K.
Quality and Safety in Health Care 2006;15:179–183;
Copyright © 2006 by the BMJ Publishing Group Ltd.

Conclusions: *By observing the clinical performance of nurses in a simulated videotaped pediatric stabilization event, we have identified some important areas in need of improvement in each step of the medication administration process. These findings indicate a need for improved education, training, and use of clinical aids or adjuncts for pediatric emergency nurses.*

1) Your abstract in draft form.

   Title: _____

   Introductory sentence or two: _____
   _____

   Methods used in the research: _____
   _____

   Results of the research: _____
   _____

   A sentence of conclusion: _____
   _____

2) Combine your sentences from the draft you have just created. Combine them in a logical, meaningful way to create your new abstract. Try to write yours in 100 words or less.

   _____
   _____
   _____
   _____
   _____

3) Now, go online to check your answers. Discover how well you have done and how close you have come to the actual abstract by Morgan, Luo, Fortner, and Frush. You can read it at http://qshc.bmj.com/cgi/content/abstract/15/3/179. Go on to read the entire article, if you like. If you cannot access it on the Internet, try your local university, medical, or nursing library. They may be able to access it for you.

Safety and Accuracy in Medication Administration

Safety and accuracy in medication administration are not simply related to knowledge of pharmaceuticals and principles of pharmacology. They include the ability to work and communicate competently in the English language. Recognizing that professional obligations, protocols, and procedures for medication administration are not the same and are not standardized worldwide, this section explores not only the terminology required to safely administer medications, but it also offers an insight into the cultural context of medication administration in the United States and Canada.

VOCABULARY ALERT: MEDICATION ADMINISTRATION In the context of health care, the term *medication administration* is used as a concept. It refers to the entire process of researching or learning about a medication, preparing to administer it, administering it to a client or patient following protocols, and engaging in all follow-up care specifically related to monitoring and evaluating the effects of that medication on the client.

Reading Selection 8-4

Read the following discussion about medication errors.

MEDICATION ADMINISTRATION: SAFE PRACTICE STRATEGIES

In the previous section, an abstract was presented that identified the very serious problem of medication errors. A thorough search of the professional literature on this subject (i.e., journal articles) will show that a good number of these errors occur as the result of transcription errors. This means that when one person copies a prescribed order onto another document or into the patient's chart, an error is made. This is also sometimes known as a data entry error. Observe the following flow chart, Figure 8-1. It illustrates a procedure known as processing an order and it, of course, includes transcription.

There is evidence in the research to show that many medication errors are the result of being unable to read a physician's handwriting. In the United States and Canada, the nurse has a legal obligation to seek clarification from the person prescribing (the prescriber) every medication order whenever in doubt. This means the nurse has the professional right and responsibility to ensure she or he is able to read and

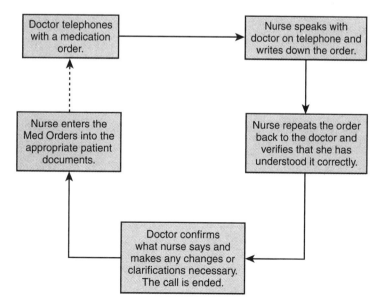

Figure 8-1

understand the order before attempting to transcribe and administer it. This can be done face-to-face or on the telephone.

When medication orders are given by a doctor by telephone, they must also be transcribed by the nurse. Safe Practice or Best Practice Protocols require that the order is written down and immediately read back to the prescriber. This verifies its accuracy. Transcription to patient documents cannot be initiated prior to this safety check.

In the case of the prescribing doctor, he or she is legally responsible for the clarity and accuracy of his or her medication orders. In the United States and Canada, physicians and surgeons are increasingly aware of the role that nurses play in questioning and clarifying medication orders. There are current societal and legal pressures on physicians throughout our two countries to ensure their writing is legible and that they are more open and receptive to the clarification sought by nurses. The safety of the patients is the highest priority.

Finally, it is important to note that medication orders are processed (transcribed and documented) by the nurse on duty or by a pharmacist. Sometimes they are processed by a medical office assistant or hospital unit clerk, but this would only be under the permission of an employer and/or a state or provincial regulation.

VOCABULARY ALERT: KARDEX Sometimes referred to as a Kardex file, this document is a very brief, concise overview of the patient's care. It functions as a quick reference for the care team, highlighting all pertinent information on current treatment and care, diagnostic tests and schedules, diagnosis, allergies, and identification. It is referred to each shift by the nurses and auxiliary care providers. It is frequently updated as changes occur. Sometimes, but not always, the Kardex also includes a list of medications. It always includes a list of known allergies, including allergies to medications.

 READING EXERCISES

You can demonstrate your understanding of a reading passage or conversation not only by answering questions but also by being able to provide a systematic, step-by-step summary of the procedures outlined, for example in a flow chart. Your enhanced skills in English will also enable you to read medication labels.

Understanding the General Meaning

Respond to the following questions with short answers.

1) This reading on medication errors deals with one particular type of error. What is that?

_____

2) Whose safety is at risk should a medication error occur?

_____

3) A flow chart is included in the reading. What is it trying to illustrate or explain?

_____

4) At which stage or stages in the process of transcribing a medication order can an error occur? Identify the stage and explain your rationale.

_____

_____

5) Does anyone have the right to question a doctor's medication orders? If so, who?

_____

6) If a doctor phones the hospital unit and wants to leave some verbal orders for medications for a client, who will he or she need to speak with?

_____

7) Create a flow chart. Illustrate the safe practice procedure for receiving a medication order by telephone from a doctor.

 BUILDING VOCABULARY

Determining Meaning from Context. The following words and terms are taken from the reading. Discover all you can about them by looking at them in these new examples. Next, go on to choose the correct meaning for the word from the choices provided. Finally, take a look at how the words expand in English.

1. Medication order (noun, proper term)

In context:
a) A medication order is also known as a prescription order.
b) A medication order is also very often referred to as a doctor's order.

Meaning: The best definition for the term *medication order* is to say it
a) identifies a drug the doctor wants the patient to take and gives instructions on how to take the drug
b) identifies a drug the pharmacist wants the patient to ingest and provides instructions on how to do so
c) is a demand from the doctor that the patient must take the medication
d) is a legal requirement that the patient must take the medication prescribed by the physician

2. Transcribe *(verb)*

In context:
a) When the handwriting is illegible, it is very difficult to try to transcribe the medication order.
b) I'd like you to transcribe these orders now, please.

Meaning: The best definition for the verb *transcribe* is to
a) translate into legal jargon
b) translate into medical terminology
c) copy and interpret something spoken or written into a document
d) repeat something spoken or written

Word expansion:
a) *Transcription* occurs when you take a medication order over the telephone and then document it. (noun)
b) I'm sorry, I can't talk right now. I am in the middle of *transcribing* (present continuous + auxiliary verb, *am*)
c) Ray *transcribed* the order as soon as he received it from the doctor. (verb, past tense)

3. Obligation *(noun)*

In context:
a) Health professionals have a legal obligation to not harm the patient.
b) I have a professional obligation to learn about new medications prior to administering them to patients.

Meaning: The best definition for the noun *obligation* is

a) duty and responsibility
b) duty and legality
c) responsibility and best practice
d) suggestion

Word expansion:

a) If the medication order states the med should be given at noon, the nurse is *obligated* to give it then. (transitive verb)
b) Membership in a professional organization *obligates* the person to abide by their rules of codes of ethics, conduct, and standards. (verb, present tense)

4. Safe practice *(term; concept in health care)*

In context:

a) The provision of safe practice is an obligation of a health professional.
b) Continuing competency education programs are a way to ensure safe practice in health care.

Meaning: The best way to explain the term *safe practice* is to say it is

a) actions that require rehearsal and repetition
b) reviewing and repeating skills before attempting to do them with patients
c) using sterile technique in all actions involving patients or clients
d) actions, knowledge, and competencies that will not harm patients or clients

Word expansion:

a) Educators ensure beginning health practitioners have the knowledge and skills necessary to be competent in providing care without harming patients or clients. This concept is known as *safety to practice*.[1]

5. Follow-up care *(adjective, term)*

In context:

a) Once discharged from the hospital, your follow-up care will include home visits from the nurse three times per week for 3 weeks.
b) Some types of follow-up care require written referrals from a member of the multidisciplinary health-care team.

Meaning: The best way to explain the term *follow-up care* is to say it is

a) an obligation of the patient to seek more treatment in the community
b) the assignment of a nurse to visit the patient in the home
c) a phase of care that continues in the community after discharge from the hospital or a series of treatments
d) care and treatment after admission to the hospital

Word expansion:

a) "Hi, Mary, I am Andrea, a nurse practitioner in the community. I *will be following up* your care now that your surgery has been completed and you are preparing to go home. Let's talk about your recovery period." (verb, future simple continuous)

6. Best practice *(term; concept in health care)*

In context:

a) Best practice refers to the use of appropriate, widely accepted, and consistently used treatments or care delivery practices that promote high standards of health care.
b) A synonym for best practice is standard of care.

---

[1]DuGas, Esson, and Ronaldson (1999), *Nursing Foundations: A Canadian Perspective.*

Meaning: The best way to explain the term *best practice* is to say it means
a) absolute excellence in treatment and care delivery
b) comprehensive, collaborative care
c) cost effective, collaborative care
d) procedures and treatments of high standards that have been proven to be effective in care delivery

Word expansion: This term does not expand, however, you might like to learn more about best practices initiatives to more clearly understand what is meant by this term. An excellent website full of examples is the On-Line Resource Center of the Appalachian Regional Commission. Type in the search words *best practices* or click the menu choice on the left side of the page: *Information by Topic – Health*. Find the page, "Best Practices in Health Care." Read through the creative, innovative best practices in eight American states at http://arc.gov/index.jsp.

READING EXERCISES

Reading Medication Labels. There is often confusion about the name of a medication as it appears in a medication order. That is because a medication may have three very different names that may legally be used to represent it. Chemical names describe the molecule(s) that make up the drug. Generic names are the official, legal names of drugs and they may specify its chemical compound. Brand names (sometimes referred to as trade names) are those names given to a drug or medication by the person or company that has developed, designed, or produced it. A brand name medication is a version or specific formulation of a generic one. This formulation is copyrighted or patented by the owner or patent/copyright holder of the product.[2] In health care, we most often see brand and generic names being used interchangeably. It is the absolute responsibility of anyone qualified to prescribe and/or administer a medication to be certain they understand exactly which drug/medication is being identified. Box 8-3 contains some examples of names that are used interchangeably in medication orders or prescriptions:

A) Here are some examples of medication labels. The brand name is fictitious, but the generic and chemical names are not. Study each label and then answer the questions.

1)

	25 tabs
PAINAWAY	
325 mg	
Acetaminophen 325-mg tablets	oral
Expiry date: 08/10 Product C8H9NO2	

a) What is the generic name of this drug? _____
b) What is the brand name of this drug? _____
c) What is the chemical name for this drug? _____

2)

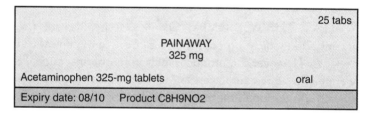

SEIZURE-FREE
100-MG CAPSULES

Contains: Phenytoin sodium 100-mg capsules

Oral preparation
Expiry: 10/10/10 $C_{15}H_{12}N_2O_2$ 252.27

a) What is the generic name of this drug?
_____
b) What is the brand name of this drug?
_____
c) What is the chemical name for this drug?
_____

---

[2]The symbol © signifies copyright, meaning the name, title, or any written material related to it is the sole property of the owners.

BOX 8-3 Generic and Brand Names of Some Common Drugs

GENERIC NAME	BRAND NAME
acetylsalicylic acid	Aspirin©
acetaminophen	Tylenol©, Panadol©, Anacin©, Acephen©
ibuprofen	Advil©, Midol©, Motrin©, Genpril©

Example of a Chemical Name: Acetaminophen is $C_8H_9NO_2$

3)

NORUNS 2-MG
GEL CAPS
50 capsules

Loperamide Hydrochloride capsules

EXPIRES: 11/12/09

Contains: 1-Piperidinebutanamide, 4-(4-chlorophenyl)-4-hydroxy-N,N-dimethyl-α,α-diphenyl-

a) What is the generic name of this drug? _____
b) What is the brand name of this drug? _____
c) What is the chemical name for this drug? _____

B) Study the labels again. They include important information for the consumer (the person who will administer or take the medication). For example, you will see the dosage of each tablet or capsule and an expiration date for the product. Answer the following questions based on that information.

1) What is the size or dosage of the Painaway tablets? _____

2) When is the expiry date for Seizure-Free? Write the numbers and then write the proper words for the date to match. _____ _____

3) How many gel caps are in the bottle of Noruns, according to the information on the label? _____

VOCABULARY ALERT: THE ABBREVIATION *MG* In health care, the abbreviation *mg* refers to milligrams. On medication orders, prescriptions, and clinical notes it is written in lower case letters, *mg*. However, on product labels from pharmaceutical companies, this abbreviation may appear in uppercase letters as *MG*. It means the same thing. Note that best practices for health professionals suggest it be written as *mg*. The abbreviation can be made plural, *mgs*.

SPEAKING EXERCISE

Find a friend or colleague with whom you can discuss your role in the administration of medication. Use new words and concepts from this section of the unit. Speak slowly to articulate your words clearly, but not so slowly that the listener becomes inattentive. Set a goal of speaking for 3–5 minutes. When you are done, ask the listener for feedback about your verbal and nonverbal behaviors. How confident did you look? How confident did you sound? How clear was your speech? The Pronunciation Hints box that follows will help.

Pharmacology and Medication Administration

PRONUNCIATION HINTS

milligrams – **mĭl'ĭ**-grămz

acetaminophen – ă-sĕt" ă-**mĭn'ō**-fĕn

acetylsalicylic acid – ăs'ētal-săl'ĭ-s'ĭl-ik **ăs"ĭd**

ibuprofen – ī"bū-**prō'fĕn**

transcription – trăn-**skrĭp'**shŭn

Kardex – **kar**-dĕks

LISTENING EXERCISE

Return again to the Internet and listen to a discussion by Dr. Harvey V. Fineberg, MD, PhD entitled, "We Can Do More to Avoid Medication Errors." It is produced by Medscape General Medicine and can be located at http://www.medscape.com or at http://www.video.google.com.

WRITING EXERCISE

This is a two-part exercise. First, read the two short scenarios below and answer the questions from an American/Canadian perspective. Second, compare your answer with the practice and protocols for safe medication administration in your country of origin. Comment on the similarities and differences.

1) A doctor phones the unit and speaks with a nurse. He wants to leave some new medication orders with her. The doctor has a heavy accent and is of a non-English speaking background.

   a) What will the nurse need to do to ensure safe practice as she processes these orders?

   _____

   b) If this scenario was to occur in your country of origin, how would it compare?

   _____

2) A nurse is transcribing some new medication orders left by the surgeon this afternoon. This surgeon has a tendency to be authoritarian and disrespectful to the nurses. Unfortunately, his written orders are very difficult to read: the handwriting is not very legible. The nurse asks another nurse to help interpret the orders, but that nurse cannot read it clearly, either.

   a) What steps will the first nurse take to ensure these medication orders are accurately transcribed?

   _____

   b) If this scenario were to occur in your country of origin, how would it compare?

   _____

   _____

Reading Selection 8-5

Read the following information about some interesting protocols and initiatives in medication administration that are aimed at protecting the client from harm during the process of medication administration.

PROTECTION FROM MEDICATION ERRORS: PREVENTATIVE ACTION

It is clear that medication errors are of grave importance and measures are being taken locally and nationally to create strategies that will reduce them. One such strategy has developed into a protocol at all major health facilities and is a core component of medication administration education and practice for nurses and others who are directly involved in giving medications. It is known as the "7 Rights." This is a systematic approach to protecting patients from medication errors. Its full name is the "7 Rights of Medication Administration." The 7 Rights involves a series of safety checks done with the patient and his or her medication prior to its administration. Each and every time a medication is to be given, the responsible health professional is obligated to protect the patient from harm by systematically going through the process of verifying the 7 criteria shown in Box 8-4.

BOX 8-4 The 7 Rights of Medication Administration

- right client
- right drug
- right dose
- right time
- right route
- right reason
- right documentation

Another example of a preventative strategy designed to reduce and/or eliminate medication errors (and more importantly, protect the patient) is the American Bar Code Label Rule implemented in 2006 by the U.S. Federal Drug Administration Agency. All prescription drugs, over-the-counter medications, and biological products, such as vaccines, blood, and blood components commonly used in hospitals are subject to this new rule.

Essentially, this new initiative means that upon admission to a hospital, the patient receives an identification wristband that includes a bar code identification component. The nurse (for example) will carry a scanner whenever administering medications. This device is used to call up identifying information on the patient from the patient's hospital records, particularly his or her name, social security number, and list of medications. The nurse then scans the patient's wristband. The two read-outs on the scanner must match before the medication is administered. If they do not, a warning box appears on the screen and the nurse is alerted to take action to clarify or remedy the situation.

Understanding the General Meaning

Answer the following questions about the text you have just read.

1) What is the main focus of this reading?

_____

2) In what types of situations are these strategies occurring?

_____

3) What is meant by the term the "7 Rights"?

_____

4) You may be familiar with bar codes on products you purchase in a store. Information such as the product number and price are embedded in a series of what appear to be black lines or bars. The reading talks about bar codes on patient wristbands. What types of information would be recorded on a hospital wristband? The reading identifies two of these things. Identify two or three more that would be relevant to patient care.

_____

5) The title of the reading mentions preventative action. What is being prevented?

_____

6) Two preventative actions are discussed in this reading. Name them.

_____

Building Vocabulary

Determining Meaning from Context.   To build vocabulary, study the following words and terms taken from the reading. Discover all you can about them by looking at them in these new examples. Next, go on to choose the correct meaning for the word from the choices provided. Finally, take a look at how the words expand in English.

1. Grave *(adjective)*

In context:
a) The patient is in grave condition. He may not survive.
b) There are grave consequences to giving too much medication to a patient.

Meaning: The best way to define the word *grave* in the context of patient care is to say
a) tombstone
b) very serious and possibly dangerous, harmful, or life threatening
c) deadly or impending death
d) gray in color

Word expansion:
a) Dr. Franklin *gravely* told the staff that the virus had spread and the facility had to be quarantined. (adverb)

2. Measures *(noun)*

In context:
a) A number of safety measures are in place when giving a patient medications. The 7 Rights are an example.
b) Disaster measures in place at the hospital include evacuation maps.

Meaning: The best way to define the word *measures* in this context and in the context of the reading is to say
a) steps in a procedure or process
b) units of size
c) standard assessment and evaluation of sizes
d) legal obligations

Word expansion:
a) The hospital administration *has measured* the risks of medication errors in their facility and implemented new directives to reduce them. (verb, present perfect tense)
b) Standardizing the *measurement* of medications nationally helps protect consumers from taking incorrect doses. For example, many over-the-counter liquid or syrup medications *are measured* by standard teaspoonfuls. (noun; then verb, past tense)

3. Verifying *(verb, present simple continuous)*

In context:
a) I am verifying that I have the right patient when I ask him to tell me his name.
b) Please wait a moment. The pharmacist is verifying the prescription with your doctor. He is on the phone with her right now.

Meaning: The best way to explain the verb *verifying* is to say it means
a) advising
b) checking the truth, accuracy, or interpretation

c) calculating

d) processing

Word expansion:

a) This medication is a controlled narcotic. I must seek *verification* for your prescription by contacting the physician that ordered it for you. (noun)

b) The patient kept telling me she wanted her "blue" pill. I had prepared to give her a pink one. I returned to her file and checked the doctor's orders. I am correct. I *verified* that her medication has been increased and that the new dosage comes in the form of a pink pill. It seems the patient doesn't know this yet. I will go back to her now and talk to her about the change in her medication before asking that she take this new one. (verb, simple past tense)

4. Wristband *(noun)*

In context:

a) Every patient is given an identifying wristband when they seek treatment in a hospital.

b) It is unwise to cut off your wristband and throw it away while you are still in the hospital.

Meaning: The best way to define the noun *wristband* in the context of medicine is to say it is a

a) bracelet

b) bracelet that wraps around the wrist that includes identifying data

c) bandage that encircles the wrist that includes your name

d) medic alert bracelet

Word expansion:

a) *Wristbands* supporting charities or philosophical perspectives are now very commonly worn around the world. An example is the HIV/AIDS awareness campaign wristband. It is made of red plastic. Peace wristbands are similar, but they are generally green. (noun, plural)

5. Systematic *(adjective)*

In context:

a) The systematic process of completing the 7 Rights protocol will facilitate best practices in medication administration.

Meaning: The best way to understand the word *systematic* is through its synonyms. Choose the best synonyms from these choices:

a) protocol and process

b) incremental steps

c) organized, methodical, step-wise

d) accumulative

Word expansion:

a) The pharmacist in the drug store *systematically* reviews each and every prescription he or she receives to ensure accuracy. (adverb)

b) A common *system* for medication administration is use of the blister pack. (noun)

> **VOCABULARY ALERT: SYSTEMATIC VERSUS SYSTEMIC** The word *systematic* should not be confused with the word *systemic*. They are very different. As you have seen, systematic refers to a process of thinking and acting. Systemic on the other hand, refers to a whole system or the whole body. For example, a blood infection is systemic: it has an effect on the whole body.
>
> Be very careful of pronunciation of these two terms.
>
> systematic – sĭs″tĕ-măt′ĭk (4 syllables)
>
> systemic – sĭs″tĕ-mĭk (3 syllables)

Following the 7 Rights Protocol. This exercise will enhance your ability to speak with your patient while you follow the steps of the 7 Rights of Medication Administration protocol (if bar codes are not used in your facility).

Study Box 8-5 and then answer the questions on page 366.

BOX 8-5 The 7 Rights of Medication Administration: Defined

STEP ONE: Verify you are speaking to the right (correct) patient.

- Ask the patient to say his or her name even if you already know it.
- Ask the patient to state his or her date of birth.
- Check the patient's wristband and read the name to ensure it matches (a) who you intend to give the medication to, (b) what the patient has told you is his or her name, and (c) the date of birth given by the patient and that on the wristband, and the information you have on your Medication Administration Record (MAR).

STEP TWO: Verify you have the right drug for the identified patient.

- Compare the MAR to the doctor's orders.
- Compare the MAR to the label on the medication supplied by the pharmacy.

STEP THREE: Verify you have the right dose of the medication.

- Check the doctor's orders.
- Check the dosage identified on the MAR with the label on the medication supplied by pharmacy. Be careful that the dose identified on the label matches the dose ordered. There may be more than one bottle or packet of the same drug available, but they are of different dosages or strengths.

STEP FOUR: Verify you have the right route for the drug.

- Check the MAR with the doctor's orders.
- Check the label on the medication and ensure it says how it is to be administered. Be careful. There may be tablets, capsules, liquids, and injectable forms of the medication available as well as topical preparations. Be sure to match the doctor's orders, MAR, and medication labels.

STEP FIVE: Verify that this is the right time to give the medication.

- Check the doctor's orders and the MAR for the times of administration: when this medication is to be given.
- Check the label on the medication supplied and ensure the same times of administration are identified.

STEP SIX: Verify the reason for the medication.

- Check the doctor's progress notes or ask him or her for the reason.
- Check with the patient. Patients in the United States and Canada are generally aware of the medications they are taking in the hospital and at home and they are able to state the reason why they are taking them. They are informed consumers. (Note: This step will alert the person administering the medications that an error may have been made in ordering or transcribing a medication if the medication in hand has no relation to the patient's health condition.)

STEP SEVEN: Document/record the administration of the medication in the appropriate patient records: the chart and the MAR.

- Check the name and other identifying information on the chart prior to entering a note.
- Sign in the appropriate place on the MAR that the medication has been administered. Sign immediately upon giving the med.
- Remember that not all medication administered is noted in the nurse's notes or progress notes. Meds given stat (immediately) and prn (as needed) are examples of special circumstances that require special notations in the client charts.

A) Answer the following questions based on the steps of the 7 Rights protocol.

1) In the context of medication administration, what is meant by the term "right route"?

_____

2) The doctor's orders have been transcribed onto a Medication Administration Record (MAR) sheet. Give one reason why the next nurse on duty must still check what is written on the MAR with the doctor's order sheet.

_____

_____

3) Where does a nurse sign or make note that she or he has given the medication?

_____

4) What is meant by "give the medication at the right time"?

_____

_____

B) Using the 7 Rights of Medication Administration, answer the questions for the following situations.

1) Mrs. Warren is an 85-year-old patient. She has a moderate degree of dementia. She is on your medical unit with a diagnosis of a broken hip. You are going to give her pain medication now.

Nurse: Hello, it's time for your medication. Please tell me your name.

Patient: Maggie Warren, dear.

Nurse: Thank you, Maggie. And when were you born?

Patient: 1965. Yes, 1965. It was a very good year!

Q: Maggie cannot have been born in 1965 if she is 85 years old today. What is your next step to ensure safe administration of medication?

_____

2) Mr. Blake, 34 years old, is in the hospital on your unit. He says he is in a great deal of pain. He rings the buzzer and calls out repeatedly, demanding medication. You go to him.

Nurse: Yes, Mr. Blake, how can I help you?

Mr. Blake: Morphine, morphine. I can't stand the pain. Give me more morphine.

Nurse: Tell me more about your pain, Mr. Blake. Where is it exactly?

Mr. Blake: Here, there . . . everywhere. Oh, never mind. Just get me the morphine, will you?

Nurse: Mr. Blake, I need a little information before I can give an analgesic. On a scale of 1–10, how would you rate your pain?

Mr. Blake: It's a 25! Now get me that morphine!

Nurse: Mr. Blake, you are prescribed acetaminophen with codeine for pain. I can get you some of that, but you are not prescribed morphine.

Mr. Blake: Who said so? I want morphine. Get it for me now!

Nurse: No sir, I cannot. It's not prescribed.

Mr. Blake: Oh yes it is. The doctor ordered it this morning. The other nurse gave it to me then. Don't lie. Just get me the morphine. Hurry up!

Nurse: Let me check that, Mr. Blake. I'll be right back.

Q: Following the 7 Rights protocol, what is the nurse's next step?

SPEAKING EXERCISE

Find a partner to work with. Read the two dialogues in the last exercise aloud. Role play: add some emotion to your voice as you speak. Work on your ability to speak naturally with your voice and your nonverbal communication as you do so. Try to make the interactions sound like normal conversation. The Pronunciation Hints box that follows will help.

> **PRONUNCIATION HINTS**
>
> morphine – **mor'**fēn
>
> wristband – **rĭst**-bănd
>
> dementia – dē-**mĕn'**shē-ă
>
> ensure – en-**shŭr**
>
> administration – ăd'mĭn'ĭ-**strā**-shŭn

LISTENING EXERCISE

Listen to a lecture entitled, "Preventing Medication Errors" produced by the Osher Lifelong Learning Institute, University of California, San Francisco, and the Department of Clinical Pharmacy at UCSF. You can find this at http://www.youtube.com.

WRITING EXERCISE

Use your new vocabulary to compare and contrast the medication error prevention strategies from your country of origin with those identified in this section of Unit 8.

_____

_____

_____

_____

_____

Reading Selection 8-6

Read the following short discussion about the problems of using abbreviations in medication administration.

INTERPRETATION OF MEDICATION ORDERS DEPENDS ON INTERPRETATION OF CAREER-SPECIFIC ABBREVIATIONS

You have seen that accuracy in medication administration very often depends on the accuracy of reading and interpreting a medication order. Commonly used abbreviations are part of the reason for this. There have been many discrepancies and differing interpretations of their meaning by all members of the health-care team over the years, despite numerous attempts to standardize medical abbreviations (in this case, specifically related to safe practices in medication administration). Currently in the United States, the Food and Drug Administration (FDA) and the Institute for Safe Medication Practices (ISMP) have come together to create a list of error-prone abbreviations that they recommend we **not** use in our professional practice.[3] ISMP Canada has a similar list.[4] The Joint Commission of the American Academy of Physical Medicine and Rehabilitation has also issued a "Do Not Use" list of abbreviations.[5] Finally, the Joint Commission on Accreditation of Health Care Organization (JCAHO) in the United States **requires** hospitals to adhere to their Do Not Use list.[6] The goal is to reduce the risk of harm to patients or clients in the community and to promote safe practices among member of the health-care team.

Despite the growing awareness about this issue of safe practice, many health professionals, particularly those new to the country, are not fully aware of the recommendations or requirements of these various organizations and commissions. Nor are they necessarily cognizant of the need for the standardization of abbreviations used in medication administration in English-speaking North America. As a health-care provider in the United States or Canada it is absolutely essential to your own level of professional competency and commitment to patient care that you know which medical abbreviations are acceptable in your clinical practice setting/place of employment. This is your responsibility to the safety and welfare of your patients.

 READING EXERCISES

Written and verbal communication among health-care professionals frequently includes the use of medical abbreviations. It is essential that all health professionals, including those for whom English is not their native language, understand know how to use these abbreviations. This section will help you do that.

Understanding the General Meaning

Respond to the following questions using short answers.

1) What is the social purpose of this text?

2) In which genre is this short discussion written?

3) Why were the words "not" and "requires" highlighted in bold type?

4) What is the full and proper name of the ISMP?

5) What is the full and proper name of the JCAHO?

6) Who may not be fully aware of which medical abbreviations are acceptable for use and which are not?

---

[3]ISMP (USA): http://www.ismp.org/tools/errorproneabbreviations.pdf or
   http://www.ismp.org/tools/abbreviations
[4] ISMP (Canada): http://www.ismp-canada.org/download/ISMPCanadaListOfDangerousAbbreviations.pdf
[5] American Academy of Physical Medicine and Rehabilitation: http://www.aapmr.org/hpl/pracguide/jcahosymbols.htm
[6] Joint Commission: http://www.jointcommission.org

7) What is the goal of creating a Do Not Use list of medical abbreviations?

_____

8) How would you find out more information about any of the organizations identified in the reading?

_____

9) Whose responsibility is it to know about approved versus nonapproved medical abbreviations?

_____

GRAMMAR ALERT: USE OF ABBREVIATIONS TO REPRESENT PROPER NAMES This reading exercise provides two examples of how the abbreviations for proper names are introduced in a text.

In all formal writing a full name must be written out the first time it appears. It is followed by its initials or abbreviated form in parentheses immediately thereafter. Any subsequent reference to the name can be simplified by using the short form. This is standard, academic protocol for written work.

Example: It is possible that at some time or another you may take the full name of this text-book, *Medical English Clear and Simple,* and abbreviate it in your own writing like this: I am working through the book *Medical English Clear and Simple* (MECS). I find it very helpful to my studies. I expect to finish MECS in a month or two.

Building Vocabulary

Using New Words in Sentences. For this exercise, write a new sentence that means the same thing, using words from the Word Bank below to replace the key word identified. You may need to reformulate the sentence to make it make sense.

WORD BANK

deviations

work

well-being

aware

at this time

even though

1) discrepancies

There have been many *discrepancies* in interpretation of the meanings of medical abbreviations.

New sentence: _____

2) despite

Despite numerous attempts to standardize medical abbreviations, many of the error-prone ones are still being used in health care today.

New sentence: _____

3) currently

Currently in the United States and Canada, agencies and organizations are researching the use of medical abbreviations and their relationship to the occurrences of medication administration errors.

New sentence: _____

4) cognizant

Nor are they necessarily *cognizant* of the need for the standardization of abbreviations used in medication administration in English-speaking North America.

New sentence: _____

5) practice

There are lists of medical abbreviations that agencies recommend we **not** use in our professional *practice.*

New sentence: _____

6) welfare

This is your responsibility to the safety and *welfare* of your patients.

New sentence: _____

Using Medical Abbreviations. We have been talking a lot about medical abbreviations used in the administration of medications. This exercise will introduce a number of them. Work with them in the next few exercises to discover all you can about them and how you will or will not use them in your own safe practice.

VOCABULARY ALERT: USE OF MEDICAL ABBREVIATIONS Remember, even though you may not use all of these abbreviations, you must be able to recognize them when you encounter them so that you can seek clarification and verification of what the prescriber of the medications really intended for the patient.

Study Box 8-6 and then proceed to the questions that follow. This exercise also requires that you use the Internet. Go online to the Joint Commission website at http://www.jointcommission.org/. Search for the menu item "Patient Safety." Click it. Select the "Do Not Use List." Then, answer the following by selecting true or false.

1) Qd is an approved, acceptable abbreviation in a medication order.

_____ true _____ false

If your answer is "false," please explain and provide an alternative method of writing what you mean: _____

2) Bid is an approved, acceptable abbreviation in a medication order.

_____ true _____ false

If your answer is "false," please explain and provide an alternative method of writing what you mean: _____

3) Tid is an approved, acceptable abbreviation in a medication order.

_____ true _____ false

If your answer is "false," please explain and provide an alternative method of writing what you mean: _____

4) Qid is an approved, acceptable abbreviation in a medication order.

_____ true _____ false

If your answer is "false," please explain and provide an alternative method of writing what you mean: _____

BOX 8-6 Common Medical Abbreviations and Their Meanings

ABBREVIATION	MEANING
qd	once per day (×1)
bid	twice per day (×2)
tid	three times per day (×3)
qid	four times per day (×4)
hs	at bedtime
ac	before meals
pc	after meals

5) hs is an approved, acceptable abbreviation in a medication order.

_____ true _____ false

If your answer is "false," please explain and provide an alternative method of writing what you mean: _____

6) ac is an approved, acceptable abbreviation in a medication order.

_____ true _____ false

If your answer is "false," please explain and provide an alternative method of writing what you mean: _____

7) pc is an approved, acceptable abbreviation in a medication order.

_____ true _____ false

If your answer is "false," please explain and provide an alternative method of writing what you mean: _____

8) @ is an approved, acceptable abbreviation in a medication order.

_____ true _____ false

If your answer is "false," please explain and provide an alternative method of writing what you mean: _____

Sentence Completion.   In the context of medication administration, use medication abbreviations correctly. Complete the sentences or answer the questions.

1) Maria needs to have heart medication once per day. How often does she need it?
She needs it _____.

2) Rufus is a diabetic. He needs his insulin before breakfast. Using a medical abbreviation, when does he need it? He needs it _____.

3) John takes a sleeping pill before bed. When does he take it? The order reads: Sleeping tablet X .375 mg at _____.

4) Some medications need to be given after meals. This is known as _____ administration.

5) Antibiotics are only given for 7 days and usually at least twice per day. Then you must stop them. Randy is to take his medication twice a day. The doctor's order reads: Antibiotic XYZ 250 mg _____ × 7 days and then stop.

SPEAKING EXERCISE

Read the following information aloud. Ask a peer or teacher to help you with pronunciation. You might want to record yourself speaking so you can listen back any time you want to self-evaluate the improvements you are making in pronunciation and fluency. The Pronunciation Hints box that follows the reading will help.

THE MEDICAL ABBREVIATION *PRN*

The medical abbreviation prn means "as needed." In a health-care setting, staff often communicate with one another using this abbreviation. They simply say the letters aloud. For example: "Bob needs a prn." Medications, treatments, and care interventions can be ordered or completed on a prn basis. This means the nurse is to use her or his medical knowledge and an assessment of the situation (including interpersonal communication with the patient to gather information) to make a clinical decision whether or not to take action. The patient chart or documentation of this will also use this abbreviation. Prn may be written with or without the periods. For example: "Given analgesic prn at 10:45 am."

Sometimes the term prn is misinterpreted to mean "give upon demand" or "give on request." This thinking puts the responsibility for care and management of an individual's pain or treatment in his or her own hands. (This popular strategy is part of the concept of empowerment, wellness, and health promotion.) Patient's wishes or desires for prns are not always health-promoting. When in the hospital or under the direct supervision of a nurse, professional nursing judgment and clinical decision-making skills take precedence over the patient's wishes. Good assessment skills by the nurse are expected to be used before action is taken. This is a safety-to-practice issue.

PRONUNCIATION ALERT Most abbreviations used in medication administration are spoken simply by saying their letters aloud. For example:

prn – pē -ar-en
bid – bē -ī-dē

PRONUNCIATION HINTS

analgesic – ăn"ăl-jē'sĭk

interpersonal – ĭn"tĕr-**pĕr**'sŏn-ăl

precedence – **pres**'ĕ-dĕns

LISTENING EXERCISE

If you have recorded yourself reading the exercise above aloud, listen to your recording now without looking at the words in this book. Listen only. Do not let the written words be your guide. Evaluate yourself.

- What do you notice about your open pronunciation?
- Are you speaking clearly?
- Are you speaking at a normal rhythm and rate?

If you have not recorded yourself, ask a peer to read any part of this section aloud to you. Do not read along with them. Listen only. What do you notice about the way they speak? What lesson do you learn from listening to another?

WRITING EXERCISE

Use a key word from the previous exercises to create new sentences. You are given these words in parentheses.

1) _____ (error-prone)

2) _____ (medication, breakfast)

3) _____ (relax, bath, bedtime)

4) _____ (occasionally, over-the-counter)

5) _____ (practice, aware, abbreviations)

Treatments, Interventions, and Assistance

Pharmacology and medication administration continue as the means for career-specific language development. Within the context of treatments, vocabulary building centers on the use of antibiotics and oral administration of medications. Interventions are explored through the example of analgesic medication; the language of intramuscular injections is also identified. Finally, within the context of assistance, communicative strategies for teaching and learning with clients about their medications are the focus; the language of blister packs is also introduced. Professional and lay terminology, modes of medication administration, and common abbreviations are highlights of this section of Unit 8.

Reading Selection 8-7

Read the following short text in preparation for the exercises that follow.

TREATMENTS INVOLVING MEDICATIONS

Medications are used in the treatment of illnesses, diseases, disorders, and injuries. They are just one part of holistic care, but they can often bring about relief from pain, speedy recovery, or the ability to think clearly again. Antibiotics are an example of medications administered to combat infections and promote healing. They can be given by injection or intravenously, taken orally (by mouth), and even administered topically (on the skin).

 ## READING EXERCISES

Understanding the General Meaning

Read the text again. Think about it. Do you understand it?

1) What is the gist of this text?

2) What kinds of medications are given to fight infections?

3) What can medications bring about?

Building Vocabulary

Fill in the Blanks. Study the Grammar Alert on this page in preparation for the exercise that follows.

> **GRAMMAR ALERT: ADVERBS THAT DESCRIBE "HOW"** Recall a distinguishing feature of adverbs is that they generally end in –ly and describe the action of a verb. An important type of adverb used to provide information about the use of medication in the treatment of the patient is the adverb of *manner*. It tells us **how** a medication is actually given. For example, when we have to take meds, we generally take them orally, meaning by mouth. Oftentimes, we apply medications to our skin. This means the meds are applied topically. From time to time we may need to get an injection. We might receive these under the skin, subcutaneously, or maybe intramuscularly, deep into the muscles of

our thighs or buttocks. And, when we are really ill or injured, medications may be given through the intravenous route, directly into our veins. In this case, we receive our medications intravenously.

A) In Table 8-1 you are to make a list of the adverbs used when describing how medications are administered. Take these from the Grammar Alert box. Identify their root words in the second column. Notice that the words from which these adverbs originate are anatomical terms you have already learned in *Medical English Clear and Simple.*

Table 8-1 Adverbs and Their Root Words	
ADVERB	ROOT

B) Complete the following by filling in the blank with an appropriate adverb.

1) When given by injection, penicillin is an example of a drug that must be given deep into the muscle tissue. This injection is given _____.

2) Surgical patients who have an intravenous line *in situ* (in place) may receive their antibiotic medication by that route. They are taking their medications _____.

3) Matilda has not lost her ability to swallow. She can take her meds _____.

4) Belinda has an infected mosquito bite. The infection is not systemic. It is localized at the site of the wound. She has been applying an over-the-counter antibiotic to it to promote healing. She is using this medication _____.

5) Benjamin has diabetes mellitus. He injects his insulin just under the skin, but not into the layers of muscles. He is taking insulin _____.

Recognizing Types of Oral Medications. Oral medications are the most common meds and the safest to take. Professional practice will necessitate that you know the difference between types of oral meds by how they are supplied. Study the following.

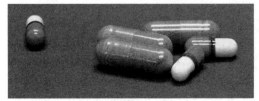

Capsules are also known as caps. Gel caps are designed to dissolve quickly. The capsules are made of a gelatin compound. Time-release caps are designed to dissolve gradually, slowly releasing the medication into the system.

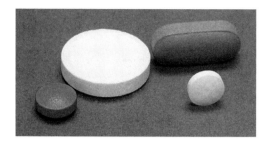

Pills are also referred to as tablets. They are round, solid, and hard. They may have an indentation across the center that allows the pill to be divided into smaller portions. When a pill is divided along the indentation line, it is said to be "scored." Some pills are also identified by the fact that they are chewable.

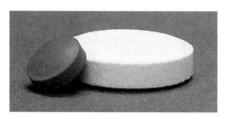

Tablets are also commonly referred to as pills; however, they may come in a wide variety of shapes. They are solid. Tablets may also appear scored and some can be designated as chewable.

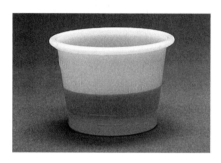

Liquid oral medications come in a variety of formulations:

- Suspensions are liquid forms of the drug itself
- Elixirs contain medications dissolved in water or alcohol
- Syrups are concentrated sugar solutions that contain the drug

Sentence Completion.   Use your new vocabulary and new understanding of how oral medications are supplied to complete the following sentences.

1) Wayne's medication comes in the form of two red, cylindrical shapes that are translucent. If you hold them up to the light you can see through them. These are likely ⸺⸺⸺⸺.

2) Arnie's medication is round, white, and has an indented line across the center of it. Arnie is taking a ⸺⸺⸺⸺.

3) Bill takes a multivitamin each morning. It is hard, solid, round, and shiny. This is a

   ⸺⸺⸺⸺.

4) Jerry is on antibiotics. He is taking a medication that is cylindrical in shape and shiny, but he cannot see through it if he holds it up to the light. He is taking a ⸺⸺⸺⸺.

5) Christian's medication is measured by the teaspoonful. He takes one teaspoon orally each night before bed. This medication is ⸺⸺⸺⸺.

6) Jamie is 5 years old. He takes a vitamin every day. It is purple and in the shape of a cartoon character. He doesn't swallow it whole. He is not supposed to. It doesn't dissolve. This type of medication is ⸺⸺⸺⸺.

SPEAKING EXERCISE

Re-read the exercise you have just completed. Read it aloud. Try the method of chaining again. It will help you put a string of sentences together in an easy, more natural way of speaking. The following Pronunciation Hints box will help.

LISTENING EXERCISE

Search the radio or television airwaves for an English-language program in which they are talking about medications. Remember, in the United States and Canada we are well-informed consumers of health-care products. The general public has a lot of knowledge about medications, but they also seek a lot of knowledge about them, too. There are numerous programs about this topic. Listen carefully to how people talk about the meds they take and the manner of how they ask questions of doctors, nurses, pharmacists, and others.

WRITING EXERCISE—A REFLECTIVE QUESTION

Do you think that medications are used as often or as frequently in the treatment of illnesses and disorders in your country of origin as they are here in the United States or Canada? Take some time now to write down your thoughts.

_____

_____

_____

_____

_____

Reading Selection 8-8

Read the following information aloud or silently to yourself.

INTERVENTIONS WITH MEDICATIONS

Medications are also used to intervene in illnesses, disorders, and situations. Pain is an excellent example of where and when medications are used to intervene. For example, during a prolonged and difficult labor and delivery, analgesic medication may be administered to the expectant mom to help alleviate her pain. Clients with long-term illnesses or conditions such as cancer or rheumatoid arthritis also endure pain. They may be prescribed an analgesic medication on a long-term basis to help them cope. When pain symptoms are diminished, quality of life becomes possible for these individuals.

Humans also experience emotional pain, such as when a loved one dies. They may experience fear of the unknown as well, and even fear of pain itself. In these instances, our care interventions may include the prescription and administration of anti-anxiety (anxiolytic) medications. Intervening with medications doesn't have the direct intent of healing. Instead, the goal is to alleviate symptoms related to illnesses, injuries, or situations in life that affect the body's and mind's ability to deal effectively with these circumstances.

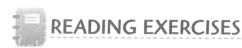

READING EXERCISES

These exercises will not only help you understand the general meaning of new words and build vocabulary, but also enable you to understand specifics about analgesics and about the ways medications can be administered.

Understanding the General Meaning

Respond to the following questions in full sentences.

1) What is the purpose of this short reading?

_____

2) What is an anxiolytic med?

_____

3) Which examples are used to illustrate when an analgesic might be used as an intervention?

_____

4) When medications are used as interventions, is cure the goal?

_____

5) For how long can analgesics be prescribed?

_____

Building Vocabulary

Analgesics are commonly used in medicine and nursing so you must be familiar with their forms and uses. In addition, you may be called upon to administer an intramuscular (IM) injection of a medication, so you must be familiar with the sites where such injections should be given. These exercises will help you become familiar with both of these topics.

Understanding the Use of Analgesics.   The reading introduced the topic of analgesics. Think very carefully about this as you answer the next few questions. Short answers are acceptable.

1) Is pain something that can be cured?

_____

2) Is there such a thing as emotional pain?

_____

3) What is the goal of analgesic use?

_____

4) The common term for an analgesic is "pain killer." Is pain really killed when these meds are taken?

_____

Understanding Intramuscular Injections.   It is possible to administer analgesics and anti-anxiety medications by some of the routes indicated in a previous exercise. Analgesics can be given by intramuscular injection, intravenously, orally, and even topically. However, anxiolytic medications can only be given orally or by intramuscular injection. The following exercises deal with intramuscular injections. First, study the graphic that locates the sites on the body where intramuscular (IM) injections may be given. Then, fill in the blanks to complete the sentences. Use the graphic of IM sites to guide you.

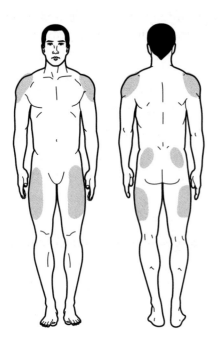

1) Roy is experiencing a great deal of pain associated with his leg amputation right now. The doctor has decided to give him an analgesic by IM injection. The patient says he wants it in his "backside." Where does Roy actually want to receive the injection?

_____

2) Gracie is in the emergency room. She is anxious, loud, and acting up. She was in a car accident and has a number of lacerations to her hands and face. One of these needs sutures. She can't concentrate on that. She says she needs "to get out of here" because she is afraid the police will arrest her for causing the accident. She agrees to take an analgesic, but only by injection. She wants it, she says, in the side of her hip. This anatomical location is known as the

_____

3) Max has multiple sclerosis. He cannot move from the neck down to his toes, but he can still feel. He is in bed right now. He tells you he is experiencing severe muscle pain from involuntary muscle spasms. You will give him an analgesic by the IM route into the front of his upper leg. This site is known as the ———————.

4) Barb has been having a lot of pain since admission to the hospital. She is being given analgesic medication by injection every 6–8 hours. She says her hips and legs look like "pin cushions" and she wants to know if she can have the next injection "anywhere else" on her body. You know that some medications can be injected intramuscularly into the upper arm. You will check the pharmaceutical compendium to see if this site is acceptable for use with this type of medication. This site is anatomically known as the

——————— .

SPEAKING EXERCISE

Go back now and read Understanding Intramuscular Injections aloud. Ask a peer or teacher to help you with pronunciation. Use the chaining method again to help you put sentences together. The Pronunciation Hints box below will help.

PRONUNCIATION HINTS

ventrogluteal – věn"trō-gloo'tē-ăl

dorsal – dōr'săl

gluteus – gloo'tē-ŭs

vastus lateralis – văs'tŭs lăt"ĕr-ā'lĭs

anxiolytic – ăng"zī-ō-lĭt'ĭk

LISTENING EXERCISE

You might want to listen to and watch instructions for giving intramuscular injections produced by *Nursing Lab, Take Two:* "Administering an Intramuscular Injection." It is available at http://www.youtube.com.

WRITING EXERCISE

Use your new vocabulary. Write a short paragraph describing your own experience and skills with giving intramuscular injections for analgesic or anti-anxiety medications.

_____

_____

_____

_____

_____

Reading Selection 8-9

ASSISTANCE WITH MEDICATION ADMINISTRATION

Medications are often the subject of teaching and learning activities that occur between a health professional and his or her client. Many of our clients/patients are on multiple medications. They may also take over-the-counter (OTC) medications, sometimes concurrently with prescribed medications, but they may not have told the doctor about this at the time the doctor was writing a prescription. Taking multiple medications at the same time is referred to as polypharmacy. It can be dangerous. As health professionals, we must be able to gain this information from clients and evaluate the situation. We must know about drug interactions. The knowledge and ability to explain medications as well as how they should be taken is crucial to the professional, moral, ethical, and legal responsibilities we have to our patients and clients. We want to keep them safe and able to experience the desired therapeutic effect of the drug(s). Additionally, we must be able to advise clients where they can find more information about their meds.

Understanding the General Meaning

Read the text again. Think about it. Respond to the following questions with complete sentences.

1) This text has a social purpose. It gives us a message. What is the gist of that message?

_____

2) Identify one type of assistance a health professional will give to a person taking medications.

_____

Comprehending Specific Information

Answer the following questions with short answers.

1) What is polypharmacy?

_____

2) What would a health professional need to gain from a client about his or her medication use?

_____

3) Do clients in the community or patients in the hospital always tell the nurses and doctors all of the medications they are taking? Explain your answer.

_____

_____

4) Give an example from the text of something a health professional would teach a client about a medication.

_____

Building Vocabulary

Becoming Familiar with Sentence Structure. Become more familiar with the vocabulary and sentence structure used in the reading. Unscramble these sentences. Write them out correctly.

1) take sometimes medications told these she prescription may over medications concurrently prescribed have doctor at a they writing time also counter the about was the but not with time the

_____

_____

2) professionals must to information the health be able as this we evaluate and situation gain

_____

Using New Vocabulary in Sentences. Use the key word or words from the reading to create new, full sentences.

1) over-the-counter, concurrently

_____

2) polypharmacy, dangerous

_____

3) assists, medication administration, client

_____

SPEAKING EXERCISE

Read the following paragraph aloud. Ask a peer or teacher to help you with pronunciation if you can. Repeat the exercise as many times as you need to in order to feel more comfortable with it. The Pronunciation Hints box following will help.

In relation to safe practice in medication administration, standards of practice for health professionals determine their practice boundaries. This means each of the health professions, acting under a law or a legislated act, ensures that their registered members have the knowledge, skills, and competencies required to safely administer medication within their scope of practice.

PRONUNCIATION HINTS

legistlated – lĕj´ĭs-lāt

scope – skōp

LISTENING EXERCISE

Go on the Internet again. Search the video sites such as *YouTube* for a short clip by Illumistream Health Production (Jan. 2008), *Professional Medication Review* entitled, "Topimax (Topiramate)." In this clip, a pharmacist clearly and succinctly explains what this anti-epileptic drug is for and how to take it. She is a Doctor of Pharmacy at the University of Southern California. She uses the language of the consumer and remains highly professional throughout. Notice that this video clip also contains some pictures of capsules, pills, and tablets. Listen for pronunciation, but also for the content of what she is teaching her clients.

WRITING EXERCISE

Consider the video clip you have watched in the last exercise. The pharmacist is speaking in the information genre. She has adjusted her linguistic choices of words, intonation, and so on to suit a very specific target audience. Who is this video clip designed for? Write the answer to this question and any comments you have about the video clip here.

_____

_____

_____

Reading Selection 8-10

This last section of Unit 8 concerns itself with communication in the context of teaching and learning for medications. It begins with a dialogue between a nurse and a patient. She is teaching him about his new prescription. Read the interaction aloud with a partner or silently to yourself. This is a very long conversation, but don't worry, you can absolutely do it.

YOUR NEW MEDICATION, MR. KOZMA

Nurse: Hi, Mr. Kozma. My name is Melinda and I am your nurse this morning.

Patient: Hello.

Nurse: I understand you are going to be discharged home from the hospital today.

Patient: Yes. I think I can leave around 11:00 a.m.

Nurse: Yes, that's correct. But first I'd like to spend a little time with you talking about your medications. As you know, Dr. Halstrom has started you on an anti-anginal medication.

Patient: Anti-anginal?

Nurse: Yes. That's a medication used to help alleviate chest pain.

Patient: (The patient doesn't speak, but he looks confused.)

Nurse: Mr. Kozma, you look confused. How can I help?

Patient: You are using words that I don't really know.

Nurse: Oh, I'm sorry. Let me start again. The doctor has started you on a medication that will give you relief from the pain you feel in your chest sometimes. That type of pain is called angina. Has the doctor explained that to you?

Patient: Yes, I understand now why I get pains in my chest. But they are awful.

Nurse: Yes, they can be quite painful and a bit scary, too, can't they?

Patient: Yeah, right! I thought I was gonna die from a heart attack. I know better now.

Nurse: Good. OK, so yesterday you started on this new med called nitroglycerine.

Patient: Yes, I took one yesterday. You only take that nitro pill once in a while; when you need it for pain, right?

Nurse: Yes, that's right. It sounds like the nurse yesterday taught you about the medication. Is that correct?

Patient: Yes, he was very nice.

Nurse: OK, and did he tell you about the side effects you might experience?

Patient: Yes, I know that I might get a headache or some dizziness and some other things. Yes, he told me all about that. I didn't get any side effects yesterday when I took one, but it's good to know this information for the next time.

Nurse: Yes, good. So let's just spend a couple of minutes talking about how you will take this medication at home and I'll tell you a couple of more things that you might like to know about it.

Patient: All right.

Nurse: Nitroglycerine is only to be taken prn—when you need it. It is not a good idea to take it at any other time. As you know, it dissolves under your tongue. The name for that is sublingual. Your nitro is sublingual.

Patient: Sublingual.

Nurse: Yes. There are two occasions when you can take it. The first is if you expect to do an activity that will cause a lot of exertion or cause your heart to work very hard. Take a tablet about 5 or 10 minutes prior to that. The second occasion for using the nitro is when you feel chest pain beginning. In that case, put a tablet under your tongue. You can repeat this twice, as long as you wait at least 5 minutes between taking a tablet, OK?

Patient: OK. If I should need to take another nitro pill, I will wait at least 5 minutes.

Nurse: Correct. But remember, you must not, MUST NOT take more than three doses of nitroglycerin. If you are still experiencing pain at that time, you need to get medical help immediately. Do you understand that, Mr. Kozma?

Patient: Yes, it sounds scary, but I understand it. If my medication doesn't relieve my pain, I need to get to the hospital as soon as possible because I might be having a heart attack.

Nurse: It's possible, Mr. Kozma. And we don't want that. It's best if you come into the hospital so we can be sure.

Patient: Yes, exactly. That is exactly what I will do. Anything else I need to know?

Nurse: Just one more thing. Nitroglycerine comes in a dark-colored container. That is because it doesn't like the light. That is to say, its chemical compound can be affected by the light. It should always be kept out of the sunlight, OK?

Patient: Yes.

Nurse: Great, Mr. Kozma. Now I need to go over your other medications just briefly with you. I see from your chart that you take a sleeping pill and a laxative at bedtime. You've been taking these for quite a long time, haven't you?

Patient: Yes, a long time. I know about them.

Nurse: They both come in pill form, don't they?

Patient: Yes.

Nurse: I know you have some arthritis in your fingers and I was wondering if your prescriptions are dispensed to you in medication bottles or if they are given to you in blister packs?

Patient: What is a blister pack?

Nurse: Oh, all right. Well, I wondered about that. If you have pills in bottles, it can sometimes be difficult for people with arthritis to open them. Many, many medications are now provided by the pharmacy in something called a blister pack. It's a cardboard (we call it a "card") about the size of a piece of writing paper. It has plastic bubbles on it. Each of these bubbles contains your exact,

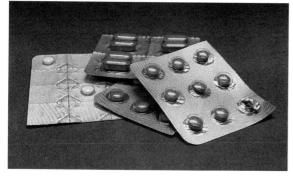

personal doses of medications prepared by the pharmacist. All you do is punch out a bubble with your thumb or finger when it is time to take the meds. If you take two meds at the same time, like you do, it may be that your pharmacist will put both of those meds into one bubble. However, your nitroglycerine will always be packed on a separate card, because you don't take it routinely.

Patient: Oh, that sounds easy. Then I don't have to worry about trying to take the cap off the pill bottles and spilling those darn pills all over the counter. Oh, that would be so helpful! How can I get a blister pack?

Nurse: Well, it's quite simple, Mr. Kozma. You just need to ask your pharmacist. He or she will be happy to help you with this.

Patient: Great! Thanks.

Nurse: OK, my pleasure. Now is there anything else you'd like to talk about or ask about your medications?

Patient: No thanks, you've been very helpful. Thanks.

Nurse: You're welcome, Mr. Kozma. If you have any other questions before you are discharged, please ask me. Otherwise, please consult with your doctor, pharmacist, or nurse-practitioner. They'll be happy to help you understand your medications. Bye-bye.

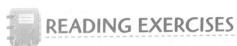

READING EXERCISES

Understanding the General Meaning

Read the dialogue again if you need to. The following questions will help you evaluate whether or not you have understood its general meaning. Short answers are acceptable.

1) What is the main purpose of the conversation between the nurse and the patient?

_____

2) Is nitroglycerine taken routinely?

_____

3) Why is the patient taking nitroglycerine?

_____

4) What is the patient's name?

_____

5) Who is teaching whom?

_____

Comprehending Specific Information

Take a moment now to review the dialogue again as you work through these exercises. Choose the best answer from the multiple choices.

1) The medical term for chest pain is
   a) heart attack.
   b) myocardial infarction.
   c) angina.
   d) anti-anginal.

2) Chest pain may occur for this patient if he
   a) sleeps.
   b) goes jogging.
   c) bends over.
   d) lays flat on his back.

3) A blister pack is
   a) a cardboard.
   b) a method of dispensing medications.
   c) a bubble board.
   d) a method of compressing angina.

4) Where is Mr. Kozma right now?
   a) at home
   b) at work
   c) in the hospital
   d) at the walk-in clinic

5) Tomorrow, if he wants to, who can Mr. Kozma ask for more information about his prescription?
   a) his clergyman
   b) this nurse
   c) his pharmacist
   d) all of the above

Pharmacology and Medication Administration

6) The nurse teaches Mr. Kozma about two separate things. The first is his nitroglycerine. What is the other thing?
   a) not to do strenuous exercise
   b) blister packs
   c) his sleeping pill and laxative
   d) calling the doctor

7) If the nitroglycerine is ineffective to treat Mr. Kozma's chest pain, what should he do?
   a) seek medical help, quickly
   b) call his doctor
   c) call his pharmacist
   d) take a fourth nitroglycerine tablet sublingually

8) What is the first action of a sublingual medication? It
   a) evaporates.
   b) dissolves.
   c) flushes.
   d) metabolizes.

9) What does sublingual mean?
   a) through the nose
   b) down the throat
   c) under the tongue
   e) orally

10) At first, the patient is confused by the nurse's
    a) vocabulary.
    b) enthusiasm.
    c) professionalism.
    d) all of the above

11) When the patient experiences angina, emotionally he finds it
    a) pleasant.
    b) confusing.
    c) scary.
    d) interesting.

Building Vocabulary

For written communications you must be able to spell the new English words you are learning. You must also be able to communicate verbally with patients and use appropriate vocabulary. These exercises will help you do both.

Improving Your Spelling of New Words. Become more familiar with new vocabulary by unscrambling these words. Write out the correct spelling.

1) lgalusbuni _____

2) tsrbiel _____

3) ddbroarac _____

4) etrgoylnrncie _____

5) gaanni _____

6) agalnniati-n _____

7) xalveati _____

8) dshgciaedr _____

9) leivaltea _____

10) palfinu _____

Answering Patients' Questions.   Follow the example set by the nurse in the teaching and learning dialogue to create your own answers to patient questions. Use full sentences to reply.

1) "Nurse, I can't open this pill bottle. I always have trouble with these bottles."

   "_____

   _____"

2) "I have some ointment for the rash on my hand but it burns me."

   "_____

   _____"

3) "Excuse me, nurse. I got a new medication yesterday. It isn't any good. It's givin' me a bad stomach. I hate it."

   "_____

   _____"

4) "Nurse, what will I do if this new sleeping pill doesn't work? I'm being discharged from the hospital today and I'm worried I won't get any sleep."

   "_____

   _____"

5) "Nurse, what is this little pink pill in the cup? I don't take pills like that. I've never seen one like that before. Did you make a mistake?"

   "_____

   _____"

6) "Oh, I know what that yellow pill is, nurse."

   "_____

   _____"

SPEAKING EXERCISE

Read the dialogue aloud again. Do so with a partner, but if that is not possible, read it aloud yourself, changing your voice for each character. Try to sound as natural as possible when talking. Remember, this is a dialogue of a communication; a conversation between two people. It should sound like that. The Pronunciation Hints box below will help.

PRONUNCIATION HINTS

anginal – ăn-jī'năl

alleviate – ăl-lēv-ē'āt

sublingual – sŭb-lĭng'gwăl

nitroglycerin – nī"trō-glĭs'ĕr-ĭn

LISTENING EXERCISE

You have just completed a lengthy dialogue between a nurse and a patient. This is a perfect opportunity for you to record yourself speaking. Record the dialogue of yourself and, if possible, with a partner. Listen back. Listen to hear how smooth or fluent the conversation sounds. Go back to those places in the dialogue that don't sound fluent and work on them until they do.

WRITING EXERCISE

Use your new vocabulary. Write a few sentences describing an experience you have had teaching a patient about his or her new medication.

_____

_____

_____

_____

ANSWER KEY

Pharmacology, Pharmacodynamics, and Pharmacokinetics

 ### READING SELECTION 1—ALL THINGS PHARMACOLOGICAL

Understanding the General Meaning

1) Two main themes in the text are to highlight the root word *pharma* and to explain the fields of pharmacology.

2) Acetylsalicylic acid (aspirin) was used to support the claim of an unexpected benefit of a drug.

Mix and Match

BOX 8-1	Mix and Match: Words Derived from *Pharma*: Answers
WORD	DEFINITION
pharmacokinetics	movement of drugs through the body
pharmatherapeutics	helping or healing effects of drugs
pharmaceuticals	synthetic or manufactured drugs
pharmacodynamics	how drugs affect cells
pharmacology	science of drugs, their actions, and interactions
pharmacist	understands and dispenses medications

Fill in the Blanks

1) pharmacist, pharmacy

2) pharmaceutical

3) therapeutic or pharmacotherapeutics

4) pharmacotherapy

5) pharmacokinetics

6) pharmaceuticals

7) pharmacodynamics

Building Vocabulary

Determining Meaning from Context

1) e, 2) e, 3) b, 4) b, 5) b, 6) a, 7) c

Mix and Match

BOX 8-2 Mix and Match: Words Derived from *Medic:* Answers	
WORD	APPROPRIATE EXPLANATION
medicate	administer
medicinal	health promoting
medical	type of school for doctors
medically	a way to speak
medicine	something you take to get better
medication	something the nurse or doctor administers
medic	performs medical duties in the armed forces
paramedic	person most often found working in an ambulance

Fill in the Blanks

1) paramedics or paramedical personnel

2) medical, medical

3) medicine

4) medication

5) medic, medical

6) medically

7) medicated

8) medicate

9) medication, medicated

10) medicines or medications

Using Common Medical Prefixes

1) An anti-epileptic medication is one that prevents seizures.

2) An antihypertensive medication is used to prevent or control high blood pressure.

3) An anticancer medication is one that prevents the growth of cancer cells or prevents the spread of cancer in the body.

4) An antitoxin medication is one that reduces or eliminates the harmful effects of a toxin.

5) An anti-anginal medication is one that alleviates angina or chest pain.

6) An antiviral medication prevents the spread of a virus.

7) An antibacterial medication eliminates bacteria.

8) An antidiarrheal medication prevents or stops diarrhea.

9) An anti-inflammatory medication is one that prevents or alleviates inflammation.

10) An antipyretic medication is one that reduces fever.

Fill in the Blanks

1) antihistamine, medication

2) antiemetic

3) medic

4) antihypertensive

5) medically, antibiotic

6) antimanic

7) antidiarrheal, medication

READING SELECTION 2—SIDE EFFECTS OR ADVERSE EFFECTS?

Understanding the General Meaning

1) Medications can affect the body in negative ways.

2) to provide clarity; to differentiate between side effects, adverse effects, and toxic effects

3) unwanted, undesirable, contrary

4) poison

5) moderate to severe

6) toxic effects

Building Vocabulary

Determining Meaning from Context

1) b, 2) c, 3) b, 4) d

Using New Vocabulary in Sentences

Examples of possible sentences:

1) Poison has a negative, toxic effect on the body.

2) Fine tremors are an adverse effect of some medications.

3) The patient is so anxious about the pending results of her lab tests that she is trembling.

4) The lady had an adverse reaction to the medication she took.

5) Swallowing a toxic substance can be fatal.

6) One of the main effects of this drug is sleepiness.

READING SELECTION 3—ABSTRACT

Understanding the General Meaning

1) *Survey of Nursing Perceptions of Medication Administration Practices, Perceived Sources of Errors and Reporting Behaviours*

2) The general intent of the research is to review the whole process of medication administration within the hospital and to develop a systematic approach to medication error control.

3) The perceived source of error most often cited was transcription (processing) and the second most frequently cited source was the legibility of handwritten medication orders (prescribing). Years of experience as a nurse did not factor into the amount of errors occurring.

4) The target audience is nurses, quality control, and administration professionals in hospitals.

5) This is a cross-sectional survey.

6) It is not clear what their credentials are. The abstract suggests the researchers and authors are part of an interdisciplinary team in a hospital, but this does not mean that each is actually a health professional.

7) If they were concerned about the number of medication errors occurring in their facility and wanted to know why they occurred and how they might prevent them.

8) medication error control, medication safety practices, medication error reporting

Understanding Specifics in the Abstract

1) The research findings say this was not significant; years of experience are not a factor in medication admission error.

2) The perceived source of error most often cited was transcription (processing), and the second most frequently cited source was the legibility of handwritten medication orders (prescribing).

3) The conclusion of this research was a need for ongoing education and information sessions on policies and procedures specific to safe medication practices for all nurses, regardless of years of experience.

Building Vocabulary

Sentence Completion

1) systematic approach

2) cross-sectional survey

3) medication variance

4) standardization

Reading and Interpreting an Abstract

1) Yes – Title, Introduction, Methods, Results, Conclusion

2) In January 2003, St. Mary's Hospital Center in Montreal, Quebec, established an interdisciplinary Committee on the Systematic Approach to Medication Error Control to review the whole process of medication administration within the hospital and to develop a systematic approach to medication error control.

3) A cross-sectional survey on medication administration practices, perceived sources of errors and medication error reporting of nurses, adapted from a nursing practice survey and medication variance report (Sim and Joyner, 2002), was conducted over a two-week period in February 2004.

4) The need for ongoing education and information sessions on policies and procedures specific to safe medication practices for all nurses, regardless of years of experience, was identified.

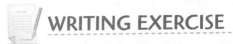

WRITING EXERCISE

Sample answer for abstract in draft form:

Title: Opportunities for performance improvement in relation to medication administration during pediatric stabilization

Introductory sentence or two: Accuracy in medication administration in pediatric stabilization is crucial to positive patient outcomes.

Methods used in the research: To assess the situation, the researchers videotaped a simulated pediatric stabilization event.

Results of the research: The researchers identified some important areas for improvement in medication administration.

A sentence of conclusion: The results of the research showed a clear need for improved education, training, and use of clinical aids or adjuncts for pediatric emergency nurses in this situation.

Safety and Accuracy in Medication Administration

READING SELECTION 4—MEDICATION ADMINISTRATION: SAFE PRACTICE STRATEGIES

Understanding the General Meaning

1) transcription error

2) the patients/clients

3) the process of transcription and verification

4) The answer is that errors can occur at every stage. Here are some examples:

- When the doctor writes a medication order there is a possibility of error in all aspects of the order: the dosage or frequency of administration might be wrong and/or the doctor may have overlooked the fact the patient is allergic to the drug, etc.

- When the nurse reads and interprets the order there is a possibility of error. The nurse may not have been able to clearly read the order and has mistaken one word for another or one abbreviation for another.

- When the nurse transcribes the doctor's order, there are many possibilities for errors. For example, when the nurse transcribes the order into the Medical Administration Record (MAR) sheet, he or she may be temporarily distracted and miscopy part or all of the order; the nurse may not have knowledge of the medication she is transcribing and without some, runs the risk of transcribing an order that had an error in it; the nurse's own handwriting may be illegible, causing mistakes to be made by other nurses who misinterpret it; the nurse may not read the order accurately (even though the writing is legible) and so writes what he or she "thinks" is the order. As a result, the wrong information (the wrong drug or related information) is written on the MAR. Similarly, when the nurse transcribes the information onto the patient's Kardex there is a possibility for error. If the Kardex information is not documented at the same time as the MAR, the medication order may be written inaccurately as immediate memory of it fades and distractions occur between the two events. Because the MAR is a smaller document in size, the nurse may want to use even more abbreviations to get the information onto it. These abbreviations may be shortcuts that are not generally understood, accepted, or approved by the care facility and the care team. In addition, there is possibility of error in the patient's chart.

- The nurse's notes need to be written in close proximity to the completion of all other transcription and documentation to avoid transcription error and miscopying for many of the reasons stated previously.

5) Yes, the nurse, the pharmacist, and the patient all have this right.

6) a nurse

7) Flow Chart

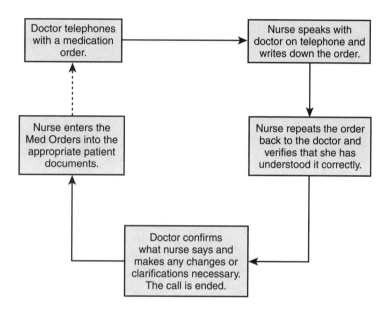

Building Vocabulary

Determining Meaning from Context

1) a, 2) c, 3) a, 4) d, 5) c, 6) d

Reading Medication Labels

A) 1) a) acetaminophen, b) Painaway, c) $C_8H_9NO_2$
   2) a) phenytoin, b) seizure-free, c) $C_{15}H_{12}N_2O_2$ 252.27
   3) a) loperamide, b) Noruns, c) 1-Piperidinebutanamide, 4-(4-chlorophenyl)-4-hydroxy-N,N-dimethyl-alpha,alpha-diphenyl-

B) Study the labels again.
   1) 325 mgs
   2) 10/10/10 October 10, 2010 or 10 October 2010
   3) 50

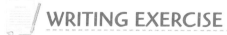

WRITING EXERCISE

1) a) The nurse should seek clarification, reading the orders back to the doctor to check the accuracy of what she or he has heard from the doctor. Unrelated to the accent, the nurse is also expected to question the accuracy of the medication order if, based on the nurse's own knowledge of pharmacology, the order seems incorrect or inappropriate.

2) a) The nurse will call or speak with the doctor person-to-person to seek clarity. This may be uncomfortable and anxiety-provoking for the nurse due to the surgeon's demeanor, but patient safety is the priority of care here. This obligates the nurse to seek clarification and ensure accuracy in transcription.

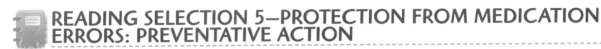

READING SELECTION 5—PROTECTION FROM MEDICATION ERRORS: PREVENTATIVE ACTION

Understanding the General Meaning

1) The main focus of this reading is prevention strategies for reducing or eliminating medication errors/protecting patients from medication errors.

2) These prevention strategies are being used wherever and whenever a qualified health professional administers medications.

3) The 7 Rights is a process, an approach, a protocol, a strategy for preventing medication errors by going through 7 specific steps of verification.

4) Examples are: patient's name, social security number (in Canada it's a social insurance number), date of birth, allergies, date of admission, diagnosis, and list of medications.

5) medication errors

6) 7 Rights of Medication Administration; Bar Code Label Rule

Building Vocabulary

Determining Meaning from Context

1) b, 2) a, 3) b, 4) b, 5) c

Following the 7 Rights Protocol

A) 1) How a medication is to be administered; for example, intravenous, injection, topical, pill, etc.
2) Because the nurse who did the transcription may not have actually given the medication. The next nurse might be the first to do so and discover an error of some sort.
3) On the MAR.
4) Medications are given once a day or throughout the day (e.g., every 4 hours or every 6 hours). Some are given before or after meals. Some are given immediately. They all vary and by order (as prescribed) must be given at the proper, indicated time for the best therapeutic effect.

B) 1) Check her wristband for her date of birth and compare that with what is on her chart.
2) Consult the doctor's orders and the MAR. It is possible that an order was written and this nurse is not aware of it, but it is also very possible that the patient is asking for a drug that is NOT ordered for him. He simply wants it, likes it, or prefers it. If the nurse makes a clinical judgment that the patient would benefit from a stronger analgesic than acetaminophen with codeine, she or he has the right to suggest this to the physician.

READING SELECTION 6—INTERPRETATION OF MEDICATION ORDERS DEPENDS ON INTERPRETATION OF CAREER-SPECIFIC ABBREVIATIONS

Understanding the General Meaning

1) to inform readers about current issues in the use of medication abbreviations related to medication administration and to advise them of agencies and organizations that affect their own clinical practice

2) information genre; telling and reporting information

3) to draw the reader's attention to them. They are important words that alert the reader to think about his or her own use of medical abbreviations

4) Institute for Safe Medication Practices

5) Joint Commission on Accreditation of Health Care Organization

6) many health professionals, particularly those new to the country

7) to reduce the risk of harm to patients or clients in the community and to promote safe practices among member of the health-care team

8) Go to their websites. The URL addresses are noted in the footnotes at the bottom of the page.

9) Health professionals have this responsibility. Rationale: The employer is supposed to adhere to directives issued by authoritative organizations and lawmakers, but this is not always the case. The health professional, as a licensed or registered member of the profession, has as the first priority of care a duty to protect the patient from harm. This includes protection from errors in transcribing or interpreting medication orders that use medical abbreviations.

Building Vocabulary

Using New Words in Sentences

Examples of possible answers are given:

1) There have been many *deviations* in interpretation of the meaning of medical abbreviations.

2) *Even though there have been* numerous attempts to standardize medical abbreviations, many of the error-prone ones are still being used in health care today.

3) *At this time* in the United States and Canada, agencies and organizations are researching the use of medical abbreviations and their relationship to the occurrences of medication administration errors.

4) Nor are they necessarily *aware* of the need for the standardization of abbreviations used in medication administration in English-speaking North America.

5) There are lists of medical abbreviations that agencies recommend we NOT use in our professional *work*.

6) This is your responsibility for the safety and *well-being* of your patients.

Using Medical Abbreviations

1) False. Qd is often mistaken for various other forms of the abbreviation, such as qid. Note: It is often misread as OD, meaning "right eye." This can be confusing and dangerous. Use the word "daily" instead of the abbreviation.

2) True

3) True

4) True. Note: Although this abbreviation has not been clearly identified on the Joint Commission's list, if you read the reasons for not using Qd, you will see that qid might also be misinterpreted. It might be preferable to write ×4 or ×4 daily. You must check with your employer.

5) True

6) True

7) True

8) False. It is sometimes mistaken for the number 2 and in electronic charting can be typed in error as this number. Use the word "at" instead.

Sentence Completion

1) daily or once per day (Note: Write out these words, do not use Qd if it is not approved in your facility, even if you see others using it.)

2) ac

3) hs

4) pc

5) bid

 # WRITING EXERCISE

Answer examples:

1) Some medical abbreviations are proven to be error-prone.

2) If you take your medication before breakfast, you take it ac.

3) At bedtime, some people like to take a warm bath and relax before going to bed.

4) Almost everyone we know takes the occasional over-the-counter medication prn.

5) The more you practice reading, writing, and using medical abbreviations, the more aware you will be of their meanings.

Treatments, Interventions, and Assistance

 ## READING SELECTION 7—TREATMENTS INVOLVING MEDICATIONS

Understanding the General Meaning

1) The gist of this text is that medications are one part of the treatment given for illnesses, injuries, disorders, and diseases.

2) antibiotics

3) Medications can bring about relief from pain, speed recovery, or restore the ability to think clearly again.

Building Vocabulary

Table 8-2 Adverbs and Their Root Words: Answers	
ADVERB	ROOT
orally	oral
topical	topic
subcutaneously	subcutaneous
intramuscularly	intramuscular
intravenously	intravenous

Fill in the Blanks

1) intramuscularly

2) intravenously

3) orally

4) topically

5) subcutaneously

Sentence Completion

1) gel caps or gel capsules

2) scored pill

3) tablet

4) capsule

5) liquid

6) chewable

READING SELECTION 8—INTERVENTIONS WITH MEDICATIONS

Understanding the General Meaning

1) The purpose of this short reading is to differentiate intervention goals with medications from treatment goals.

2) An anxiolytic is an anti-anxiety medication used to reduce anxiety or fear (of the unknown or fear of pain, for example).

3) The examples used are the case of a prolonged and difficult labor and delivery and rheumatoid arthritis and cancer.

4) No, the goal is alleviation of symptoms.

5) They can be prescribed for short or long periods of time. Rationale: It depends on the status of the illness or health situation that is causing the pain.

Building Vocabulary

Understanding the Use of Analgesics

1) No, pain is alleviated, dissipated, or diminished.

2) Yes, there is such a thing as emotional pain.

3) The goal of analgesic use is to alleviate physical pain and discomfort.

4) No. The underlying symptom that caused the pain is still not treated. Remember, pain is a symptom. It is how the body tells you something is wrong and needs your attention.

Understanding Intramuscular Injections

1) At the dorsal gluteal site (also known as the gluteus medius or gluteus maximus). Note: This site is no longer a preferred site for an intramuscular injection. However, many older patients and immigrants are familiar with it and will request that it be used. Clinical judgment by the health professional (usually the nurse in this situation) will determine if the patient can or cannot have the medication here and why. The patient's choice must always be considered.

2) ventrogluteal site. Note: Today, this is the preferred site of deep muscle injection. Note that many of the elderly and individuals from other countries are not familiar with this site. They may be apprehensive about receiving an injection here and even concerned about the nurse's knowledge and skills related to this choice of site. The health professional involved will need to be aware of the patient's concerns and provide some teaching.

3) vastus lateralis site. Note: This injection site is often taught to home care patients who give their own intramuscular injections. This might be, for example, a person living with cancer.

4) dorsal gluteal

READING SELECTION 9—ASSISTANCE WITH MEDICATION ADMINISTRATION

Understanding the General Meaning

1) The gist of the message is that health professionals need to be knowledgeable about medications not only to be able to teach clients about them, but also to ascertain if the meds the client is taking now are safe to be taken together.

2) They will assist the patient with education, teaching them about their meds.

Comprehending Specific Information

1) The administration or taking of many drugs concurrently (at the same time)

2) Data or information about what medications the client is currently taking

3) No. Many people either don't think of OTC medications as chemical compounds that might interact with prescribed drugs or they don't want their doctor to know about them. Sometimes when a person takes a contraception pill or minor analgesic every day, it becomes so normal for them that it doesn't occur to them to mention it.

4) An example of this from the text is how to take the medication.

Building Vocabulary

Becoming Familiar with Sentence Structure

1) They may also take over-the-counter medications, sometimes concurrently with pre-scribed medications, but have not told the doctor about these at the time he or she was writing a prescription.

2) As health professionals, we must explain to our clients that polypharmacy can be dangerous.

Using New Vocabulary in Sentences

Sample answer sentences are given:

1) Sometimes people take over-the-counter medications concurrently with prescribed med-ications (or prescription medications).

2) Polypharmacy can be dangerous.

3) The nurse assists the client with learning about how his medication is to be administered.

READING SELECTION 10—YOUR NEW MEDICATION, MR. KOZMA

Understanding the General Meaning

1) Teaching and learning about a new medication

2) No

3) For angina; chest pain. Rationale: We have no specific information about his cardiac health, so we cannot comment on that.

4) Mr. Kozma

5) The nurse is teaching Mr. Kozma.

Comprehending Specific Information

1) c, 2) b, 3) b, 4) c, 5) c, 6) b, 7) a, 8) b, 9) c, 10) a, 11) c

Building Vocabulary

Improving Your Spelling of New Words

1) sublingual

2) blister

3) cardboard

4) nitroglycerine

5) angina

6) anti-anginal

7) laxative

8) discharged

9) alleviate

10) painful

Answering Patients' Questions

Sample answers given:

1) "Here, let me help you. You say you have trouble opening these bottles. Have you considered getting your medications prepared in blister packs?"

2) "You may be experiencing a side effect of the med. I'll let the doctor know."

3) "You think your new medication is giving you a stomach ache. I'll let the doctor know."

4) "If you aren't able to sleep by the second night, please call your doctor and advise her. She might want to order something else for you."

5) "The doctor ordered this new medication for you. Let me teach you a little bit about it and why it has been prescribed for you."

6) "It sounds like another nurse has explained your new medication to you."

Photo Credits

Unit 1

Page 31, bottom: Schuster, PM: *Communication: The Key to the Therapeutic Relationship.* FA Davis, Philadelphia, 2000.
Page 40, 2nd and 3rd from top: Effgen, SK: *Meeting the Physical Therapy Needs of Children.* FA Davis, Philadelphia, 2005.

Unit 2

Page 67, 1st and 2nd from left; page 77, bottom; page 78, top: Effgen, SK: *Meeting the Physical Therapy Needs of Children.* FA Davis, Philadelphia, 2005.
Page 67, 3rd from left: Williams, L, and Hopper, P: *Understanding Medical Surgical Nursing,* ed 3. FA Davis, Philadelphia, 2007.
Page 67, 4th from left: Wilkinson, JM, and Van Leuven, K: *Fundamentals of Nursing: Theory, Concepts, and Applications,* Vol. 1. FA Davis, Philadelphia, 2007.
Page 70, middle, bottom; page 71, 1st, 2nd, 4th, and 5th from top: Starkey, C, and Ryan, J: *Orthopedic and Athletic Injury Evaluation Handbook.* FA Davis, Philadelphia, 2003.
Page 72, 2nd from top: Dillon, PM: *Nursing Health Assessment: A Critical Thinking Case Studies Approach,* ed 2. FA Davis, Philadelphia, 2007, p 307.
Page 77, middle: Schuster, PM: *Communication: The Key to the Therapeutic Relationship,* FA Davis, Philadelphia, 2000.
Page 87: Scanlon, VC, and Sanders, T: *Essentials of Anatomy and Physiology,* ed 5. FA Davis, Philadelphia, 2007.

Unit 3

Page 97: Scanlon, VC, and Sanders, T: *Essentials of Anatomy and Physiology,* ed 5. FA Davis, Philadelphia, 2007.
Page 107, top and bottom: Dillon, PM: *Nursing Health Assessment: A Critical Thinking Case Studies Approach,* ed 2. FA Davis, Philadelphia, 2007.

Unit 4

Page 144; page 175: Scanlon, VC, and Sanders, T: *Essentials of Anatomy and Physiology,* ed 5. FA Davis, Philadelphia, 2007.

Unit 5

Page 187; page 220: Scanlon, VC, and Sanders, T: *Essentials of Anatomy and Physiology,* ed 5. FA Davis, Philadelphia, 2007.

Unit 6

Page 234; page 242; page 274; page 277, top row, 2nd from left: Scanlon, VC, and Sanders, T: *Essentials of Anatomy and Physiology,* ed 5. FA Davis, Philadelphia, 2007.
Page 252, top row, 2nd from left; middle row, 4th from left; bottom row, 2nd from left: Schuster, PM: *Communication: The Key to the Therapeutic Relationship.* FA Davis, Philadelphia, 2000.

Page 252, middle row, 1st from left; page 252, middle row, 4th from left; page 252, bottom row, 2nd from left; page 277, top row, 4th from left: *Catalano: Nursing Now: Today's Issues, Tomorrow's Trends,* ed 5. FA Davis, Philadelphia, 2009.

Page 252, top row, 1st from left; page 277, middle row, 3rd from left: Anderson, MA: *Nursing Leadership, Management, and Professional Practice from the LPN/LVN: In Nursing School and Beyond.* ed 4. FA Davis, Philadelphia, 2009.

Page 267: From Hockenberry, MJ, and Winkelstein, ML: *Wong's Essentials of Pediatric Nursing,* ed 7. Mosby, St. Louis, 2005, p 1269. Used with permission.

Unit 7

Page 287, top row, 1st from left: Singer, AS, Burstein, JL, and Schiavone, FM: *Emergency Medicine Pearls,* ed 2. FA Davis, Philadelphia, 2001, p 209. Used with permission.

Page 287, top row, 2nd from left: Williams, L, and Hopper, P: *Understanding Medical Surgical Nursing,* ed 3. FA Davis, Philadelphia.

Page 287, bottom row, 2nd from left; page 287, bottom row, 3rd from left: Dillon, PM: *Nursing Health Assessment: A Critical Thinking Case Studies Approach,* ed 2. FA Davis, Philadelphia, 2007.

Page 287, bottom row, 2nd from left: Singer, AJ, and Hollander, JE: *Lacerations and Acute Wounds: An Evidence-Based Guide.* FA Davis, Philadelphia, 2003.

Page 316, top: Singer, AS, Burstein, JL, and Schiavone, FM: *Emergency Medicine Pearls*, ed 2. FA Davis, Philadelphia, 2001, p 78. Used with permission.

Page 316, middle; page 333: Wilkinson, JM, and Van Leuven, K: *Fundamentals of Nursing: Theory, Concepts, and Applications,* Vol. 1. FA Davis, Philadelphia, 2007.

Index

emergency department admission, 127–130
  head-to-toe assessment, 125–127
care priorities, 76
cartilage, 63
cases, 95
CAT scan, 259
cause, verb tenses of, 22
cavities, 54
cells, 53
Center for Disease Control and Prevention, 311
central nervous system (CNS), 231–232, 237, 244
cerebellum, 244
cerebrovascular accident (CVA), 263–267
cervical cancer, 292
chain of infection, 310–315, 332–334
charting guidelines, 299
charts, 238–239
chemotherapy, 159
chest pain, 113
chewing, 185
chickenpox, 303
chronic, 149
chronic disease, 148
chronicity, 147
chronic obstructive pulmonary disease (COPD), 148–151
"chunks" of language, 150
circulatory system, 96–99
  See also cardiovascular system
  assessing function and failure of, 99–114
circumduction, 68
clinical pathways, 256–257, 295–296
closed questions, 117–118
Clostridium difficile, 198
CNS. *See* central nervous system (CNS)
coagulate, 318
colds, 300
cold symptoms, 164
collaborate, 5
colon, 185
coma, 259, 261
coma scale, 259
comminuted fractures, 258
communication scripts, 304
compendium, 341, 350
competent, 11
comprises, 59–60
compromised, 285–286
concussion, 258
condyloid joints, 68
congested, 166–167
congestive heart failure (CHF), 107–113
connective tissue, 53, 55, 56
conscience, 12
constipation, 203–206, 210
consumer, 3
contagious, 299, 301
contracted, 302
contraction, 109
contusions, 68, 258
COPD. *See* chronic obstructive pulmonary disease
copula, 189
coronary, 94–95
coronary artery bypass surgery (CABG), 95

coronary artery disease, 93, 108
CPR (cardiopulmonary resuscitation), 171
cranial cavity, 56
cranial nerves, 231
cranium, 244
creative writing, 67
critical thinking, 209, 245, 258, 266–267
CT scan, 269
cultural competency, 11
cure, 5
cyanosis, 151–152

damaged, 109
debilitating, 265
decongestant, 167
decubitus, 286
decubitus ulcer, 284, 293–295, 325–327
deep puncture wounds, 284
defecate, 188
defecation, 195
deficiencies, 248
degrees, 25
demographic, 94
dendrites, 231
depressed fractures, 258
deprived, 114
descriptive reports, 100
descriptors, 257, 283
devastating, 264
diagnosis
  making simple, 165–166
  working, 208
diagnostic tools, pain scales, 267–269
diaphragm, 142
diarrhea, 198, 210
diastolic pressure, 104
dietician, 193
digestion, 185–186, 188
digestive system. *See* gastrointestinal system
digital, 204
diminished capacity, 150
disabling, 248
disease, 5
disease-causing microorganisms, 289–292
disease prevention, 1
dislocations, 68
dispenses, 26
distribution, 338
dizziness, 253
do, verb tenses of, 22
doctor's office, calling, 35–41, 50–52
Do Not Use list, 368
dormant, 306
droplets, 306
drugs, 338
drugstores, 24–35
  filling prescriptions, 28–33
  prescriptions, 33–35
dys-, 266
dysarthria, 265
dysphagia, 265
dysphasia, 265

musculoskeletal system, 53–92
   anatomy and physiology, 53–63
   body movement, posture, gait, ambulation, and position, 63–73
   bones, 63–67
   common medical complaints of, 76–77
   components of, 57
   joints, 68–73
   treatments, interventions, and assistance, 74–84
      emergency rooms, 74–79
      walk-in clinics, 79–84
myocardial infarction, 93, 108, 113–115
myocardial tissues, 96

nail, 37–38
nausea, 198
needs, 3
nerve cells, 231
nervous system. *See* neurological system
nervous tissue, 53, 56
neurological, 248
neurological system, 231–282
   anatomy and physiology, 231–245
   brain, 241–245
   common complaints and disorders of, 245–258
      epilepsy, 254–258
      neurological dysfunction, 246–250
      pain and headaches, 250–254
   components of, 231–232
   divisions of, 237–240
   medical prefixes for, 248–249
   treatments, interventions, and assistance, 258–269
      cerebrovascular accident (CVA), 263–267
      head injuries, 258–263
      pain scales, 267–269
neurologist, 249
neuronal, 248
neurons, 231
neuropathway, 248, 249
neurosis, 249
neurosurgeon, 249
neurosurgery, 249
neurotransmitter, 249
neuro-vitals, 249
nitrogenous, 196
norepinephrine, 237
Norwalk virus, 300
nouns, ending with -*ing*, 73
nucleus, 53
nurses, responsibilities of, 10
Nursing Certification Licensing Examination (NCLEX), 8
nutrients, 193–195
nutrition, 193, 198
nutritional deficits, 246
nutritional history interview, 198, 201–202
nutritionist, 193

obligation, 357–358
occipital lobe, 241
occupational therapist (OT), 18
oral cavity, 56
oral medications, 374–375
organizational charts, 238–239

organs, 53
osteoarthritis, 68
over-the-counter (OTC) medications, 24, 26, 379
oxygen, 97, 114, 141
   lack of, 168–172

pain, 250–254, 376
pain scales, 267–269
palpated, 101
pancreas, 185
parasympathetic nervous system, 237
parenchymal injury, 258
parietal lobe, 241
Parkinson's disease, 249
participles, 307
passive-receiver, 4
pathological, 159
pathology, 198
pathophysiology, 283–292, 321–325
pathways, 256–257, 295–296
patient complaints, 76–77, 164–168, 200
peer-reviewed journals, 350
pelvic cavity, 56
penetrating wounds, 68
perceptivity, 259
peripheral nervous system, 231, 237
personal narrative, 115
personal reflection, 127, 130
pesticides, 246, 247
pharmaceutical industry, 337
pharmaceuticals, 339
pharmaceutics, 337
pharmacies, 24–35
pharmacists, 24, 30–31, 339
pharmacodynamics, 337–354
pharmacokinetics, 337–354
pharmacological vs. pharmalogical, 339
pharmacology, 337–354
   See also medications for GI disorders, 210–213
pharmatherapeutics, 339
pharynx, 142, 185
pH balance, 155, 195
phlegm, 155
physician's handwriting, 355
physiotherapist (PT), 18
pills, 375
pivot joints, 68
plasma, 110
poison, 347–348
pollutants, 143
position, 63–73
posture, 63–73
potential, 347
potentiating, 261
prefixes, 338–339, 345
prepositions, of place, 83
prescriptions, 24, 30
   clarity of, 355–356
   content of, 33
   filling, 28–33
   interpretation of, 367–372
   writing, 33–35